Interpersonal Psychotherapy
A Clinician's Guide

Interpersonal Psychotherapy
A Clinician's Guide

Scott Stuart MD
Associate Professor of Psychiatry and Psychology
at the University of Iowa, Iowa City, Iowa, USA

Michael Robertson FRANZCP
Director of the Mayo Wesley Centre for Mental Health,
Taree, New South Wales, Australia

A member of the Hodder Headline Group
LONDON

First published in Great Britain in 2003 by
Arnold, a member of the Hodder Headline Group,
338 Euston Road, London NW1 3BH

http://www.arnoldpublishers.com

Distributed in the United States of America by
Oxford University Press Inc.,
198 Madison Avenue, New York, NY10016
Oxford is a registered trademark of Oxford University Press

Whilst the advice and information in this book are believed to be true and
accurate at the date of going to press, neither the authors nor the publisher
can accept any legal responsibility or liability for any errors or omissions
that may be made. In particular (but without limiting the generality of the
preceding disclaimer) every effort has been made to check drug dosages;
however, it is still possible that errors have been missed. Furthermore,
dosage schedules are constantly being revised and new side-effects
recognized. For these reasons the reader is strongly urged to consult the
drug companies' printed instructions before administering any of the drugs
recommended in this book.

British Library Cataloguing in Publication Data
A catalogue record for this book is available from the British Library

Library of Congress Cataloging-in-Publication Data
A catalog record for this book is available from the Library of Congress

ISBN 0 340 80923 X

1 2 3 4 5 6 7 8 9 10

Commissioning Editor: Serena Bureau
Production Editor: Anke Ueberberg
Production Controller: Bryan Eccleshall
Cover Design: Terry Griffiths

Typeset in 10/12pt Minion by Phoenix Photosetting, Chatham, Kent
Printed and bound in Malta by Gutenberg Press

What do you think about this book? Or any other Arnold title?
Please send your comments to feedback.arnold@hodder.co.uk

To Shana, Kaela, Ryson, Darra, and Logan – *SS*
To my family – *MR*

Acknowledgments

We are indebted to many for their help with this project. We are particularly grateful to Mike O'Hara and the staff of the Iowa Depression and Research Center. We thank Bryanne Barnett for her assistance on some aspects of the discussion of Attachment theory as well as Richard White, Jackie Curtis and Kay Wilhelm for their support and helpful reviews of the 'Problem Area' chapters in particular. We would also like to thank Georgina Bentliff and Serena Bureau of Arnold publishers for their advocacy and patience over the life of the project.

Finally, we are grateful to our spouses Shana and Amanda, for their unfailing support, encouragement and friendship through what has been a much larger undertaking than any of us anticipated.

Scott Stuart
Iowa City, USA

Michael Roberson
Sydney, Australia

Contents

Preface

We present herein a guide to conducting Interpersonal Psychotherapy. Our use of the term 'guide' is intended to convey that Interpersonal Psychotherapy is best conceptualized as a treatment which is grounded in empirical research, theory, and clinical experience, and which should be applied using a healthy dose of clinical judgment. It is not a treatment which is best delivered in formulaic fashion or by rote.

Our primary goal is to assist therapists in their endeavors with the unique individuals with whom they work, with the belief that Interpersonal Psychotherapy (IPT) is an extremely useful framework for both clinicians and their patients to accomplish the goals that they have mutually set forth. Our objective aim is to provide a guide to the conduct of IPT, but our subjective aim is to help therapists better understand their patients. This mirrors the goals of IPT – namely that therapists should aim to help their patients alleviate their objective suffering, always keeping in mind the necessity of subjectively understanding their individual patients, while helping their patients to better understand themselves.

We are greatly indebted to the pioneering work of Gerald Klerman, Myrna Weissman, and the other authors of the 1984 text, *Interpersonal Psychotherapy of Depression*.[1] Nearly all of the research that has been conducted regarding IPT has been based on this manual, as have numerous adaptations of IPT which have been developed for disorders other than depression.[2,3] This research has had an important impact on the field of psychotherapy as a whole, and the treatment of depression in particular.

However, while IPT enjoys empirical support for its *efficacy*, there is no research to date evaluating its *effectiveness* in typical clinical settings.[a] In other words, IPT has been empirically demonstrated to be of benefit when used:

- In an academic setting with therapists specifically devoted to its application.
- With subjects (as opposed to patients) who meet carefully selected diagnostic criteria and who do not have comorbid diagnoses.
- With subjects who agree to be involved in a randomized clinical trial.
- With subjects who are not typically required to pay for their treatment.
- Following a tightly controlled protocol which dictates strict adherence to a manual.

---

[a]The same criticism can be made for all of the other psychotherapies – there are virtually no empirical data available about the application of 'manualized' therapies in 'real-world' clinical settings.

In contrast, most clinicians work in settings in which it would be nearly inconceivable to be able to meet weekly with a patient[b] for sixteen consecutive weeks as is required by most research protocols. Most clinicians are paid on the basis of the number of patients they treat each day, rather than being paid by a research grant. Most clinicians do not have the luxury of working with patients with 'classic' major depression without any comorbid diagnoses – a typical 'real-life' patient may have symptoms of both depression and anxiety, and have dysfunctional personality traits and substance abuse problems as well. And most patients who request treatment do so with some idea about the kind of treatment they would like to receive, whether it be medication, therapy, or something else entirely – they are simply different from the subjects seen in research studies who agree to be randomly assigned to treatment.[4]

While we hold that empirical research regarding the *efficacy* of a treatment is essential (e.g., the benefit of a treatment when applied in a strict research setting in a randomized, controlled study), we also firmly believe that the *effectiveness* of the treatment (e.g., the benefit of the treatment when applied in clinical settings) is the ultimate measure of its clinical utility.[4,5] Though empirical research regarding the clinical use of IPT is lacking at present, there is a great deal of clinical wisdom and experience which addresses these issues. *We believe that the practice of IPT should be based on both empirical data and this clinical experience.*

This belief leads to a fundamental conclusion about manualized forms of IPT and about manualized treatments in general. *Requiring strict adherence to a manual outside of a research protocol is likely to diminish the effectiveness of the treatment because it discourages therapists from exercising their clinical judgment.* The data that a therapist obtains from a patient during the course of therapy, such as the degree of insight the patient is developing, the degree to which he or she is motivated to change, or the effect of the transference on their interaction, should assist the therapist to better decide whether the patient might benefit from a homework assignment, might develop more insight with a well-timed therapist self-disclosure, or might improve more with twenty as opposed to sixteen sessions of therapy. These decisions should be mutually determined within each therapeutic dyad, not dictated 'a priori' by a manual.[6–9] Thus this book should serve primarily as a guide rather than a manual – it should provide a set of principles which serve as a framework for the conduct of therapy rather than a set of rules which constrain therapy.

This is reflected in our presentation of IPT in this text. For instance, clinical experience with IPT has made clear that some patients benefit greatly from homework assignments, whereas the efficacy studies of IPT have prohibited the explicit assignment of homework. Clinical experience has demonstrated that conducting consecutive weekly sessions of IPT, then terminating treatment abruptly after twelve or sixteen sessions, is not the way to conduct IPT most effectively in a clinical setting. In contrast, all of the efficacy studies evaluating acute treatment with IPT have required that consecutive weekly sessions be provided. It is usually much more *effective* clinically to negotiate the scheduling of sessions with the patient, and to meet for several biweekly or monthly sessions prior to finishing therapy. Clinical experience has been that utilizing clinical judgment within the framework of IPT is much more *effective* than strict adherence to a manual.

---

[b]We have used the term 'patient' rather than 'client', recognizing that both are used interchangeably and that both are used by mental health professionals to signify the people who seek psychotherapeutic treatment. This convention should not, however, convey any intent to see such people as anything less than unique individuals.

Clinical experience with IPT has also made clear that the *primary means for understanding the people who seek treatment with IPT, and for conceptualizing their problems, is best based upon a biopsychosocial model.* Manualized treatments often imply (or even require) that patients must be 'diagnosed' with a psychopathologic disease, and that treatment be conceptualized as a medical intervention.[10,11] It is our position that human psychological functioning is complex, multifactorial, and far beyond characterization as a simple medical 'disorder.' Even the term 'biopsychosocial,' which has been in vogue for more than a decade to describe the etiology of psychological suffering, recognizes that we are more than the sum of our genes or our 'medical' selves.[12-15]

It is our belief that strict adherence to a medical model of psychopathology dehumanizes both the therapist and the person with whom he or she is working. The medical model requires that *patients*, not *people*, must be *diagnosed* with a specific medical disorder, usually as defined by DSM[16] or ICD[17] criteria. This approach not only categorizes and defines the people with whom we work by their 'symptoms' or 'diagnoses,' it limits the ability of therapists to understand them as unique individuals, and to work creatively with them to develop solutions to the problems they are experiencing. As the primary goal of therapy in general, and IPT specifically, is to understand the person seeking treatment, using only strict medical diagnoses to develop that understanding and reflect it to the patient clearly detracts from that goal.

Therefore, although there is great value in using a medically-based diagnostic system as one way to understand patients, it should not be used as the primary basis for conceptualizing the patient's problems, nor as the basis for treatment. The door should be open to the clinical use of IPT for those patients who present with interpersonal problems in general. Some of these people will be depressed, some will be anxious, some will have personality issues, many will have combinations of these factors. Some will be old, some adolescents; some will be male, some female; some will be from cultural backgrounds different from their therapists'; some will be poor, some wealthy; but all will be individuals who can be understood in part as social beings who are intimately involved in a social network, and are thus potential candidates for IPT. The question of whether the treatment should be applied in a clinical setting if the patient does not meet strict diagnostic criteria for major depression is not relevant; it is the individual's unique problems and social context that should be used to make a determination regarding his or her suitability for IPT.

In summary, the available empirical evidence should form the foundation for IPT, should be built upon by clinical experience, and should be supplemented by clinical judgment.

THE HISTORY OF IPT

The developmental trajectory of IPT has been somewhat different from most of the other 'brands' of psychotherapy currently practiced. Most psychotherapies have been derived from clinical observations which gradually coalesced into more or less coherently articulated theories explaining how the treatments 'worked.' In many cases, exemplified by behavioral therapy, these theoretical hypotheses about the mechanisms of change also led to the introduction of specific therapeutic techniques. Over time, additional insights from continuing clinical observations were incorporated into these theories, which were seen (by some at least) as dynamic and evolving formulations rather than as a static set of principles. Resistance to changes in these therapies and their supporting theories was, and still is, frequent; those individuals who added to or modified treatments were often branded iconoclasts and were 'excommunicated' from the previously established and well-entrenched psychotherapeutic school. Psychoanalysis is an excellent example of this kind of development (both in terms of its gradual and highly politicized evolution and the rigidity of its various schools).

Cognitive Behavior Therapy (CBT)[18] stands as another notable example of psychotherapy development, though in contrast to psychoanalysis, CBT serves as a prototype for psychotherapy evolution over the last two decades, in which the dictates of 'evidence based' medicine have required the empirical validation of psychotherapeutic treatments. Largely influenced by psychopharmacologic trials, the randomized and well-controlled efficacy treatment trial has become the 'sine qua non' method for 'proving' that a psychotherapy works.[19] Thus the typical progression of psychotherapy development, epitomized by CBT, currently moves from clinical observation to theory to empirical testing of efficacy. Ideally, empirical results are disseminated and influence clinical practice, and as additional experience is gained and additional observations accumulate, both theory and clinical techniques are modified and improved.

IPT, in contrast, evolved in a strikingly different fashion. Rather than beginning as a set of clinical observations which were used as the basis for the development of a coherent theory of psychopathology, and which in turn suggested specific techniques to bring about change, IPT began as a manualized treatment developed for an empirical research protocol. In fact, IPT was initially developed not as a clinical treatment for depression, but for the express purpose of serving as a manualized 'placebo condition' for a psychopharmacologic treatment trial for depression.[20–22] It was largely accidental that IPT was discovered to be of benefit.

IPT was developed in the 1970s,[20] during which time the medical model of psychopathology reigned supreme. Further, there was an increasing emphasis on empirical testing of treatments, particularly psychotropic medications, fueled both by the pharmaceutical industry and the desire of many psychiatrists to be seen as a legitimate, empirically-based 'medical' specialists.[23,24] It was widely held within this paradigm that psychotherapy was not a particularly effective treatment, and that it should largely be subsumed by psychopharmacologic treatments.

Nonetheless, some early studies of the treatment of depression with medication included psychotherapy as a treatment component, as the trials were designed to mirror the clinical practice of the time, which generally included some form of psychodynamic psychotherapy along with medication. Klerman, Weissman, and their colleagues incorporated a manualized form of psychotherapy in their trials of medication as a maintenance treatment for depression. This manualized treatment, which later became Interpersonal Psychotherapy, was initially called a 'high contact' condition in the treatment trials,[25] the presumption being that there may be some benefit from the non-specific effects of contact with a therapist, but none that would be attributable to any specific techniques.[22]

Explicitly following the medical model established by pharmacologic treatment trials, a codified manual describing the procedures and techniques to be used in the psychotherapy condition was developed, so that fidelity to treatment could be preserved. The primary concern of the investigators was that the therapeutic treatment be reproducible – the specific techniques to be used and the theoretical basis for the psychotherapeutic interventions were of secondary importance.[22]

In contrast to the investigators' expectations, the early studies of IPT demonstrated that it had a therapeutic effect.[20,26] Klerman *et al.* subsequently described the treatment more fully,[1] and began to develop a theory to explain why it worked. As IPT was largely conceived of as a 'social work' or 'social support' intervention, it was hypothesized that change in social circumstances and social relationships was largely the driving force behind improvement. Empirical data have since provided evidence for this hypothesis. The original investigators' enthusiasm to continue to empirically test IPT in rigorously controlled trials has largely propelled the widespread adoption of IPT in research settings.

In essence, IPT was constructed in 'retrograde' fashion rather than being derived from clinical observations which were then developed into a theory and subsequently tested empirically. IPT began as a manualized form of therapy which was believed to be an inert treatment, or at most was simply a codification of 'non-specific' therapeutic factors common to all psychotherapies. The original purpose of IPT was to serve as a credible and reproducible placebo psychotherapy. It was not originally developed from clinical observations, and it has been only recently that much attention has been paid to its theoretical foundations.

The pervasive influence of this model of development has had two profound effects on the current use of the therapy. First, 'manualized' IPT was constructed first and foremost to meet the demands of an empirical research protocol; IPT was not designed to meet the demands of clinical settings. Consequently, the use of IPT has been largely restricted to academic settings and efficacy studies, with clinical dissemination lagging behind empirical research. Second, the historical emphasis on reproducibility in efficacy research studies has led to an insistence that IPT must follow the dictates of the research manual, rather than making allowances for clinical judgment when it is adapted to clinical settings.

These two effects were magnified by the inclusion of IPT as one of the two psychotherapeutic treatments investigated in the National Institute of Mental Health Treatment of Depression Collaborative Research Project (NIMH-TDCRP).[27] The NIMH-TDCRP, which utilized what is still considered to be the gold-standard methodology for psychotherapy efficacy studies, was designed to definitively answer how efficacious psychotherapy (IPT and CBT specifically) and medication were as acute treatments for depression. The rigorous design of the NIMH-TDCRP dictated that IPT be adapted to the research protocol, rather than adapting the protocol design to reflect good clinical use of IPT.[28] This further solidified the notion that IPT was a 'research' therapy and that the reproducibility of IPT, as opposed to the clinical modification of IPT for individual patients, was paramount. The emphasis on reproducibility and adherence to the IPT manual, as was required in the initial efficacy studies and the NIMH-TDCRP, led to an insistence that it continue to be conduced exactly as specified in the 1984 manual.[1] Rather than being conceptualized as a dynamically developing treatment which should incorporate new clinical observations and clinical experience, the way in which IPT was described in the NIMH-TDCRP study became the singular and 'correct' way to conduct it.

Another ramification of the inclusion of IPT in the NIMH-TDCRP was that some of the elements specific to IPT were included (or excluded) primarily as a means of distinguishing it from CBT. The NIMH-TDCRP was designed to include only empirically tested treatments, and by intent, the two psychotherapies to be compared were to be as different as possible in hypothesized effects, therapeutic stance, and specific interventions.[27] Specific techniques, such as the assignment of homework, which is intrinsic to CBT, were overtly excluded from IPT. IPT came to be described as relying largely on 'non-specific' techniques such as non-directive exploration and clarification in order to distinguish it from the behavioral components of CBT. Thus the exclusion of homework in IPT, for example, is largely the result of research expedience rather than being supported by a specific theoretical rationale or being based on clinical experience. The lack of techniques specific to IPT, or of techniques which follow from a theoretical base supporting IPT, has led some critics to describe IPT as being nothing more than a 'time-limited psychodynamic psychotherapy,' or as sophisticated means of encouraging social support.[28]

IPT has since been viewed by many solely as a 'research-based' treatment. The way in which IPT was adapted to the NIMH-TDCRP protocol simply furthered this impression amongst practicing clinicians. While IPT has been adapted to a number of different disorders, it has remained within the efficacy research paradigm – i.e., it has consistently been applied in a manualized form only to reified diagnostic entities following a strict medical model.[28] Although the clinical use of IPT has been increasing in Europe and Australasia, it has until recently largely been confined to academic centers in North America. Clinical dissemination, despite an impressive array of efficacy research, has been underwhelming. This is, in our opinion, due primarily to the fact that IPT has not yet evolved beyond the narrow constraints imposed by efficacy research, rather than being continually refined by clinical experience.

A METAPHOR FOR IPT

Learning psychotherapy is like learning to play chess. If you want to learn how to play chess well, you need to do two things: read books which explain how to play, and play a lot of games against the best competition you can find.

Nearly all chess textbooks divide chess games into opening, middle, and endgame phases. There are always extremely detailed discussions about how to begin the game, ranging from simple descriptions of the movements of the various pieces to elaborate opening defenses with names such as the Italian Game or the Vienna Game. Many, just like the variants of psychotherapy, are named after the experts who first described them.

Chess manuals also have detailed descriptions of the conclusions of games, and it is expected that good players will study the endgames of the great masters. As with the opening phases, elaborate descriptions and analyses are offered for the few moves which conclude a game.

In contrast, there isn't much information about what happens in the middle of games. This is particularly striking considering how much of the game actually takes place in this 'middle' phase. The middle part of the game is somewhat shrouded in mystery – a black box which connects the input of the opening phase to the endgame output.

Psychotherapy manuals are like chess textbooks. Most provide detailed information about how to select patients for the specific brand of therapy being described, how to begin treatment, and how to introduce the treatment model to the patient. This is usually followed by a brief description of techniques that might be used (a simple description of how the pieces move outside of the context of the actual game), and then a detailed description of the end of therapy is given.

There is reason to be critical of this approach, which clearly neglects the importance of understanding techniques in the context of the whole of treatment. However, much of the reason that disproportionate time is spent on the opening phases of the chess game and the psychotherapy treatment, and the reason that so much effort is expended on the end of the game/treatment, is that these are the two times in the process during which things can be described with any preciseness. There are simply too many permutations and too many possibilities to even begin to describe what happens in the middle of the game or the middle of the therapy. In contrast, the fewer number of possibilities of move and countermove, statement and response, during the opening phase makes it more amenable to precise description. When only a few pieces are left at the end, or when only a session or two is left, it again becomes possible to offer more precise descriptions – there aren't so many moves that they defy analysis.

This is where playing a lot of games with the best competition – or working with the most challenging patients – comes into the picture. Experience is the best way to learn to conduct the middle phase – even more so if there is a chess master or psychotherapy supervisor to offer further insights and tips along the way. You've got to play the game, or conduct the therapy, to become proficient. Learning the middle phase, and becoming familiar with what moves to make, depends not on rigidly following a manual but on developing intuition and judgment. The master chess players, and the master therapists, are those who have developed an intuitive sense of what will work best in a particular game with a particular client, and who have the judgment to decide when and how to do it. The master chess players and therapist are artisans, not technicians. And as one can devote a lifetime to mastering chess, expert clinicians do the same with continual study, self-reflection, and constant practice.

After working through the 'how-to' manuals and getting some experience, chess players move on to the 'case-study' books that essentially describe the great games of the masters. Rather than getting technical information, these case studies are read to hone the chess player's sense of judgment, timing and intuition – in essence to get inside the mind of the great chess masters. Similarly, at a certain level of development, therapists also learn from case reports which describe individual cases from which general principles can be gleaned.

Master psychotherapists are those who work to understand the craft of psychotherapy as well as specific techniques. While the eponymous opening defenses and the various brands of psychotherapy, such as IPT, CBT, hypnotherapy and the like, are important tools to have at one's disposal, they do not constitute the whole of the experience or the process of therapy. Just as chess masters intimately understand the various opening strategies, psychotherapy masters should understand and practice a variety of approaches. The art of both chess and psychotherapy is in knowing, often intuitively, when to use which specific strategy, and in having the ability to do so.

Master clinicians, like master chess players, recognize that textbooks and manuals are limited. Though helpful in providing a framework for treatment, clinical practice demands that therapists be flexible and that they use clinical judgment in applying the therapy to individual patients.

CONCLUSION

This text is designed to guide clinicians who wish to practice IPT. Our primary goal is to make IPT available and applicable – to encourage the dissemination of what we believe to be an extraordinary treatment for a variety of interpersonal problems and psychiatric syndromes. We offer a new paradigm, in which IPT can be used as a foundation for a treatment which is conducted by individual therapists, exercising their clinical judgment within each unique clinical relationship. IPT should be grounded in theory, empirical research, and clinical experience, and should always incorporate clinical judgment. The question that clinicians should be asking themselves as they conduct IPT is not, 'is this the "correct" approach according to the manual,' but rather, 'is this approach the best for this particular patient.'

INTERPERSONAL PSYCHOTHERAPY: A NEW PARADIGM

1 The practice of IPT should be based on both empirical data and clinical experience.
2 Incorporating new empirical evidence and clinical experience into the IPT model will continue to improve the treatment.
3 IPT therapists should be guided by descriptions of treatment rather than by manuals which dictate treatment.
4 Utilizing clinical judgment within an IPT framework will improve outcome.
5 IPT need not be restricted to specific diagnostic entities, but can be applied to a variety of interpersonal problems.

REFERENCES

1. Klerman, G.L., Weissman, M.M., Rounsaville, B.J., Chevron, E.S. 1984 . *Interpersonal Psychotherapy of Depression*. New York: Basic Books.
2. Klerman, G.L., Weissman, M.M. 1993. *New Applications of Interpersonal Psychotherapy*. Washington, D.C.: American Psychiatric Press.
3. Weissman, M.M., Markowitz, J.W., Klerman, G.L. 2000. *Comprehensive Guide to Interpersonal Psychotherapy*. New York: Basic Books.
4. Nathan, P.E., Stuart, S., Dolan, S. 2000. Research on psychotherapy efficacy and effectiveness: between Scylla and Charybdis? *Psychological Bulletin*; **126**, 964–81.
5. Barlow, D.H. 1996. Health care policy, psychotherapy research, and the future of psychotherapy. *American Psychologist*; **51**, 1050–8.
6. Edelson, M. 1994. Can psychotherapy research answer this psychotherapist's questions? In: Talley, P.F., Strupp, H.H., Butler, S.F. (eds), *Psychotherapy Research and Practice: Bridging the Gap*. New York: Basic Books.
7. Garfield, S.L. 1996. Some problems associated with 'validated' forms of psychotherapy. *Clinical Psychology: Science and Practice* 3, 218–29.
8. Strauss, B.M., Kaechele, H. 1998. The writing on the wall- comments on the current discussion about empirically validated treatments in Germany. *Psychotherapy Research* 8, 158–70.
9. Henry, W.P., Strupp, H.H., Butler, S.F., Schacht, T.E., Binder, J.L. 1993. The effects of training in time-limited dynamic psychotherapy. Changes in therapist behavior. *Journal of Consulting and Clinical Psychology* 61, 434–40.

10. Henry, W.P. 1998. Science, politics, and the politics of science: the use and misuse of empirically validated treatment research. *Psychotherapy Research* **8**, 126–40.
11. Horowitz, M.J. 1994. Psychotherapy integration: implications for research standards. *Psychotherapy and Rehabilitation Research Bulletin* **3**, 8–9.
12. Engel, G.L. 1980. The clinical application of biopsychosocial models. *American Journal of Psychiatry* **137**, 535–44.
13. Engel, G.L. 1982. The biopsychosocial model and medical education: who are to be the teachers? *New England Journal of Medicine* **306**, 802–5.
14. Sadler, J.Z., Hulgus, Y.F. 1992. Clinical problem solving and the biopsychosocial model. *American Journal of Psychiatry* **149**, 1315–23.
15. Hartmann, L. 1992. Presidential address: reflections on humane values and biopsychosocial integration. *American Journal of Psychiatry* **149**, 1135–41.
16. American Psychiatric Association. 1994. Diagnostic and Statistical Manual of Mental Disorders, 4th edition. Washington, DC: *American Psychiatric Association*.
17. World Health Organization 1992. International Statistical Classification of Diseases and Related Health Problems : ICD-10. 10th edition. Geneva: World Health Organization.
18. Beck, A.T., Rush, A.J., Shaw, B.F., Emery, G. 1979. *Cognitive Therapy of Depression*. New York: Guilford Press.
19. Parloff, M.B. 1986. Placebo controls in psychotherapy research a sine qua non or a placebo for research problems? *Journal of Consulting and Clinical Psychology* **54**, 79–87.
20. Klerman, G.L., DiMascio, A., Weissman, M.M., Prusoff, B.A., Paykel, E.S. 1974. Treatment of depression by drugs and psychotherapy. *American Journal of Psychiatry* **131**, 186–91.
21. Weissman, M.M., Klerman, G.L., Prusoff, B.A., Sholomskas, D., Padian, N. 1981. Depressed outpatients: results after one year of treatment with drugs and/or interpersonal psychotherapy. *Archives of General Psychiatry* **38**, 51–5.
22. Weissman, M.M. 2001. International Society of Interpersonal Psychotherapists web site (interpersonalpsychotherapy.org).
23. Detre, T. 1987. The future of psychiatry. *American Journal of Psychiatry* **144**, 621–25.
24. Detre, T., McDonald, M.C. 1997. Managed care and the future of psychiatry. *Archives of General Psychiatry* **54**, 201–204.
25. DiMascio, A., Weissman, M.M., Prusoff, B.A. 1979. Differential symptom reduction by drugs and psychotherapy in acute depression. *Archives of General Psychiatry* **36**, 1450–6.
26. Weissman, M.M., Prusoff, B.A., DiMascio, A. 1979 The efficacy of drugs and psychotherapy in the treatment of acute depressive episodes. *American Journal of Psychiatry* **136**, 555–8.
27. Elkin, I., Parloff, M.B., Hadley, S.W., Autry, J.H. 1985. NIMH Treatment of Depression Collaborative Treatment Program: background and research plan. *Archives of General Psychiatry* **42**, 305–16.
28. Markowitz, J.C., Svartberg, M., Swartz, H.A. 1998. Is IPT time-limited psychodynamic psychotherapy? *Journal of Psychotherapy Research and Practice* **7**, 185–95.

Section 1

Introduction

1

Introduction

Interpersonal psychotherapy (IPT) is a time-limited, dynamically informed psychotherapy which aims to alleviate patients' suffering and improve their interpersonal functioning. IPT focuses specifically on interpersonal relationships as a means of bringing about change, with the goal of helping patients to either improve their interpersonal relationships or change their expectations about them. In addition, the treatment also aims to assist patients to improve their social support networks so that they can better manage their current interpersonal distress.

IPT was originally developed in a research context as a treatment for major depression and was codified in a manual developed by Klerman *et al.* in 1984.[1] Since that time, a great deal of empirical evidence supporting its use has accumulated. In addition, as clinical experience with the treatment has increased, the use of IPT has broadened to include not only the treatment of patients with a variety of well-specified diagnoses as described in DSM-IV,[2] but also the treatment of patients presenting with a variety of interpersonal problems.

The prevailing view among researchers and clinicians using IPT is that it should reflect the best of both empirical research and clinical experience, and that it should continue to incorporate changes as additional data (both quantitative and qualitative) and experience continue to accumulate. Rather than being a static and fixed treatment, clinical experience and research have informed the adaptations which have been made to IPT. These continuing improvements have allowed IPT to be disseminated and utilized in general clinical settings rather than being used exclusively in reified academic research settings. Moreover, the ability of clinicians to apply their clinical judgment when providing IPT in a clinical setting has also increased its effectiveness and allowed it to be applied to a more widespread group of patients.

Consequently, this book is written to reflect the current 'state of the art' of IPT, recognizing that future research and clinical experience will lead to further refinements in the treatment, and that IPT will continue to evolve over time. Both empirical data based on the manualized forms of IPT and clinical experience have contributed to the description of IPT as it is used at present.

CHARACTERISTICS OF IPT

IPT is characterized by three primary elements.

Table 1.1 *Characteristics of IPT*

1 IPT focuses specifically on **interpersonal relationships** as a point of intervention.
2 IPT is **time limited** when used as an acute treatment.
3 **The interventions used in IPT do not directly address the patient–therapist relationship** as it develops in therapy.

In addition, IPT is based on a *Biopsychosocial Model* of psychological functioning.[3] Rather than narrowly viewing psychological distress or psychiatric problems as medical problems, the IPT approach is to view the patient's functioning in broad terms as a product of his or her temperament, personality, and attachment style, based upon a foundation of biological factors such as genetics and physiological functioning, placed in the context of social relationships and broad social support.

Although even this model has limitations, it is the most appropriate for IPT for three reasons. First, it is congruent with the theoretical basis for IPT, in which attachments in relationships and the individual's ability to communicate effectively are hypothesized to be intimately linked with psychological functioning. Second, the biopsychosocial model leads directly to the specific techniques and interventions that are used in IPT. This includes not only psychological interventions, but is consistent with the use of IPT in combination with psychotropic medication when indicated. Third, the biopsychosocial model makes clear that the patient needs to be active and to take responsibility for change – rather than simply 'sitting and waiting' for a biological agent to take effect, the patient should be active in generating change within his or her social environment, and should take charge of making changes in specific interpersonal relationships.

I. Interpersonal orientation of IPT

IPT is based on the premise that interpersonal distress is intimately connected with psychological symptoms. Thus, the foci of treatment are two-fold.

- *One focus is the conflicts and transitions in relationships in which the patient is engaged*: the aim is to help the patient to either improve communication within those relationships, or to change his or her expectations about those relationships.
- *The second focus is helping the patient to build or better utilize his or her extended social support network* so that he or she is better able to muster the interpersonal support needed to deal with the crises which precipitated the distress.

This approach is extremely well suited, for instance, to the treatment of women who may be experiencing an episode of postpartum depression.[4,5] Many women in these circumstances describe that their distress is linked to conflicts in their relationships with their partners. In addition, many also report that they have difficulty making the transition from 'working woman' to 'mother,' and that this change in social circumstances and social support has contributed to their problems. A therapist using IPT would help the patient to resolve the conflicts with her partner over issues such as division of child-care labor, and would also assist the woman to garner more support from her social network. This might include connecting with and asking for support from other friends who have had children, extended family members, or colleagues at work. It could also include encouraging the patient to become involved in a new mothers' support group. Resolution of the particular interpersonal conflict, along with improved interpersonal support while the role transition is being negotiated, then leads to symptomatic improvement.

IPT is therefore clearly distinct from treatments such as Cognitive Behavior Therapy (CBT)[6] and psychoanalytically oriented psychotherapy. In contrast to CBT, in which the focus of treatment is the patient's internally based cognitions, IPT focuses on the patient's interpersonal communications with others in his or her interpersonal sphere. In contrast to analytically oriented treatments, in which the focus of treatment is on understanding the contribution of early life experiences to psychological functioning, IPT focuses on helping the patient to improve his or her communication and social support in the present. Past experiences, while clearly influencing current functioning, are not a major focus of intervention.

This latter point leads to a corollary of the IPT approach – by virtue of its time limit and its focus on here-and-now interpersonal functioning, IPT is designed to resolve psychiatric symptoms and improve interpersonal functioning rather than to change underlying dynamic structures. While ego strength, defense mechanisms, and personality characteristics are all important in assessing suitability for treatment, change in these constructs is not presumed to occur in IPT. Rather, they are taken as given for a particular patient, and the question that drives the therapist's interventions is: 'given this patient's personality style, ego strength, defense mechanisms, and early life experiences, how can he or she be helped to improve here-and-now interpersonal relationships and build a more effective social support network?'

II. Time limit for acute treatment with IPT

IPT is characterized by a time-limited acute treatment phase, and a contract should be established with the patient to complete acute treatment after a specified number of sessions. Clinical experience has shown that having a definitive endpoint for the acute phase of therapy often 'pushes' patients to make changes in their relationships more quickly,[1] a point emphasized by the authors of other time-limited therapies.[7,8] In addition, the time limit also influences both patient and therapist to maintain their focus on the matter at hand, namely improving the patient's interpersonal functioning in his or her current relationships.

The time frame is also extremely important in helping to prevent the therapy from moving from a symptom-focused treatment to one that is based on the use of the transference relationship. IPT is focused on the rapid resolution of interpersonal crises, and on the problems that patients are experiencing in their current interpersonal relationships.

Shifting this focus to one in which the patient–therapist relationship becomes primary makes it more difficult to generate immediate change in patients' social networks and their relationships outside of therapy. Thus, encouraging the development of transference, which is fostered by increasing the duration and intensity of sessions, is likely to shift the work from relationship change to intrapsychic exploration.[9] (See footnote a.) Maintaining a time-limited approach helps to keep this from happening.

In general, a course of ten to twenty sessions is used for the acute treatment of interpersonal problems, depression, or other major psychiatric illnesses. While empirical research regarding acute treatment is at present limited to controlled studies in which weekly therapy is provided and then abruptly stopped, clinical experience has been that tapering sessions over time is generally a more effective way of utilizing the treatment. In other words, weekly therapy may be provided for six to ten weeks, followed by a gradual increase in the time between sessions as the patient improves, such that weekly sessions are followed by biweekly and monthly meetings. Though acute treatment should be time-limited, both empirical research and clinical experience with IPT have clearly demonstrated that maintenance treatment – particularly for those patients with recurrent disorders such as depression – should be provided for patients who have responded to acute treatment in order to reduce the risk of relapse.[10] This maintenance treatment should be distinguished from the acute phase of treatment in IPT, and a specific contract for the maintenance phase must also be negotiated with the patient for this phase.[9] Thus, even though the acute phase of treatment is time-limited, the therapist will often explicitly negotiate a contract in which some form of future contact is specified. There is no need in IPT to 'terminate' at the end of acute treatment, especially as it is clearly not in the interest of most patients to do so.

III. Interventions in IPT do not directly address the patient–therapist relationship

IPT is characterized by the absence of interventions which directly address the therapeutic relationship. Though sharing this characteristic with CBT and several other solution-focused therapies, IPT clearly differs in this way from the dynamically oriented therapies. A more thorough explanation of the use of the treatment relationship in IPT is necessary to appreciate fully this element of the treatment.

Both Bowlby[11] and Sullivan[12] have written extensively about the ways in which an individual's life experiences lead them to interact in subsequent relationships. Sullivan used the term 'parataxic distortion' to describe the phenomena in which individuals impose characteristics of previous relationships upon new relationships.[12] In other words, individuals' experiences in previous relationships inform what they expect in new ones. This expectation then leads them to 'impose' characteristics upon new individuals with whom they come into contact. These imposed characteristics are often not accurate, but represent instead the sum of their previous relationship experiences. New relationships are 'distorted' by these imposed and inaccurate expectations.

---

[a]This is in no way to imply that transference-based psychotherapies are not useful – in fact, they are likely more beneficial than IPT for patients with severe personality disorders. Rather, the use of interventions which address the transference aspects of the therapeutic relationship is simply outside of the scope of IPT.

For example, if an individual has had previous abusive relationships, he or she will tend to react to new people as if they too will be abusive. The previous experience is superimposed upon the new. New relationships will be distorted because the expectation is that new significant others will be abusive, even if in reality that is not the case. Similarly, if an individual has had experiences of being deceived, then he or she will also superimpose that lack of trust upon new relationships, and will act 'as if' the new person should not be trusted.

Though Sullivan believed that these formative experiences were largely the result of early life experiences, the parataxic distortion characteristically imposed by an individual could be modified over time by experiences in adulthood. For instance, a severe trauma, such as an assault, could profoundly change the expectations that an otherwise trusting individual might have about new relationships. Further, Sullivan also argued that the distortions could be modified in both positive and negative ways. While the above examples are indicative of negative modification, the distortions could also be modified positively in productive, intimate, and trusting relationships.

Bowlby[13] described a similar phenomena using the term 'working model of relationships' to describe the ways in which individuals behave in new relationships. This mental construct, like Sullivan's concept of parataxic distortion, represents the accumulated experience of an individual in all of his or her relationships. The purpose of the working model is to organize interpersonal behavior – it allows an individual to predict the behavior of others and to act accordingly. In a fashion similar to Sullivan's concept of parataxic distortion, this working model reflects all of an individual's experiences, with a heavy, but not exclusive, emphasis on early life interactions. The working model of attachment forms the basis for the development of new relationships, as the individual imposes the old working model upon new relationships with the expectation that new acquaintances will behave similarly to people in past relationships.

The problem with this, according to both Sullivan and Bowlby, is that while parataxic distortions and working models may be accurate representations of earlier relationships, and may in fact have served to protect an individual from potentially abusive situations, they severely restrict the development of new intimate relationships. New relationships become constrained by the model or the distortion, as opposed to being allowed to develop unfettered. Working models which reflect an accurate view of others as abusive during childhood are no longer accurate in adulthood with all new relationships, yet the imposition of the model prevents an individual from trusting others or developing any sense of intimacy, and also prevents the realistic appraisal of good and bad relationships. Distortions may reflect a distrust of others which developed honestly as a consequence of real breaches of trust in early relationships, but when they are superimposed upon new relationships in which the development of trust and intimacy would otherwise be possible, they severely limit the individual's ability to function interpersonally.

Because these distortions and working models are imposed upon all relationships, they also occur within therapeutic relationships. Given enough time, a patient will display behavior towards his or her therapist which is reflective of his or her parataxic distortions or working model of attachment. This is in essence the theoretical basis for transference. Thus, the therapist is in a unique position to experience and examine the way in which a patient develops and maintains relationships, because the therapist is in a relationship in which he or she is the person upon whom the distortions or working models are imposed.

Both Sullivan and Bowlby, in the tradition of Freud and other psychoanalysts, believed that one of the most powerful ways to work on correcting these distortions was to examine in detail the relationship between therapist and patient. This was done overtly and explicitly, using techniques such as interpretation, in which the transference was directly discussed, and clarification, in which the therapist would directly ask the patient for his or her reactions to the therapist.

Moreover, in psychoanalytic treatments in particular, the therapy is structured in such a way that the transference is magnified so that it may be more closely examined. Psychoanalytic therapy is designed to facilitate the patient's projection of his or her parataxic distortions or working model of relationships onto the 'blank screen' of the therapist. This is enhanced by therapist opacity, by high-frequency sessions (four to five times per week), and by open-ended treatment which may last several years. All serve to intensify the patient–therapist relationship, with the goal of examining the transference as it is displayed in the therapeutic relationship.

Transference, parataxic distortions, and the imposition of working models are universal phenomena in all psychotherapy, including IPT. However, while in IPT the therapist's experience of patient–therapist relationship is used to provide information about the patient and his or her interpersonal world, the transference elements of this relationship are not addressed directly by the therapist as a part of the treatment. The use of the therapeutic relationship in IPT to understand the patient's interpersonal functioning, and to assess the patient's attachment style is crucial. The use of the therapeutic relationship in IPT to formulate questions about the patient's interpersonal relationships outside of therapy is also extraordinarily important. The use of transference to inform the therapist about potential points of resistance and potential problems in therapy – to predict the likely outcome of treatment – is also paramount.

Table 1.2 *Use of the Patient–Therapist Relationship in IPT*

- To assess the patient's attachment style.
- To formulate questions about the patient's interpersonal relationships outside of therapy.
- To understand the patient's interpersonal functioning outside of the therapeutic relationship.
- To inform the therapist about potential points of resistance.
- To inform the therapist about potential problems in therapy.
- To plan for the conclusion of therapy.
- To predict the likely outcome of treatment.

The direct examination of the patient–therapist relationship is not encouraged in IPT, however, because it switches the focus of treatment from more immediate work on the patient's current social relationships to an intense experience with, and analysis of, the relationship with the therapist. Addressing the patent–therapist relationship directly as a primary technique shifts the therapy from one that is oriented towards improvement in symptoms and immediate interpersonal functioning to a therapy that is oriented towards intrapsychic insight.

While this may be quite helpful for well-selected patients, the majority of patients that are seen in general psychotherapy practice are generally much more concerned with immediate symptom relief than with self-actualization – they simply are not operating at the top of Maslow's hierarchy of needs.[14] Usually, self-actualization is not even 'on the radar screen;' instead, patients are distressed and come to therapy because they lack a sense of intimacy, acceptance, or self-esteem. In other words, they are experiencing interpersonal distress, and their goal is to relieve that distress as quickly as possible. Talk of transference, an expensive and lengthy course of therapy, and treatment with a therapist who may be perceived as being unsupportive, is neither what they want nor need.

IPT is therefore structured in such a way that transference problems are less likely to develop. First and foremost, the patient is not explicitly encouraged to discuss the patient–therapist relationship. In addition, the IPT therapist generally takes a supportive stance, rather than being neutral. The acute phase of therapy is time-limited, and the treatment is specifically focused on interpersonal issues in the patient's social relationships.

While IPT is specifically designed to delay or diminish the effect of parataxic distortions on the conduct of therapy, it would be a grave mistake to ignore the extraordinary trove of information about the patient which can be gleaned from the therapeutic relationship. Though the patient–therapist relationship is not directly addressed in sessions, the clinician can – using his or her observational skills and finely honed intuitive sense of the relationship that is developing – gather a vast amount of information about the patient. This is because the way in which the patient behaves in therapy is a direct reflection of the way in which he or she behaves and communicates in relationships outside of therapy. Gathering this information is crucial, as it informs the therapist about the patient's suitability for treatment, the prognosis for therapy, potential roadblocks that may occur, and also informs the specific techniques that should be used during therapy. Understanding the transference, recognizing the distortions that the patient brings to therapy, and developing hypotheses about the patient's interpersonal working model, are all essential to IPT.

As an illustration of this use of information about the parataxic distortions that occur in therapy, consider a patient who forms a relationship with his or her therapist that is dependent in nature. The patient may manifest this dependency as difficulty in ending sessions, calls to the therapist between sessions, or in more subtle pleas to the therapist for help or reassurance. This transferential relationship should inform the therapist about several aspects of the patient's functioning:

1 The patient is likely to have similar problems in relating to others in a dependent fashion.
2 The patient is likely to have difficulty ending relationships with others.
3 The patient has likely exhausted others with persistent calls for help.

A hypochondriacal patient would be an excellent example of this kind of behavior, manifest in the ways described. This information is then used by the therapist to formulate hypotheses about the patient's difficulties with others, and would lead the therapist to ask questions about how the patient asks others for help, ends relationships, and feels when others are not responsive to his or her needs. These questions are directed outside of the therapy relationship, however, to interpersonal relationships in which the patient is currently engaged, rather than directed to the relationship between therapist and patient.

Further, this information should be used by the therapist to predict potential problems that may arise in treatment, and to modify the therapy accordingly. For instance, the therapist might hypothesize that the patient's dependency is likely to cause a problem when concluding therapy, and may begin discussing the ending of therapy much earlier in the treatment than with less dependent patients. The therapist may also want to emphasize to a dependent patient the need for the patient to build an effective social support network, so that the patient's attachment needs are more fully met outside of therapy rather than fostering a dependent or regressive relationship in the therapy itself. Appropriate modifications would also be made with patients who are avoidant or who manifest other personality characteristics.

In addition, data gleaned from the therapeutic relationship should provide the therapist with information about the patient's prognosis in therapy. More severe parataxic distortions, and those which are manifest earlier in treatment, suggest a poor outcome. This information should not be used nihilistically, but rather should lead the therapist to more realistic expectations for the treatment.

In summary, the patient–therapist relationship – and particularly the patient-generated distortions in that relationship – are extremely important in IPT, but are not addressed directly in therapy. To do so detracts from the focus on symptom reduction and rapid improvement in interpersonal functioning that is the basis of IPT, and also typically leads to a much longer course of treatment than is required for IPT. The goal in IPT is literally to work with the patient to quickly resolve his or her interpersonal distress before problematic transference develops and becomes the focus of treatment.

A METAPHOR FOR IPT

The Sydney Harbor Bridge was completed in 1932, and even today is considered an engineering marvel. The single arch, more than 500 meters in length, spans one of the most beautiful harbors in the world, with a magnificent view of the Sydney Opera House, the Rocks, and downtown Sydney. On clear days the view extends all the way to the Pacific Ocean and beyond. It is simply one of the most spectacular sights in the world.

Since 1998, people have been allowed to climb up a very narrow catwalk to the top of the bridge. The arch, which is 134 meters above the harbor, is the highest point on the bridge. It is completely exposed, and on a windy day the whole bridge literally sways back and forth, giving climbers the queasy feeling that they will be pitched over the side and plummet each of those 134 long meters to the water below.

Those who are more adventurous and decide to climb the bridge are able to see one of the most breathtaking views in the world. It is attainable, it is magnificent – but it requires taking a risk. It requires suspending one's sense of psychological safety. It requires extending oneself beyond what many people are willing to do. The gain to be had is there, it is concrete, and it is palpable, but it requires physical and psychological effort.

Imagine what it would be like to climb the Sydney Harbor Bridge. For some people who are adventurous or who are genetically or temperamentally endowed with a predisposition to risk-taking, the Sydney Harbor Bridge climb is an exhilarating experience. No fear, no anxiety, just the thrill of the adrenaline rush that comes with being suspended over 120 meters (400 feet) in the air.

For others, the climb is a bit more anxiety-provoking. Some of these mildly anxious people have the psychological resources to literally 'talk themselves' into climbing the bridge. This self-talk might include rationalizations that the climb is really safe (despite appearances to the contrary), or it might include continued self-reminders that the effort and risk will be well worth the rewards. Terms such as ego strength and a capacity for delayed gratification might be used when describing these people.

Others, because of life experience, biological, temperamental, or other factors, need some help to manage the climb. For some, cognitive reassurance is sufficient. A reminder – *from a trusted significant other* – of an accurate cognitive appraisal of the situation is needed. 'After all,' the significant other might say, 'the Sydney Harbor Bridge has stood since 1932 without falling down. Hundreds of thousands of people have climbed it without mishap.' And in Socratic fashion, such an amateur clinician might rhetorically ask, 'When was the last time you read in the Sydney Morning Herald about someone falling off the bridge? What do you think the realistic chance is that something bad will happen to you if you do the climb?' Thus cognitively reassured, these moderately anxious people are able to ascend.

For those who are yet more anxious, or who are somewhat more dependent in personality, such cognitive reassurance is not sufficient. It is not simply cognitive reappraisal that they require, it is *interpersonal reassurance*. Such people are looking for someone to literally take their hand, and figuratively to be with and support them psychologically. Such a person, though feeling very anxious about the climb, might be able to say, 'I'll do it if you go with me.'

Some people requiring this kind of reassurance are able to ask for it directly, and as a result are generally pretty successful in getting the support they need. Their significant others can respond to them easily, and are both available and willing to provide interpersonal and emotional support. In contrast, other people faced with the Sydney Harbor Bridge climb 'crisis' have personality or communication styles in which their needs are conveyed either indirectly or in a way that is counterproductive. Whining, complaining, being passive–aggressive, and dependently clinging are not good ways to get someone to hold your hand while climbing the bridge.

Finally, there are those that go to Sydney, look at the bridge, and say to themselves, 'I could never do that.' And for a variety of psychological, physical, temperamental, and social reasons, they don't.

The Sydney Harbor Bridge climb is a crisis. It is literally a transcendent experience which can be obtained by taking a risk. The approach that people take to this crisis is based largely on their biopsychosocial makeup. Genetics, temperament, early life experience, attachment, personality, social support, and adult experience all play a role in determining who will attempt – and who will succeed – in climbing the bridge.

IPT is designed to help those people who get hung up because they need interpersonal support in order to accomplish the climb. IPT is designed to help people recognize their interpersonal needs for attachment and reassurance, and to express those needs to others in a way to which they can productively respond. IPT is not designed for everyone, nor does everyone need it. Many are able to deal with their particular crises without professional help. A few have problems so severe that they need much more extensive help. But there are a significant number of people who need help to resolve a specific crisis, and who need assistance in generating or using their social support system to negotiate it.

IPT is designed to help people face their bridge crises, reach new heights, and to bring someone along with whom to enjoy the view.

CONCLUSION

The defining characteristics of IPT are its three primary elements: *interpersonal orientation; time limit;* and *the avoidance of interventions which directly address the patient–therapist relationship.* IPT is also based on the *biopsychosocial model* of psychological functioning, which allows the therapist to conceptualize patients' problems broadly as stemming from biological factors, early and later life experiences, temperament and attachment styles, and current social support. It is an extremely useful intervention for well-selected patients who face acute crises which they cannot manage alone.

REFERENCES

1. Klerman, G.L., Weissman, M.M., Rounsaville, B.J., Chevron, E.S. 1984. *Interpersonal Psychotherapy of Depression.* New York: Basic Books.
2. American Psychiatric Association. 1994. *Diagnostic and Statistical Manual of Mental Disorders.* 4th edition. Washington, DC: American Psychiatric Association.
3. Engel, G.L. 1980. The clinical application of biopsychosocial models. *American Journal of Psychiatry* 137, 535–44.
4. O'Hara, M.W., Stuart, S., Gorman, L., Wenzel, A. 2000. Efficacy of interpersonal psychotherapy for postpartum depression. *Archives of General Psychiatry* 57, 1039–45.
5. Stuart, S., O'Hara, M.W. 1995. Interpersonal psychotherapy for postpartum depression: a treatment program. *Journal of Psychotherapy Practice and Research* 4, 18–29.
6. Beck, A.T., Rush, A.J., Shaw, B.F., Emery, G. 1979. *Cognitive Therapy of Depression.* New York: Guilford Press.
7. Malan, D.H. 1976. *The Frontier of Brief Psychotherapy.* New York: Plenum.
8. Sifneos, P. 1972. *Short-term Psychotherapy and Emotional Crisis.* Cambridge: Harvard University Press.
9. Stuart, S. (in press) Interpersonal psychotherapy. In: Dewan, M., Steenbarger, B., Greenberg, R. (eds), *The Art and Science of Brief Psychotherapies: A Practitioner's Guide.* Washington, DC: American Psychiatric Press.
10. Frank, E., Kupfer, D.J., Perel, J.M. *et al.* 1990. Three-year outcomes for maintenance therapies in recurrent depression. *Archives of General Psychiatry* 47, 1093–9.
11. Bowlby, J. 1988. Developmental psychiatry comes of age. *American Journal of Psychiatry* 145, 1–10.
12. Sullivan, H.S. 1953. *The Interpersonal Theory of Psychiatry.* New York: Norton.
13. Bowlby, J. 1977. The making and breaking of affectional bonds: etiology and psychopathology in the light of attachment theory. *British Journal of Psychiatry* 130, 201–10.
14. Maslow, A. 1943. A theory of human motivation. *Psychological Review* 50, 370–96.

2

Theory and Clinical Applications

INTRODUCTION

IPT rests on a triad of theoretical underpinnings. The first and most important is *attachment theory*, which forms the basis for formulating patients' relationship difficulties and informs clinicians about the modifications they may need to make during the course of therapy. The second, *communication theory*, describes the ways in which patients' maladaptive communication patterns may lead to difficulty in their here-and-now interpersonal relationships. Communication is one manifestation of the attachment behavior that occurs in individuals, but it is an extremely important particular in IPT, as it is the point of intervention for many IPT techniques. The third, *social theory* is the basis for understanding the interpersonal context in which people interact with others, and the effect their social networks have on their interpersonal functioning.

IPT is based on the concept that psychiatric and interpersonal difficulties result from a combination of interpersonal and biological factors, following the biopsychosocial model of psychiatric illness.[1] Individuals with a genetic predisposition or biological diathesis for psychological difficulties will be more likely to have problems when stressed interpersonally. Upon this foundation rests the individual's temperament, personality traits, and early life experiences, which in turn are reflected in a particular attachment style. The attachment style may be more or less adaptive, and has effects upon the person's current social support network and his or her ability to enlist the support of significant others. Interpersonal functioning is determined by the severity of current stressors in the context of this social support.

IPT is therefore designed to treat psychiatric symptoms by focusing specifically on patients' primary interpersonal relationships, particularly in the problem areas of *grief and loss, interpersonal disputes, role transitions,* and *interpersonal sensitivity.* Although fundamental change in either personality or attachment style is unlikely during short-term treatment, symptom resolution is made possible when patients are assisted in repairing their disrupted interpersonal relationships, and when they learn new ways to communicate their needs for emotional support.

A comprehensive and well-articulated theory which supports IPT is necessary for several reasons. *The most important is that it informs the clinician about the nature of the patient's problems, and informs the clinician about the kinds of interventions that may be helpful to resolve those problems.* Thus, a comprehensive theory forms the basis for the clinician's formulation of a case, and for the determination of which specific therapeutic interventions are likely to be most helpful. It should also provide guidance in anticipating potential problems with a given individual during the course of therapy (such as problems with resistance or forming a therapeutic alliance), and should inform the therapist about the ways in which he or she can prevent or effectively manage these roadblocks.

The theoretical foundation for IPT has the following features:

1 It is based on the available empirical evidence.
2 It reflects clinical experience and clinical observations as accurately as possible.
3 It forms the basis for hypotheses that can be examined clinically with specific individuals.
4 It forms the basis for hypotheses that can be empirically tested in traditional scientific fashion with groups of patients.
5 It is subject to modifications as new empirical and clinical evidence accumulates.

The theory supporting IPT is, therefore, not a set of static ideas, but a constantly evolving set of hypotheses which are open to investigation and modification as clinical and research experience accumulates (Figure 2.1).

ATTACHMENT THEORY

Attachment theory serves as the foundation for IPT, as it describes the ways in which individuals form, maintain, and end relationships, as well as the ways in which they develop problems within them. John Bowlby among others has articulated the principles of attachment theory,[2-7] which is based on the premise that humans have an intrinsic instinctual drive to form interpersonal relationships with others. This drive is biologically grounded, a concept which is supported by both ethological research and evolutionary theory,[5] as the capacity and drive to form intimate bonds is crucial to human survival. Humans function optimally when their attachments needs are met; they develop problems, often manifest as psychiatric symptoms, when their attachment needs go unmet.

Simply put, attachment organizes behavior in interpersonal relationships. It forms the basis for a relatively enduring pattern of inner experience and interpersonal behavior which leads an individual to seek care and comfort in a characteristic way. Though always operative, it is activated to a greater degree when an individual is stressed and his or her sense of security is threatened. Attachment behavior then drives the person to seek care.

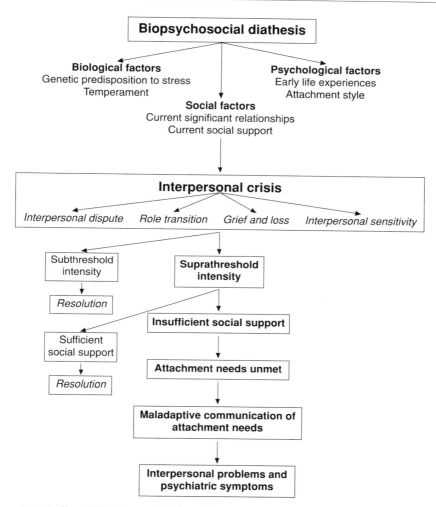

Figure 2.1 *Outline of IPT Theory*. *The biopsychosocial diathesis is the foundation upon which interpersonal crises are laid. A sufficiently intense crisis in the context of insufficient social support leads to interpersonal problems and psychiatric symptoms because attachment needs are unmet and the patient is unable to communicate them effectively.*

Bowlby described it succinctly by stating 'attachment behavior is conceived as any form of behavior that results in a person attaining or retaining proximity to some other differentiated and preferred individual. While especially evident during childhood, attachment behavior is held to characterize human beings from the cradle to the grave. In adults it is especially evident when a person is distressed, ill, or afraid. The particular patterns of attachment behavior shown by an individual turn partly on his present age, sex, and circumstances and partly on the experiences he has had with attachment figures earlier in his life' (p. 203).[3] 'The desire to be loved and cared for is an integral part of human nature throughout adult life as well as earlier, and the expression of such desires is to be expected in every grown-up, especially in times of sickness or calamity' (p. 428).[4]

Thus, attachment behavior is a part of the normal repertoire of human behavior, and is generated when an individual is stressed either physically or psychologically. Wanting to be loved and cared for is an intrinsic part of being human; the drive to seek care is magnified when an individual is feeling sick, lonely, tired, depressed, anxious, or in need of affection. In IPT, psychological problems occur, and interpersonal relationships break down, when an individual's needs for attachment are not being met. This can occur both when the individual cannot effectively communicate his or her needs to others, or when his or her social support network is incapable of responding adequately to his or her needs.

Bowlby hypothesized that particular attachment styles derive largely from early childhood experiences, as a child engages in attachment relationships with his or her primary caregivers.[2] These formative experiences lead to the development of a working model of relationships, so that the actual attachment experiences of an individual are transposed into expectations about relationships in general and new relationships in particular. In other words, the cumulative relationship experiences of an individual inform his or her views about what subsequent new relationships will be like. This model allows an individual to function interpersonally, because it gives him or her a template upon which to predict how others will behave in different circumstances.

This model, in essence, frames for the individual the statement, 'When I am stressed and in need of care and support, others will typically react towards me by doing . . . .' The response to this statement forms the basis for the way in which the individual seeks to meet his or her attachment needs. If the expectation is that these needs will be met by others, then the individual will act by directly asking for support. If the expectation, based on real life experiences to date, is that the request for support will be met with rejection, then the individual may avoid asking for help, or demand it in ways that may be self-defeating.

The working model of relationships which develops is based on real life experiences. Thus, an individual who has had experiences of abuse will understandably expect similar treatment in the new relationships that he or she forms; an individual who has experienced rejection will expect more of the same; and an individual who has had productive and trusting relationships will anticipate that new relationships will be the same. The effects of these expectations are evident during childhood, but have also been extended to adult behavior.[8,9]

Bowlby's concept of a working model of attachment bears much similarity to Sullivan's concept of parataxic distortion, in which the cumulative experiences of an individual inform the way in which he or she relates to other individuals.[10] Both Sullivan and Bowlby argued that the working model of relationships, and the subsequent distortions that occurred as a result of the model, are based largely (though not exclusively) on early life relationships with the individual's primary caregiver. Both also hypothesized that individuals experience interpersonal problems not because their working models are inaccurate reflections of their past experiences, but because the models are imposed inappropriately onto new relationships in which the individuals' assumptions about the ways others will behave towards them are not warranted.

For instance, a patient with a history of abuse is quite understandably likely to develop a working model of relationships which suggests that people are not to be trusted, or that others will take advantage of him or her – it is imposed consistently upon all relationships. While adaptive when faced with potential abuse, this model impairs the ability of the patient to function interpersonally when in situations in which abuse is not likely to occur. Such an individual is likely to have difficulty developing intimate relationships because his or her model of relationships dictates that people cannot be trusted – even those who are impeccably trustworthy are pushed away. Therapeutic examples abound, in which patients with distorted models of relationships impose them upon others in situations in which the models are inaccurate, leading ultimately to self-defeating behavior and distress. This parataxic distortion impairs the ability of the patient to function and feel secure within all relationships, including the therapeutic relationship.

An individual's working model of relationships is generally consistent both within and across relationships, coalescing to form a characteristic attachment style. That is, individuals tend to maintain the same attachment style over time in a given relationship, and also tend to form new relationships in the same fashion with consistent styles of attachment. This phenomenon is dramatically illustrated with hypochondriacal patients, for instance, who form dependent relationships with family members, significant others, and healthcare professionals that are all based on a dependent attachment style – they do not suddenly change their way of attaching to others within a given relationship, nor upon entering a new relationship.

This consistency in attachment style also forms the theoretical basis for the development of transference, i.e., given enough time, a patient will manifest the same attachment style with the therapist that he or she manifests with others outside of therapy. Thus, a sensitivity to the therapeutic relationship allows the therapist to tap into this extremely important information about the patient's attachment style and model of relationships, and allows the therapist to begin to develop hypotheses about the kinds of interpersonal problems the patient is likely to experience, and the ways in which others may be perceiving the patient. Though not addressed directly in IPT, this information is crucial to understanding the attachment and communication problems experienced by the patient in his or her current relationships.

It is also absolutely essential for the therapist to keep in mind that the attachment difficulties experienced by the patient and the distortions that the patient imposes upon new relationships are all a product of his or her real experiences. People come by their relationship models honestly. Their models and distortions reflect real attempts to cope with earlier stressors, abuse, or deprivations, and the tragedy is that these past experiences continue to haunt patients through their continuing effect on attachment and interpersonal functioning. Such tragedies call for empathy rather than pathological labels.

Bowlby[2] described three basic styles of attachment: (i) secure; (ii) anxious ambivalent; and (iii) anxious avoidant,[a] all of which bear directly upon the clinical application of IPT. *Securely attached* individuals base their relationships on working models which are healthy and flexible – in other words, they generally trust others, believe that their needs will be met, and are able to 'explore' the world and seek out new relationships and experiences with a sense of security. They manifest, as Bowlby described, the characteristics of good mental health: they are able to effectively ask for care from others when it is needed, and are able to provide care to others when asked to do so as well. Their

[a]Other authors have described additional styles. Disorganized attachment has been added by some theorists to the styles described by Bowlby, and a model incorporating four styles has also been proposed (Main, 1986, p. 944; Bartholomew, 1991, p. 945; Pilkonis, 1988, p. 946; Brennan, 1998, p. 947). Our clinical experience with IPT has led us to describe a 'compulsive caregiver' style of attachment as well, which has proved helpful in working with some patients. This style was also noted by Bowlby and others, though not incorporated into his primary model. We believe Bowlby's original description has great clinical utility and has been selected for discussion because of its conciseness.

relationships are generally satisfactory and productive, they have extensive social support networks, and are thus able to effectively manage most life crises.

Individuals with *anxious ambivalent* attachment styles, in contrast, are constantly preoccupied with ensuring that their attachment needs will be met. Their working model of relationships is such that they assume that others will not adequately care for them, and that in order to have their attachment needs met, they must constantly seek care and reassurance. Hypochondriacal patients are classic examples of this kind of attachment behavior – they are constantly seeking reassurance, and are so preoccupied with obtaining sufficient care in their attachment relationships that they lack any capacity to provide care for others.[11] Moreover, their constant reassurance-seeking behavior eventually 'wears out' their care providers, ultimately resulting in rejection. As a result, the intimate relationships that these individuals are able to develop are unstable, and they are very vulnerable to conflicts or losses which threaten their attachments. Further, since they are unable to develop mutually supportive relationships, their social support network is very poor.

Those individuals with *anxious avoidant* attachment styles often have early life experiences in which care was never adequately provided. As a result, they develop working models of relationships in which they come to believe that care will never be sufficient or perhaps even provided at all, and that their attachment needs will never be met. Interpersonal behaviors such as avoidance or compulsive self-reliance are consistent with this attachment style. Anxious avoidant individuals, lacking the belief that they will be cared for in relationships, form either superficial bonds with others or avoid them altogether. Their social support network tends to be very poor as a result. Patients with social phobia or schizoid personality disorders often fit into this category.

Individuals with both types of insecure attachment styles are twice cursed, so to speak. First, their life experiences have led them to develop working models of relationships in which they are convinced that care will not be available to them when needed. Second, because they typically lack the capacity to care for others or to develop intimate relationships, their social support networks are usually very poor. Neither their internal world, nor their external world, is adapted to deal with interpersonal stress.

In summary, attachment theory hypothesizes that individuals have difficulty when they experience disruptions in their attachments with others. This is both because of the specific loss of the attachment relationship and because their social support network is not able to sustain them during the loss, conflict, or transition. Insecurely attached individuals are much more vulnerable to difficulties with personal conflicts, such as divorce or relationship disruptions, and to role transitions such as moving or loss of a job, both because of their tenuous primary relationships and because of their poor social support networks.[12] In addition, they are also more likely to develop problems when faced with a major loss such as the death of a primary attachment figure.[13,14] These problem areas – interpersonal disputes, role transitions, and grief and loss – are specifically addressed in IPT.

The vulnerability of insecurely attached individuals is a result not only of their internal insecurity, but also stems from the fact that their social support networks are poorly constructed and poorly responsive to their needs. Further, insecurely attached individuals are largely unable to communicate their interpersonal and attachment needs directly,[15] making it unlikely that others, even if so inclined, will be able to respond to their needs effectively.

Even securely attached individuals can develop psychiatric symptoms or interpersonal problems if faced with a stressor that is great enough (e.g., the death of a spouse), but their threshold for the development of problems is higher than for those with insecure styles of attachment. Both their internal sense of security and their superior social support systems can sustain securely attached individuals in situations in which others might have difficulties. Those securely attached are also able to ask effectively for support from others when it is needed – their previous experience and internal working models indicate that it is likely to be provided – and can communicate their specific needs for support.

Attachment theory is consistent with the clearly established biological diatheses for depression and other illnesses. Genetic contributions combine with attachment style to influence the vulnerability of an individual to stress, which, when combined with a sufficient psychosocial crisis, leads to psychiatric symptoms. Given that maladaptive attachment styles often develop because an individual grows up with parents who have psychiatric problems that influence their parenting behavior, and consequently that such an individual has both a heritable biological predisposition to develop psychiatric problems as well as a maladaptive attachment style, it is not surprising that difficulties develop. Thus, the foundation of IPT is a broad-based understanding of an individual based on a biopsychosocial model.

Attachment theory suggests that one way to improve a patient's functioning would be to change his or her basic attachment style. This implies therapeutic goals of helping the patient to recognize his or her patterns of attachment, to understand how their attachment style developed, and to modify their internal model of attachment. This reworking of attachment patterns requires the development of insight through the examination of early childhood experiences, as well as an overt discussion of the therapeutic relationship to examine patterns of interaction. The patient's interaction with the therapist would be examined in detail, with the goal of using it as the vehicle for change. A primary technique would be interpretation of the transferential experience. This is essentially an open-ended psychodynamic approach to treatment.

While there is great utility in this approach with suitable patients, the time required to bring about such a fundamental change is often great, and the treatment must often be quite intensive. Bowlby himself stated that, 'a restructuring of a person's representational models and his re-evaluation of some aspects of human relationships, with a corresponding change in his modes of treating people, is likely to be both slow and patchy' (p. 427).[4] Therapy which aims to bring about such deep and lasting changes requires a great degree of motivation, insight, time, financial resources, and a patient and therapist who are able to devote themselves to the task without the need for immediate gratification. The key is to determine 'how much therapy' is appropriate for a given patient considering these factors.

In addition, focusing therapy on a patient's internal model of attachment is likely to detract temporally from a focus on the rapid resolution of his or her symptoms. Most of the therapeutic action is in the patient–therapist relationship and the interactions which flow from it. By definition, a therapy that is constructed to look more intensively at the therapeutic relationship will devote less time to working to resolve the patient's current interpersonal problems. Further, the psychodynamic therapist must always be aware of the fact that, given enough time, despite his or her best efforts to support the patient, he or she will ultimately fail to meet the patient's attachment needs as they are manifested in therapy. Thus, to continue therapy in an intense and open-ended fashion will eventually require that the therapeutic relationship be discussed as a central feature of the therapy.

In contrast, rather than attempting to change the patient's fundamental attachment style, IPT focuses on the ways in which the patient communicates his or her attachment needs, and on the way in which he or she can construct a more supportive social network. Taking the patient's attachment style as a constant, IPT works in real-time relationships to help the patient communicate his or her needs more effectively. It is not designed to change the patient's internal structures, ego functioning, or defense mechanisms, but rather to help the patient identify or develop social supports, and to help with the communication of his or her attachment needs in that context. The experience of having his or her attachment needs met may help to restructure the patient's internal model in a way that more accurately reflects reality, but this is not the primary goal of treatment. Rather, priority is given to rapid symptom resolution and improvement in interpersonal functioning, and treatment can therefore be short-term (Figure 2.2).

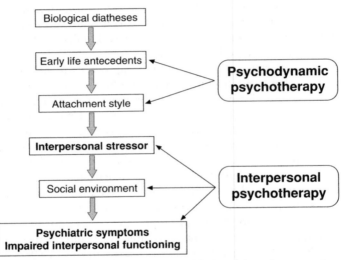

Figure 2.2 IPT and Psychodynamic Psychotherapy: Differing Points of Intervention. *IPT intervenes at the level of the acute interpersonal stressor and the current social environment with the goal of alleviating symptoms and improving social functioning. Psychodynamic psychotherapy is designed to facilitate change in fundamental attachment style by examining early life experiences and transference.*

Therapeutic implications of attachment theory

Attachment theory forms *the basis for conceptualizing a patient's distress as stemming from attachment needs which are unmet.* This may be because the patient has a maladaptive style of attaching to others which leads him or her to believe that care from others is insufficient or unavailable. It may also occur when a securely attached individual is faced with an overwhelming interpersonal crisis. In IPT, the emphasis is on quickly assisting the patient to get his or her needs met more effectively by focusing on communication within the patient's attachment relationships, and on his or her social support system, taking the attachment style as given. In long-term psychodynamic psychotherapy, the emphasis is on modifying the underlying attachment style itself.

Attachment theory also informs the *interventions* which are likely to be helpful in IPT. Exploration and clarification of the patient's current interpersonal relationships, and recent transitions in those relationships, are of help in understanding his or her attachment style. Exploring patterns of relationships, such as the ways in which the patient asks for help from others, feels that he or she is understood by others, and the typical ways in which relationships end, should also be beneficial.

Recognizing the ways in which the patient attaches to the therapist during the course of therapy is extremely helpful, as it informs the therapist about the ways in which the patient attaches to significant others. Though the patient–therapist relationship is not directly addressed in IPT, this understanding should assist the therapist to develop hypotheses about the patient's interpersonal functioning, and the ways in which it is causing the patient problems, and should direct the therapist to ask even more specifically directed questions about the patient's relationships outside of therapy.

Attachment theory forms *the basis for informing the therapist about potential therapeutic resistance, and informs the therapist about ways in which to counter it.* Patients with avoidant attachments, for example, are likely to have more difficulty in forming a therapeutic alliance with the therapist; hence, the therapist may want to take more time engaging the patient and expressing empathy early in the course of therapy. Patients with ambivalent attachments are likely to have difficulty concluding therapy and ending their relationship with the therapist; thus the therapist may want to spend more time discussing the end of treatment earlier in therapy, and may place special emphasis on helping these patients to establish external social supports that they can use in lieu of the therapeutic relationship when treatment is concluded. Securely attached patients, on the other hand, may benefit from therapist self-disclosure, and are much more likely to be able to constructively use homework assignments or direct advice from the clinician.

Attachment theory informs prognosis. The more securely attached a patient is, the better the prognosis for therapy, and this is true for a number of reasons. A more securely attached patient generally has better social support, and also has a greater capacity to ask for help when it is needed. A more securely attached patient is also able to form a more productive alliance with the therapist, and enters therapy with the expectation that it will be helpful. Such a patient is also less likely to have difficulty ending therapy, as his or her attachments outside of therapy are more satisfying than those of patients who are less securely attached.

Attachment style appears to be a powerful predictor of outcome in all varieties of psychotherapy. The reality is that in therapy 'the rich get richer' – those patients with more interpersonal and intrapsychic resources, with better social support networks, and with more adaptive attachment styles and personalities, get more from therapy.

Despite the fact that attachment appears to be intimately related to outcome in therapy, clinicians should not be nihilistic about their work with patients with more maladaptive attachment styles. There are many patients with varying styles of attachment who do quite well in treatment, and such patients should not be excluded from therapy on that basis. Further, there is no evidence that patients with more maladaptive attachment styles do better in therapies other than IPT – in fact, a reasonable argument could be made that for acute problems, IPT is well suited for many such patients because the treatment is focal and less intense than more dynamically oriented therapies. The bottom line is that the therapist should recognize that attachment style does influence outcome, and should adjust his or her expectations about what therapy is likely to achieve on that basis.

Table 2.1 *Therapeutic Implications of Attachment Theory*

Attachment theory forms the basis for:

- Conceptualization of the patient's interpersonal problems.
- Interventions to be used in therapy.
- Understanding the patient–therapist relationship.
- Predicting potential problems in therapy.
- Predicting prognosis.

COMMUNICATION THEORY

Communication theory, as articulated by Kiesler[16–19] and Benjamin[20,21] among others, is intimately connected to attachment theory, and can be understood in an IPT framework as describing the way in which individuals communicate their attachment needs to specific significant others. Attachment theory is connected to the broad, or macro, social context, while communication theory informs individual relationships on a micro level within that setting. Attachment is the template upon which specific communication occurs.

According to Kiesler,[16] human personality can be understood as an enduring pattern of recurrent interpersonal interactions. This pattern is played out across a wide variety of relationships in the individual's social network. Disordered or dysfunctional interpersonal relationships are characterized by disordered interpersonal communications, which in turn are influenced by the individual's expectations about how relationships in general are formed and maintained. This expectation, or belief, about relationships, is built upon the attachment-based 'working model' of relationships described by Bowlby.[5] The parataxic distortions imposed upon relationships as a result of inaccurate working models dramatically influences the ways in which interpersonal communication occurs.

Within every relationship, Kiesler[16] posits that individuals negotiate three specific aspects of the relationship. Because these aspects are a product of the communication between individuals, they are termed 'metacommunications' – they are communications about the qualities of the relationships itself, and reflect what the relationship is like. The elements are:

- *Affiliation*, i.e., the degree to which individuals have positive (*high affiliation*) or negative (*low affiliation*) feelings about one another.
- *Dominance*, i.e., the degree to which one or the other person is 'in charge' of decisions made within the relationship and the agenda for the relationship (*dominant versus submissive*).
- *Inclusion*, i.e., the degree to which the relationship stands as important to each individual (*high versus low inclusion*).

These three aspects of relationships can be portrayed graphically using a three-dimensional system of axes, and an individual's communication at any given moment can be graphically displayed on this grid. These three axes are shown in Figure 2.3.

The metacommunication of an individual can be plotted on this grid for any given communication. For instance, the statement, 'I love you' spoken to an intimate partner

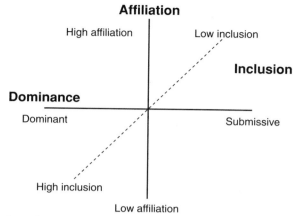

Figure 2.3 *Dimensions of Interpersonal Relationships*. *The various axes represent the elements of the relationship: the X-axis describes the level of dominance, the Y-axis the degree of affiliation, and the Z-axis the degree of inclusion.*

would convey a very high degree of affiliation, a high degree of inclusion reflective of the importance of the relationship, and a neutral degree of dominance. A statement such as, 'this project is unacceptable,' spoken by a boss to an employee, would convey a high degree of dominance along with low affiliation. And if the employee wanted to keep his job, such a statement would also convey a high degree of inclusion, as the relationship carries a great deal of significance and the employee had better strongly heed the message. A passing comment between strangers, such as, 'nice day today,' though fairly high in affiliation, would have a low degree of inclusion as the relationship is not particularly important to either participant.

On a micro-level, this communication occurs on a moment-by-moment, or statement-by-statement, basis.[22] The cumulative effect of these metacommunications determines the nature of a relationship, and is a manifestation of the attachment styles of both individuals in the relationship.

In addition to the direct communication which occurs in relationships, affiliative, dominance, and inclusion metacommunications also evoke specific responses from others.[16] These reciprocal responses follow a predictable pattern. Communication which is high in dominance tends to evoke submissive responses; communication which is high in affiliation typically evokes highly affiliative responses; and those high in inclusion naturally evoke highly inclusive responses. This is illustrated in Figure 2.4.

According to Kiesler, interpersonal problems occur because patients unintentionally elicit negative reciprocal responses from others.[22] Maladaptive attachment styles are therefore reflected on a micro level as specific communications that elicit responses which do not effectively meet the individual's attachment needs. The accumulation of these communications establishes a relationship which is reflective of the attachment styles of both participants. As noted above, attachment patterns tend to be consistent both within relationships and across relationships over time, and individuals also tend to communicate their attachment needs in a consistent fashion over time.

Anxious individuals' attachment needs are not met effectively because they tend to elicit reciprocal responses from others which are antithetical to their needs. Consider, for example, an individual who communicates a desire for care in a hostile fashion.

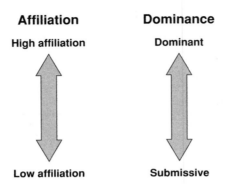

Figure 2.4 *Reciprocal Communication*. *Reciprocal responses are elicited by specific interpersonal communications. An affiliative communication from individual A tends to elicit a similar response from person B, whereas a dominant response from individual A tends to elicit the opposite response from person B: submissiveness pulls for a dominant response, and vice versa. Inclusive communications from individual A also pull for similar reponses from person B: high inclusion pulls for a similarly highly inclusive response.*

Rather than eliciting a response which is high in affiliation, this kind of communication is almost certain to evoke a response from others which is low in affiliation – in essence, potential care providers are driven away by the hostility. Demanding communications which are high in dominance are also likely to be met with resistance, as the passive response they tend to evoke will also tend to push others away.

This type of maladaptive interpersonal communication has been observed in patients with somatizing disorders,[11] who tend to be classic examples of this type of communication pattern. Such patients may, for example, frequently manifest an anxious avoidant attachment style, believing that others will never be able to meet their attachment needs. Their communication of this fear and attachment distress, however, comes in the form of statements conveying anger at not being cared for, not being understood, and not being taken seriously. This ultimately results in both the caregiver's rejecting of the somatizer, as well as the somatizing patient's rejection of help from others. Medical professionals with whom these patients come in contact are usually quite happy to have the patient move on, as the patient's persistent hostile communication has long quashed any desire of the care provider to help. The patient's hostile communications elicit hostility and rejection in return.

Hypochondriacal patients, as another example, often have anxious ambivalent attachment styles which are manifested as persistent help-seeking behavior. Unlike somatizing patients, however, their attachment needs are communicated in a way that is high in affiliation but which is very submissive. Initially, they tend to evoke caring responses from others – many hypochondriacal patients are quite pleasant to work with initially. Over time, however, the persistent help-seeking behavior, combined with a very passive and submissive pattern of communication, and an inability to be reassured by any intervention, lead others to become frustrated and ultimately reject the hypochondriac.

As a final example, consider a patient with a more schizoid personality style. With an anxious avoidant attachment style, such a patient will typically communicate in a fashion which is low in affiliation and inclusion – though not hostile, the patient may be unable to tolerate a close relationship and will remain distant. This distancing behavior and communication consistently elicits a distancing or low affiliative response from others. A lack of social skills may also inhibit the communication, leading to a frustration of attachment needs when they are communicated ineffectively to others. As this poor communication and avoidance is generalized, such a patient will likely have a very poor social support network.

In summary, maladaptive attachment styles lead to inappropriate or inadequate interpersonal communication which prevents individuals' attachment needs from being met. The continual and rigid verbal and non-verbal pattern of communication elicits a rigidly restricted range of responses from others, usually culminating in a rejecting response from others. These maladaptive attachment styles and communications are characterized by their rigidity and by the limited and rejecting responses they evoke.

In addition, patients' maladaptive attachment styles and communication patterns are reinforced by the responses which they provoke. Since those with insecure attachments tend to push others away or evoke rejecting responses as a result of their ineffective communication, their parataxic distortions or working model of relationships is reinforced. The very rejection which their behavior and communication has evoked becomes further proof that they will never receive adequate care. Since their ability to convey a need for care is greatly restricted, the threat to the minimal care they are able to obtain is met with an even more intense use of the same maladaptive communication, perpetuating and escalating the cycle. Angry somatizing patients, upon the elicitation of a rejecting response from a care provider, will communicate even more anger and hostility at being rejected in their next encounter with a medical professional. This makes it even less likely that their attachment needs will be met, and further reinforces their interpersonal working model and their maladaptive attachment style[11] (Figure 2.5).

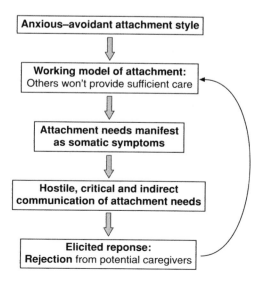

Figure 2.5 *The Interpersonal Communication of Somatizers.*

Adding insult to injury, patients displaying maladaptive communication patterns typically lack insight into their communication difficulties.[16] In other words, they are at a loss to understand why others are not providing care for them, and to understand why others ultimately also reject them. They are quite aware of the fact that they are distressed, and that their needs are not being met, but do not appreciate the fact that it is in large part the way that they are communicating that is leading to their distress. They do not understand that they are not communicating their needs effectively, nor communicating them in a way that others can respond to effectively.

SOCIAL THEORY

Research into depression and anxiety has consistently emphasized the role of interpersonal factors such as loss, poor or disrupted social support and maladaptive responses to life events.[23] The social milieu in which a patient develops interpersonal relationships, and his or her social support in particular, strongly influence the way in which he or she is able to cope with interpersonal stress.

Social theory has been described by Henderson *et al.*,[24] among others. In essence, social theory posits that a deficiency in social relationships is a causal factor in the genesis of psychological distress, and that the causal effect of these deficits holds whether an individual is exposed to high or low levels of adversity. Henderson *et al.* go on to state that it is the effect of the individual's *current* environment that is crucial.[24] While past relationships and early life environment may 'contribute to the picture by distorting the individual's perception of contemporary conditions,' it is not invoked in social theory as a necessary causal agent.[24] In summary, stress in current social relationships is an independent causative factor in the genesis of psychological distress.

Social theory therefore stands in sharp contrast to psychoanalytic theory, and clearly differentiates IPT from more psychoanalytic and psychodynamic approaches. Psychoanalysis rests on two fundamental principles: psychic determinism and the proposition that unconscious mental processes are the foundation for an individual's conscious thoughts and behaviors. In other words, according to psychoanalytic theory, individuals are largely unaware of the processes that drive their behavior, and it is these unconscious factors that lead to neurosis and psychopathology.[25]

In contrast, social theory invokes neither of these principles. The fundamental basis for social theory is that current interpersonal stressors lead to psychopathology – there is no need to rely on either unconscious processes nor psychic determinism as causal factors in psychological dysfunction. The implications of this difference are also clear – psychoanalysis is designed to elicit the unconscious determinants of psychopathology, while social theory suggests that interventions which affect current social relationships will lead to improved functioning. The latter approach is completely consistent with IPT.

Another important concept in social theory is that of qualitative responses to social stress. Rather than viewing psychiatric illness as a dichotomous proposition – i.e., one either has an illness or does not have an illness – many social theorists have argued that the distinction between emotional distress and illness is simply one of degree.[26] In other words, there is a spectrum of responses to untoward social stressors which ranges from mild distress to severe distress; psychiatric illness is simply defined as crossing an arbitrary line of severity. Further, the differences in individuals' experiences of depression are strongly influenced by psychosocial factors[27] – these experiential differences are not reflected in diagnoses, which include only symptoms. Incorporating this concept into IPT is important because it allows for the treatment of individuals who are distressed rather than limiting treatment to those who meet 'diagnostic criteria' for a particular illness.

A number of studies demonstrating an association between quality of social support and psychological problems have been conducted, including a series of studies by Henderson et al.,[24,28] who demonstrated that poor social support is associated with depression and other 'neurotic' illnesses.[29,30] Henderson also hypothesized that an individual's personality and quality of attachments, among other factors, may be responsible for the difficulties that some individuals have in obtaining care and support from others.[31]

The concept of 'social support networks' has been shown to be relevant to interpersonal and psychological distress. Studies confirm that social isolation or limited social interaction places individuals at greater risk for mental illness. The quality of the interaction, however, appears to be more important than the absolute number of relationships. This perceived social support is a function of the subjective evaluation by the individual of the dependability of the social network, the ease of interaction within the network, the individual's sense of belonging to the network, and his or her sense of intimacy with network members.[32]

Studies conducted by Brown and colleagues have also consistently demonstrated a correlation between adverse social events and the incidence of psychiatric disorders.[33,34] Both current social stressors and childhood experiences of neglect and abuse have been correlated with anxiety and depression in women.[35]

Marital conflict appears to be one of the most consistent risk factors for psychological distress. Rates of major depressive disorder are highest among separated and divorced persons and lowest among single and married persons. Recent widowhood is associated with higher rates of major depressive disorder across the life cycle,[36] and the absence of a spouse is a risk factor for major depressive disorder.[37] Grief and loss have been associated with depressive symptoms in both men and women, particularly those with poor social supports.[38,39] In contrast, the presence of attachments that can help sustain individuals during the loss appears to be helpful in preventing episodes of depression.[40]

The association of major depressive disorder and absence of a confidant exemplifies the relation between inadequate social support and psychological difficulties. Brown's studies have shown that losses in socioeconomically disadvantaged women who lack supportive relationships is a key factor in the development of depression.[37] Several longitudinal studies of social support networks and neuroses have also shown that the most important predictors of depression are not the objective characteristics of the network itself but rather the individual's perception of the adequacy of social support.[32]

In summary, an individual's social support network greatly influences the likelihood that he or she will have psychiatric difficulties. This relationship appears to be even stronger when an individual is faced with a significant psychosocial stressor. Those individuals who do not have, or do not perceive that they have, confidants or a sufficient social network are much more likely to have difficulty.

IPT: FROM THEORY TO INTERVENTION

Attachment, communication, and social theory all inform the conduct of IPT. Based on this theoretical model, the IPT therapist has four essential tasks when conducting IPT:

1 To create a therapeutic environment in which there is a high degree of inclusion and affiliation.
2 To develop an understanding or conceptualization of the patient's communication problems by recognizing the pattern of interpersonal communication as it occurs both in the patient's interpersonal sphere outside of treatment, and in the therapeutic relationship.
3 To identify the patient's maladaptive patterns of communication, and to help the patient become aware of them, so that his or her communications can be modified.
4 To assist the patient in building a better social support network, and to utilize the social supports that are currently available.

TASK 1

First and foremost, the clinician must *create a therapeutic environment* in which there is a high degree of inclusion and affiliation. Put simply, *a good therapeutic alliance is absolutely essential in IPT*, and the burden to create one is on the therapist! The therapeutic relationship needs to be developed in such a way that it holds importance for both the therapist and patient – both are actively engaged, and are attentive to the communication from the other. If this does not occur, feedback from the therapist (and from the patient) will be too easily dismissed, and the therapy itself will be jeopardized because the patient will simply abandon it. If a productive therapeutic alliance is not established, the therapeutic relationship will be such that the patient can easily devalue it and consequently ignore any input from the therapist, rendering moot all of the specific techniques the therapist might use in the treatment.

Creating a meaningful therapeutic relationship is, of course, a necessary condition of all psychotherapies. It is of particular importance in IPT, however, as the therapy is time limited. It is incumbent upon the therapist quickly to establish a therapeutic alliance, so that the 'work' of therapy can be accomplished. Thus in IPT, particular attention must be paid to all of the 'non-specific elements' of therapy: warmth, empathy, affective attunement, positive regard – all of the elements described by Rogers[41] as necessary to bring about psychotherapeutic change. It is crucial that IPT therapists be more than technicians – without establishing a productive therapeutic alliance, none of the IPT techniques and strategies will be effective.

The therapist should also constantly remember that the quality of the alliance is the primary predictor of psychotherapy outcome. Research has consistently demonstrated this to be the case in literally every form of therapy in which the alliance has been examined.[42-45] This is not to say, of course, that the specific techniques and therapeutic approaches advocated by different therapies are not important, but rather that they pale in comparison to the effects of the alliance.

The therapeutic alliance is of even more importance with patients who have maladaptive attachment styles, as they will make it difficult for their therapists to respond consistently in empathic and therapeutic ways. Rather than eliciting a sympathetic and care-giving response from their therapists, such patients will evoke hostility and rejection. The therapist must be aware of this tendency on the part of such patients, and be even more active in conveying empathy and positive regard to those patients who do not naturally evoke such responses. A patient with an avoidant style, for instance, may evoke feelings of boredom or rejection in the therapist, which will destroy the therapeutic relationship if the therapist responds in kind to this provocation. With such a patient, the therapist must recognize the interpersonal response that is being evoked by the patient, understand the communication that is eliciting it, and adapt his or her responses to create a more productive therapeutic relationship. With such a patient, the therapist may choose to use more empathic statements, or may choose to let the patient set the agenda in early sessions rather than imposing the therapist's agenda too early and risk having the patient feel rejected.

Conversely, a patient with an ambivalent style may 'wear down' the therapist with repeated requests for reassurance, so that over time, the responses that are naturally evoked by the patient are exasperation and rejection. Again, the therapist must be recognize the communication pattern, be aware of the responses that the patient evokes, and move to counter the patient's provocation by being consistently caring despite being drawn to do otherwise. With this type of patient, the therapist, recognizing the greater likelihood that the patient may become dependent on the therapist and have difficulty ending the time-limited therapeutic relationship, can counter this trend by placing even greater emphasis on the need for the patient to develop a more supportive social network outside of therapy.

Some patients, fortunately, are relatively secure in their attachments, and can communicate their needs effectively, including those in the therapeutic relationship. Such patients require little adjustment on the part of the therapist, are able to receive feedback from the therapist and use it productively, and are also able to make adjustments within their extended support network. In these cases, the therapist can move to the intermediate phase of IPT more quickly, and can begin giving feedback to the patient much more quickly, as it will be seen by the patient as helpful rather than as rejecting.

Herein lies a crucial difference between IPT and transference-based psychodynamic psychotherapies. In IPT, the therapist attempts to recognize the patient's underlying attachment needs and works to help the patient meet those needs outside of therapy. In transference-based psychotherapy, the therapist attempts to become a 'blank screen' upon which the patient projects his or her transference neurosis – this reaction is stimulated by intent as the therapist actively resists meeting the patient's attachment needs in therapy.

TASK 2

The second task of the IPT therapist is *to develop an understanding or conceptualization of the patient's communication problems by recognizing the pattern of interpersonal communication as it occurs both in the patient's interpersonal sphere outside of treatment, and in the therapeutic relationship.* Attachment theory suggests that attachment styles will be manifest across relationships, including of course the relationship that develops between therapist and patient. The patient–therapist relationship, in other words, must be attended to very carefully by the IPT therapist, as it provides extremely valuable information about the way in which the patient typically attaches to and communicates with others. The difficulties experienced by the patient in communicating within the therapeutic relationship will be manifest in his or her other relationships; the attachment style which becomes apparent in therapy will be manifest in all of the patient's other relationships, and the ways in which the therapist is drawn to respond to the patient's communications, particularly those communications involving care-eliciting behavior, will be the ways in which others outside of therapy are also drawn to respond. Thus understanding transference in IPT is paramount in developing an accurate formulation of the patient's attachment behavior and interpersonal communication.

In IPT, however, this information is used to ask questions about relationships outside of therapy rather than being used to address the relationship between the patient and the therapist. The experience of transference leads the IPT therapist to ask questions about the way the patient communicates in his or her relationships outside of therapy; the therapeutic relationship itself is not addressed as a point of intervention in IPT. When the therapist experiences the patient as passive, for instance, it should lead the therapist to ask questions about the ways in which the patient may be passive in his or her extra-therapy relationships. When the therapist feels drawn to respond in hostile ways to the patient, this should lead to queries about incidents when the patient has experienced others outside of therapy reacting in hostile ways. When the therapist is feeling frustrated, questions which investigate the possibility that others also feel frustrated by the patient should be asked.

IPT, as noted above, is characterized by a time limit and a focus on symptom resolution. While understanding that the transference which develops in IPT is crucial to its conduct, as it informs the therapist about the ways in which the patient forms and maintains relationships outside of therapy, IPT – in contrast to psychodynamic psychotherapies – does not intervene by raising transference or the therapeutic relationship as a point of discussion in therapy. The reason for this is that to do so is likely to move the patient away from a here-and-now focus on symptom resolution and into a therapy designed to modify personality or deep-seated attachment problems. While such therapies may be quite helpful for many patients, and may even be the first choice of intervention for those with severe personality or attachment difficulties, they are outside of the scope of IPT. In IPT, the focus is rapid symptom resolution; hence, the therapeutic relationship is not used as a point of discussion or intervention, because it draws the patient away from resolving his or her symptoms or interpersonal problems as quickly as possible.

Because the point of the therapy is symptom resolution rather than an examination of transference as it develops, the IPT therapist has some latitude in positioning him or herself in therapy. In transference-based therapies, the therapist ideally is a 'blank screen' upon which the patient has maximum opportunity to project and make clear his or her transference reactions. Transference-based therapies are designed in such a way that the therapist encourages the development of transference, not only by asking questions about it, but by being non-disclosing and neutral. In contrast, because IPT is designed to focus on relationships outside of therapy and therefore need not encourage the development of transference, the therapist can position him or herself in the role of a 'coach' or 'mentor.' In technical terms, the therapist's stance is to be a constant and consistent care-provider, encouraging a positive transferential relationship with the patient in which the therapist is seen as an expert who is willing and able to be of help.

On a practical level, this means that *the IPT therapist has more freedom to use techniques which might otherwise obscure the development of transference.* Self-disclosure, for instance, may be very useful with some patients who are more securely attached. The therapist may wish to speak about solutions that other patients with similar problems have found helpful (taking care to maintain confidentiality). The IPT therapist may also be active in helping the patient to extend his or her social support network, making direct suggestions to attend groups such as Alcoholics Anonymous, religious groups, new mothers' support groups, and the like, going as far, if needed, as helping the patient find resources for transportation to such groups.

In essence, the goal of the IPT therapist is to use the patient–therapist relationship to gather information which contributes to an understanding of the patient's attachment style, and as a means of understanding his or her difficulties in communication. Within therapy, rather than examining the transference with the patient, the therapist should position him or herself as an expert help-provider. The idea is to literally 'get in and get out' of therapy before problematic transference develops; thus, the paramount importance of the time limit in IPT, and the need to focus on here-and-now relationships outside of therapy in the service of the primary goal of symptom resolution.

TASK 3

The third task of the IPT therapist is *to identify the patient's maladaptive patterns of communication, and to make the patient aware of them as well so that the patient can modify his or her communication behaviors*. Put simply, the goal is *to help the patient develop insight into his or her communication style*. The therapist needs to understand the ways in which the patient communicates, the responses that the patient's communication evokes, and the ways in which the patient's style of communication is perpetuated. In addition, the therapist must assist the patient to appreciate that his or her communication is not effective – i.e., that it is not effectively achieving the patient's goal of meeting his or her attachment needs. Finally, the therapist must help the patient to change his or her communication by developing and practicing new behaviors.

The goal of treatment with IPT is change in the patient's communication and behavior so that his or her attachment needs are more fully met. In most cases, this requires at least a limited degree of insight by the patient. This is insight in which the patient recognizes his or her communication style and the responses that it evokes. It does not necessarily require insight into the genesis of the patient's attachment or communication styles. The insight need only be enough that the patient recognizes the consequences of his or her here-and-now communications with others, and in doing so, is motivated to change.

Ideally, the patient would in essence say: 'I have a tendency to communicate in a specific way. My communications tend to draw others to respond in a characteristic way as well. The responses I elicit from others aren't helpful to me, and tend to produce a response which leaves me even more frustrated. I now recognize that I can get my needs met more fully by communicating differently in a way to which others respond more positively.'

The importance of creating a therapeutic relationship in which feedback about his or her communication can be received by the patient has been discussed, as has the importance of understanding the transference that occurs in therapy. Although the transference experience provides much information about the patient's style of attachment and communication, it is by no means the only information that the therapist should use. In fact, the primary source of information for understanding the patient's communications should be incidents in which the patient has attempted to communicate his or her needs with significant others. Patterns in relationships should be explored to a great extent, both to assist the patient to see these patterns and to help the therapist understand the patient more fully. Thus, the Interpersonal Inventory, in addition to providing information about the patient's social support, should be used as a means of beginning to understand the patient's patterns of relationships. Asking questions about the ways in which the patient typically forms relationships, ends relationships, or common disappointments that he or she experiences in relationships can also be extremely helpful.

Asking questions about specific interpersonal interactions is also very useful in understanding the patient's style of communication. The technique of examining Interpersonal Incidents, described in Chapter 10, is a wonderful method to examine in detail the ways in which the patient is not effectively communicating his or her needs within relationships. IPT techniques such as problem solving can assist the patient both to recognize and to change communications, so that his or her attachment needs are met more fully. Role playing provides the opportunity to solidify the newly established ways of communicating. The goal is to help the patient recognize communication patterns, modify those patterns so that his or her needs are more effectively met, and maintain the new communication once it is established.

TASK 4

The fourth task of the IPT therapist is *to assist the patient to build a better social support network, and to utilize the social supports that are currently available.* The social milieu is intimately connected to the patient's ability to deal with interpersonal crises. The greater the support, the more likely the patient is to weather the storm. Thus, it is the therapist's task to encourage the patient to identify both existing and potential sources of support, as well as to begin to utilize them constructively.

CONCLUSION

IPT rests on a triad of theoretical underpinnings: attachment theory, interpersonal theory, and social theory. All coalesce within a biopsychosocial model as a means of conceptualizing the reasons which underlie a patient's distress as well as to direct the interventions which are used in the therapy. An acute psychosocial stressor, in a patient with biological and attachment predispositions, in the context of insufficient social support, leads to the development of symptoms and psychological distress. IPT is specifically designed to help patients by assisting them to improve their interpersonal communication and more fully develop and utilize their social support system.

REFERENCES

1. Engel, G.L. 1980. The clinical application of biopsychosocial models. *American Journal of Psychiatry* **137**, 535–44.
2. Bowlby, J. 1969. *Attachment*. New York: Basic Books.

3. Bowlby, J. 1977. The making and breaking of affectional bonds: etiology and psychopathology in the light of attachment theory. *British Journal of Psychiatry* **130**, 201–10.
4. Bowlby, J. 1977. The making and breaking of affectional bonds, II: some principles of psychotherapy. *British Journal of Psychiatry* **130**, 421–31.
5. Bowlby, J. 1988. Developmental psychiatry comes of age. *American Journal of Psychiatry* **145**, 1–10.
6. Ainsworth, M.D. 1969. Object relations, dependency, and attachment: a theoretical view of the infant–mother relationship. *Child Development* **40**, 969–1027.
7. Ainsworth, M.S., Blehar, M.C., Waters, E., Wall, S. 1978. *Patterns of Attachment: A Psychological Study of the Strange Situation*. MahWah, NJ: Erlbaum.
8. George, C., Kaplan, N., Main, M. 1985. *Adult Attachment Interview*. 2nd edition. Berkely, CA: University of California at Berkely Press.
9. Hazan, C., Shaver, P.R. 1987. Romantic love conceptualized as an attachment process. *Journal of Personality and Social Psychology* **52**, 511–24.
10. Sullivan, H.S. 1953. *The Interpersonal Theory of Psychiatry*. New York: Norton.
11. Stuart, S., Noyes, R. 1999. Attachment and interpersonal communication in somatization disorder. *Psychosomatics* **40**, 34–43.
12. Parkes, C.M. 1971. Psycho-social transitions: a field of study. *Social Science and Medicine* **5**, 101–15.
13. Bowlby, J. 1973. *Attachment and Loss: Volume 2. Separation*. New York: Basic Books.
14. Parkes, C.M. 1965. Bereavement and mental illness. *British Journal of Medical Psychology* **38**, 1–26.
15. Henderson, S. 1974. Care-eliciting behavior in man. *Journal of Nervous and Mental Disease* **159**, 172–81.
16. Kiesler, D.J., Watkins, L.M. 1989. Interpersonal complimentarity and the therapeutic alliance: a study of the relationship in psychotherapy. *Psychotherapy* **26**, 183–94.
17. Kiesler, D.J. 1996. *Contemporary Interpersonal Theory and Research: Personality, Psychopathology, and Psychotherapy*. New York: John Wiley & Sons.
18. Kiesler, D.J. 1992. Interpersonal circle inventories: pantheoretical applications to psychotherapy research and practice. *Journal of Psychotherapy Integration* **2**, 77–99.
19. Kiesler, D.J. 1991. Interpersonal methods of assessment and diagnosis. In: Snyder, C.R., Forsyth, D.R. (eds), *Handbook of Social and Clinical Psychology: The Health Perspective*. Elmsford, NY: Pergamon Press.
20. Benjamin, L.S. 1996. *Interpersonal Diagnosis and Treatment of Personality Disorders*. 2nd edition. New York: Guilford.
21. Benjamin, L.S. 1996. Introduction to the special section on structural analysis of social behavior. *Journal of Consulting and Clinical Psychology* **64**, 1203–12.
22. Kiesler, D.J. 1979. An interpersonal communication analysis of relationship in psychotherapy. *Journal for the Study of Interpersonal Processes* **42**, 299–311.
23. Weissman, M.M., Paykel, E.S. 1974. *The Depressed Woman: A Study of Social Relationships*. Chicago: University of Chicago Press.
24. Henderson, S., Byrne, D.G., Duncan-Jones, P. 1982. *Neurosis and the Social Environment*. Sydney: Academic Press.
25. Brenner, C. 1973. *An Elementary Textbook of Psychoanalysis*. New York: Anchor Press.
26. Bebbington, P.E. 1984. Inferring causes: some constraints in the social psychiatry of depressive disorders. *Integrative Psychiatry* 2, 69–72.
27. Brown, G.W. 1998. Genetic and population perspectives on life events and depression. *Social Psychiatry and Psychiatric Epidemiology* **33**, 363–72.

28. Henderson, S., Duncan-Jones, P., Byrne, D.G., Scott, R., Adcock, S. 1979. Psychiatric disorder in Canberra: a standardized study of prevalence. *Acta Psychiatrica Scandinavica* **60**, 355–74.

29. Henderson, S., Byrne, D.G., Duncan-Jones, P., Adcock, S., Scott, R., Steele, G.P. 1978. Social bonds in the epidemiology of neurosis. *British Journal of Psychiatry* **132**, 463–6.

30. Henderson, S., Byrne, D.G., Duncan-Jones, P., Scott, R., Adcock, S. 1980. Social relationships, adversity and neurosis: a study of associations in a general population sample. *British Journal of Psychiatry* **136**, 574–83.

31. Henderson, S. 1977. The social network, support, and neurosis: the function of attachment in adult life. *British Journal of Psychiatry* **131**, 185–91.

32. Henderson, A.S. 1984. Interpreting the evidence on social support. *Social Psychiatry* **19**, 49–52.

33. Brown, G.W., Bifulco, A., Harris, T., Bridge, L. 1986. Life stress, chronic subclinical symptoms and vulnerability to clinical depression. *Journal of Affective Disorders* **11**, 1–19.

34. Andrews, B., Brown, G.W. 1988. Social support, onset of depression and personality: an exploratory analysis. *Social Psychiatry and Psychiatric Epidemiology* **23**, 99–108.

35. Brown, G.W., Harris, T., Eales, M.J. 1996. Social factors and comorbidity of depressive and anxiety disorders. *British Journal of Psychiatry* **168** (suppl. 30), 50–7.

36. Paykel, E.S. 1974. Life stress and psychiatric disorder. In: Dohrenwend, B.S., Dohrenwend, B.P. (eds). *Stressful Life Events: Their Nature and Effects*. New York: Wiley.

37. Brown, G.W., Harris, T.O. 1978. *Social Origins of Depression: A Study of Psychiatric Disorders in Women*. London: Tavistock.

38. Walker, K., MacBride, A., Vachon, M. 1977. Social support networks and the crisis of bereavement. *Social Sciences in Medicine* **11**, 35–41.

39. Maddison, D., Walker, W. 1967. Factors affecting the outcome of conjugal bereavement. *British Journal of Psychiatry* **113**, 1057–67.

40. Parker, G. 1978. *The Bonds of Depression*. Sydney: Angus and Robertson.

41. Rogers, C.R. 1957. The necessary and sufficient conditions of therapeutic personality change. *Journal of Consulting Psychology* **21**, 95–103.

42. Lambert, M.J. 1992. Psychotherapy outcome research: implications for integrative and eclectic theories. In: Norcross, J.C., Goldfried, M.R. (eds), *Handbook of Psychotherapy Integration*. New York: Basic Books.

43. Barber, J.P., Connolly, M.B., Crits-Christoph, P., Gladis, L., Siqueland, L. 2000. Alliance predicts patients' outcome beyond in-treatment change in symptoms. *Journal of Consulting and Clinical Psychology* **68**, 1027–32.

44. Martin, D.J., Garske, J.P., Davis, M.K. 2000. Relation of the therapeutic alliance with outcome and other variables: a meta-analytic review. *Journal of Consulting and Clinical Psychology* **68**, 438–50.

45. Zuroff, D.C., Blatt, S.J., Sotsky, S.M., *et al.* 2000. Relation of therapeutic alliance and perfectionism to outcome in brief outpatient treatment of depression. *Journal of Consulting and Clinical Psychology* **68**, 114–24.

Section 2

Initial Sessions

3

The Structure of IPT

INTRODUCTION

This chapter is designed to provide a brief overview of the structure of IPT, emphasizing a view of the forest rather than the trees. IPT can be divided into various phases, including *assessment*, the *initial phase* of treatment, the *intermediate phase* of treatment, and the *conclusion of acute treatment*. The individual components of the structure of IPT each involve specific tasks to be undertaken by both the patient and the therapist (Figure 3.1).

PHASES OF IPT

Assessment

The purpose of the assessment phase of IPT is to determine whether or not the patient is a suitable candidate for IPT, and to determine whether IPT, if appropriate, is the best treatment available. During the assessment the therapist should focus on the patient's presenting problems and attachment style, and should ask about specific episodes of interpersonal interaction in order to begin to understand the patient's typical style of communication. The assessment ends with an agreement to proceed with IPT if it is the therapist's judgment that IPT is the treatment best suited to the needs of the individual patient (Table 3.1).

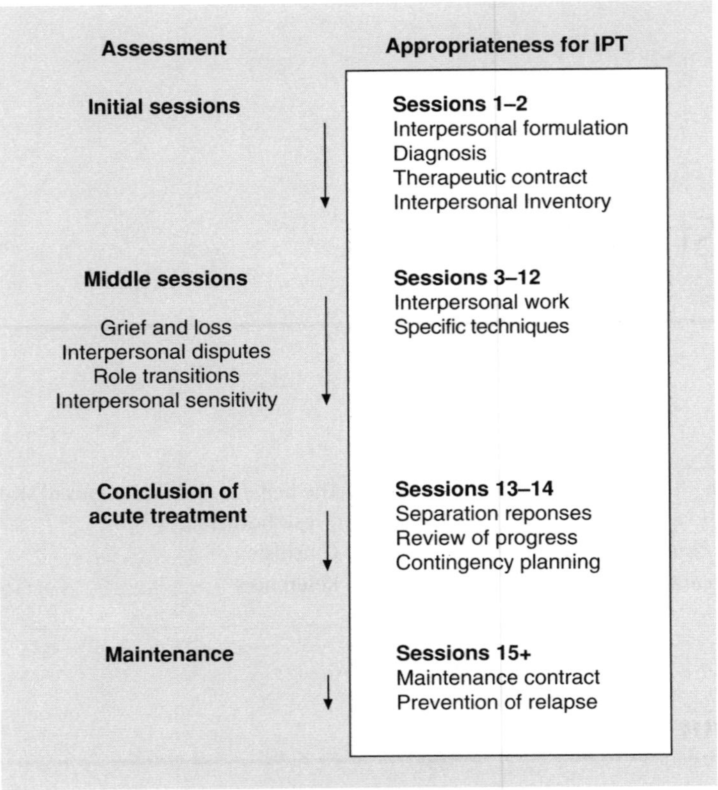

Assessment	Appropriateness for IPT
Initial sessions	**Sessions 1–2** Interpersonal formulation Diagnosis Therapeutic contract Interpersonal Inventory
Middle sessions Grief and loss Interpersonal disputes Role transitions Interpersonal sensitivity	**Sessions 3–12** Interpersonal work Specific techniques
Conclusion of acute treatment	**Sessions 13–14** Separation reponses Review of progress Contingency planning
Maintenance	**Sessions 15+** Maintenance contract Prevention of relapse

Figure 3.1 *The Structure of IPT*. *In the assessment phase, the therapist makes a determination about the patient's suitability for IPT. If IPT is indicated, the therapist develops an interpersonal formulation and negotiates a contract with the patient. In the early sessions the Interpersonal Inventory is completed. In the middle sessions, the therapist and patient work at resolving the relationship problems using the four problem areas and IPT techniques. When concluding acute treatment, the therapist and patient review progress in the problem areas as well as planning for future problems. If maintenance IPT is indicated, the patient and therapist contract for additional sessions that are usually less frequent, but maintain the interpersonal focus.*

Initial phase

The initial phase of IPT includes a number of specific tasks. The primary goals are to develop an interpersonal formulation, which is a detailed hypothesis describing and explaining the patient's interpersonal difficulties, and to gauge the patient's social support in general. Intrinsic to this process is the development of an Interpersonal Inventory. A contract should be established with the patient to proceed with IPT, and to work on several specific interpersonal problems.

Table 3.1 *The Components of IPT*

Assessment

I   Evaluate the suitability of the patient for IPT
II Evaluate the suitability of IPT for the patient

Initial sessions

I   Fully assess psychiatric and interpersonal problems
II   Develop an Interpersonal Formulation
III Conduct an Interpersonal Inventory: *Listing the patient's key current relationships and the problems associated with them*
IV   Identify problem areas: *disputes, role translations, grief and loss and interpersonal sensitivity*
V   Explain the rationale and purpose of IPT
VI   Establish a Treatment Contract with the patient: *emphasizing the focus of treatment, the time-frame, and the expectations for both the patient and therapist*

Middle sessions

I   Attend to the therapeutic relationship
II   Maintain the focus of discussion on the specific IPT problem area
III Explore the patient's expectations and perceptions of a specific interpersonal problem
IV   IPT Interventions: *techniques such as clarification, interpersonal incidents, encouragement of affect*
V   Problem solving
     Specific clarification of interpersonal problem
     Brainstorming possible solutions
     Implementation of the proposed solutions
     Monitoring outcomes, refinement of attempted solution

Conclusion of acute treatment

I   Review the patient's progress: *returning to the Interpersonal Inventory and tracking progress through the problem areas*
II   Anticipate future problems
III Positively reinforce the patient's gains
IV   Establish a specific contract for maintenance treatment if indicated

Maintenance treatment

I   Establish a specific contract
II   Focus on problem areas: *working with original problems or exploring emergent interpersonal problems*
III Monitor progress

Intermediate phase

The intermediate phase of IPT is that in which the therapist and patient work together to solve the patient's interpersonal disputes, to help the patient to adjust to his or her role transitions, or to deal with grief and loss issues. In general, after identifying several problem areas during the assessment and initial phases, the therapist gathers more information about the patient's specific interpersonal problems. Both patient and therapist then work to develop solutions to each problem, such as improving the patient's communication skills or modifying his or her expectations about a relationship conflict.

A suitable option is selected, and then the patient ideally attempts to implement it between sessions. The patient and therapist then work in subsequent sessions to refine the solution and to further assist the patient to implement the solution if he or she has had difficulty in carrying it out completely.

Concluding acute treatment

The conclusion of acute treatment is a mutually negotiated at the end of the intensive time-limited part of IPT. It includes a review of the patient's progress in resolving the interpersonal problems first identified in the interpersonal inventory, anticipating the emergence of new interpersonal problems, and planning for these and other problems which may arise in the future. The patient's (and the therapist's) reactions to the conclusion of acute treatment should be acknowledged so that they can be discussed further if needed.

Maintenance treatment

A specific contract regarding the provision or availability of maintenance treatment may be negotiated, if indicated and if suitable for the patient and therapist. In cases where a patient's problems are likely to be recurrent, the patient and therapist should develop a contract to meet for a series of maintenance sessions, meeting at prescribed intervals to monitor ongoing interpersonal problems and to help the patient continue to work on his or her interpersonal skills. This should be a structured course of treatment, in the same way the acute phase of treatment is structured. The scheduling of maintenance IPT sessions requires clinical judgement, as prolonged treatment increases the possibility that problematic transferential processes will occur. Contracting for maintenance sessions also requires careful consideration of the patient's attachment style, as longitudinal treatment may foster increased dependency with some insecurely attached patients. The complexities of this aspect of IPT are discussed in a later chapter.

IPT AND THE BIOPSYCHOSOCIAL MODEL

IPT is based on the biopsychosocial model of psychological functioning.[1] Biological diatheses in conjunction with early life experiences and attachment style lead to vulnerabilities in individual patients. Coupled with a sufficiently intense interpersonal stressor, individuals without adequate social support are likely to develop interpersonal difficulties.

The interventions used in IPT, and the framework of the therapy itself, are directly linked to attachment and interpersonal theory. The IPT therapist focuses on the patient's interpersonal relationships – particularly the way in which the patient's attachment is manifest in these relationships. The therapist is also concerned with the communication style that the patient uses in both initiating, maintaining, and disengaging from relationships. This occurs within the time-limited format of IPT, and focuses on here-and-now resolution of symptoms rather than on the patient–therapist relationship.

IPT PROBLEM AREAS

IPT focuses on four specific problem areas which reflect the interpersonal nature of the treatment. These are: (i) Grief and Loss; (ii) Interpersonal Disputes; (iii) Role Transitions; and (iv) Interpersonal Sensitivity. Psychosocial stressors from any of the problem areas, when combined with an attachment disruption in the context of poor social support, can lead to interpersonal problems or psychiatric syndromes.

- *Grief and Loss*: though commonly understood as a reaction to the literal death of a significant other, grief in IPT can best be conceptualized as a loss experienced by the patient. In addition to death, a loss such as divorce may be seen by the patient as a grief issue. Loss of physical functioning, such as that following a heart attack or traumatic injury, may also appropriately be considered in the grief and loss problem area.[2]
- *Interpersonal Disputes*: these involve a conflict between the patient and another person, and may result from either communication problems or unrealistic expectations on the part of either party.
- *Role Transitions*: as the name suggests, these involve changes in a patient's social role and the changes in social support which may accompany such transitions. These include not only life-phase transitions, such as adolescence, childbirth, and aging, but also include many social changes such as leaving home, getting married, and change in school or job status.
- *Interpersonal Sensitivity*: this is best understood as a characteristic style of relating in which the patient has difficulty forming satisfying interpersonal relationships. The poor social support network which is a consequence of this style may lead the patient to develop interpersonal problems or depression, particularly if a social stressor occurs. Often, interpersonal sensitivity reflects an insecure and avoidant attachment style, and it is also frequently associated with avoidant personality traits. In essence, patients whose problems fit into this category are overly sensitive to rejection, have difficulty forming relationships with others, and are unable to meet their attachment needs as a result.

While these categories are very helpful as a means of focusing the patient on specific interpersonal problems, it is important for the therapist to be flexible when using them. Rather than providing the patient with the proper problem area 'diagnosis,' the problem areas should be used primarily as tools to maintain focus upon one or two interpersonal problems, particularly as the time available in IPT is limited by definition. In general, the patient's view of the nature of the problem should be accepted – for example, if the patient feels that his or her recent divorce is a grief issue rather than a role transition, then the grief and loss problem area should be used. The therapeutic alliance should not be sacrificed in order to impose the 'correct' problem area 'diagnosis' upon the patient.

The therapist should also be mindful that the interpersonal problems experienced by patients are similar in that they are all derived from the combination of an acute interpersonal stressor combined with a social support system that does not sufficiently sustain the patient. In addition to addressing the specific problem, effort should always be directed towards improving the patient's social supports.

THE BENEFITS AND LIMITATIONS OF STRUCTURED PSYCHOTHERAPIES

One of the more useful ways to describe various psychotherapeutic approaches is to draw a distinction between 'structured' and 'unstructured' psychotherapies. Psychotherapeutic interventions can be placed along a spectrum on this dimension, with most of the time-limited treatments at the more structured end of the scale, and most of the analytically oriented therapies at the other. There are obvious benefits and limitations to both structured and unstructured approaches – the point is to consider how specific treatments best meet the needs of a given patient. Table 3.2 contains a comparison of 'structured' and 'unstructured' psychotherapies.

A helpful way of conceptualizing the place of IPT and other more structured psychotherapies in clinical practice is to compare them with pharmacological treatments for somatic problems. From this point of view, IPT can literally be 'prescribed' as an appropriate and indicated treatment for the specific problem with which the patient presents.

For example, the structure of IPT lends itself to a prescriptive treatment in a fashion analogous to the use of antibiotic therapy for pneumonia. Most patients with pneumonia require a structured course of antibiotics that is time-limited and specific to one bacterial pathogen; this treatment is usually highly effective in resolving the illness. There are, however, patients who are prone to recurrent infections or who are immunosuppressed. These patients require longer-term use of these or multiple agents, with marked variations in dosing and time course. While such patients are in the minority, their needs require significant use of clinical resources.

Similarly, many patients who present for mental healthcare tend to have acute and specific problems, and will benefit from an acute intervention. In these cases, a structured and prescriptive intervention such as IPT is likely to offer the greatest benefit in a limited time frame. Those patients who require ongoing and less structured interventions, such as those with severe and complex trauma experiences, profound disturbance in personality functioning, or severely debilitating mood or psychotic disorders, will likely require longer term and more flexible psychological treatments.

Borrowing further from this analogy, the concepts of 'dose–response' and 'compliance' can also be applied to the more structured psychotherapies. There is evidence that benefits to the patient accrue exponentially during the first five to ten sessions of psychological interventions, with an attenuation of benefit thereafter.[3] Though there continue to be benefits with continuing sessions, the amount of additional benefit appears to diminish with each additional session. Thus, the benefit or 'response' to treatment must

Table 3.2 Characteristics of Structured and Unstructured Therapies

	Structured	Unstructured
Examples	IPT, CBT	Psychoanalysis, self-psychology
Time frame	Time-limited	Open-ended
Focus	Improved functioning	Psychodynamic change and insight
Therapeutic relationship	Supportive, Active	Non-transparent, Passive
Discussions	Directed primarily by therapist	Directed primarily by patient
Transference	Not a point of intervention	Primary point of intervention

be considered in light of the 'dose' or number of sessions that are provided, particularly as each additional session carries the burden of cost and inconvenience for the patient.

Research has also suggested that there is a rapid decline in clinic attendance and compliance with psychotherapeutic treatments after five to ten sessions.[4] This is further supported by recent studies in Australia suggesting that 40 per cent of appointments with psychiatrists are 'one-off' (i.e., only one session), and that the average number of visits to a psychiatrist for a given patient is approximately seven.[5] This finding has also been noted in the US.[6,7] There seems to be a 'window of opportunity' for most patients within a brief time frame; it follows that this window is often best exploited using a structured treatment.

Research aside, it is an unfortunate fact that the current climate of rationalized healthcare and the emphasis on cost-effective treatments has had a profound effect on the healthcare system. While there are many advantages to more open-ended and less structured treatments, IPT and other more structured interventions can often be provided within the constraints of managed care systems. Further, IPT is also well suited to this climate because there is evidence supporting its efficacy, a point of emphasis for managed care.

CONCLUSION

In the final analysis, there should not be any contest between the 'structured' and 'unstructured' psychotherapies; each treatment has its own vital place in helping patients to overcome their psychological distress. The structure of IPT is one of its key virtues, however maintaining structure should not supercede the fact that the patient's unique needs are of primary concern. A course of IPT that adheres concretely to a manual at the expense of the patient's needs is almost certain to be a less effective treatment than that provided by a therapist who follows the principles of IPT with flexible use of clinical judgment.

REFERENCES

1. Engel, G.L. 1980. The clinical application of biopsychosocial models. *American Journal of Psychiatry* **137**, 535–44.
2. Stuart, S., Cole, V. 1996. Treatment of depression following myocardial infarction with interpersonal psychotherapy. *Annals of Clinical Psychiatry* **8**, 203–6.
3. Howard, K.I., Kopta, S.M., Krause, M.S., Orlinsky, D.E. 1986. The dose–effect relationship in psychotherapy. *American Psychologist* **41**, 159–64.
4. McKenzie, K.R. 1997. *Time Limited Group Psychotherapy in Managed Care*. Washington, DC: American Psychiatric Press.
5. Goldberg, D. 2000. Impressions of psychiatry in Australia. *Australasian Psychiatry* **8**, 307.
6. Howard, K.I., Davidson, C.V., O'Mahoney, M.T., Orlinsky, D.E. 1989. Patterns of psychotherapy utilization. *American Journal of Psychiatry* **146**, 775–8.
7. Howard, K.I., Vessey, J.T., Lueger, R., Schank, D. 1992. The psychotherapeutic service delivery system. *Psychotherapy Research* **2**, 164–80.

4

Assessment and Patient Selection

INTRODUCTION

The primary purpose of conducting an assessment is simply to determine when IPT should be used, and to whom it should be applied. The treatment and patient must be compatible to ensure the greatest likelihood of resolving the patient's interpersonal problems. When making this determination, the therapist should be guided by several factors, including the patient's attachment style, communication style, motivation and insight, and the available empirical evidence regarding IPT. All of these factors should be integrated using clinical judgment.

A therapist should never offer IPT to a patient without a proper evaluation. This is one of the few absolutes in this book, and it is based on clinical experience which has proven time and again that a therapist should always conduct his or her own evaluation. Referrals may not be accurate, the patient's clinical presentation may change between the referral and the initial evaluation, or the therapist may have a different opinion about what treatment is most appropriate for the patient.

An evaluation to determine the suitability of IPT for the patient should always be completed before a treatment contract is established. To offer a treatment contract to a patient, only to withdraw it later after discovering that IPT is not an appropriate treatment, is obviously not good clinical practice. Referrals – whether self-referrals by the patient or referrals from other professionals – should always be handled by indicating that an evaluation for IPT will be conducted, rather than implying or directly stating that IPT will be definitively provided.

In addition, an evaluation for IPT should not be conducted hastily. In a clinical setting, there is no reason why the therapist cannot take several sessions to complete the evaluation, if his or her clinical judgment so dictates that this should be done. It is naive to think that a relevant and appropriate contract for IPT (or any other therapy) can be established for all patients after only one session – it takes time to listen and understand, not to mention to develop a meaningful relationship in therapy.

Therefore, although assessment is an intrinsic part of IPT, the assessment should not be framed in a way that obligates the therapist to proceed with IPT unless it is warranted. The assessment should set the stage, so to speak, for the conduct of IPT when indicated, but should not obligate the therapist to provide IPT, nor lead the patient to expect IPT, unless it is the most appropriate treatment.

The assessment should essentially answer two simple questions:

1   Will this particular patient benefit from IPT?
2   Is IPT the best treatment that can be provided to this particular patient?

ASSESSMENT PROCESS

Rather than reiterate the entire process of conducting an assessment, this chapter will describe the elements of the assessment that are unique to IPT. However, this should not diminish the fact that conducting a thorough psychological assessment of each and every patient – including psychiatric history, family history, medical history, and a complete social assessment – is extremely important. The elements of IPT that should also be considered in the assessment include the patient's attachment and communication style, ability to provide narrative, motivation for treatment, and psychological mindedness. The empirical evidence supporting the efficacy of IPT for particular disorders should also be considered when making a determination about the suitability of IPT.

Attachment style and communication style

A good psychological or psychiatric assessment allows the therapist to see both the forest and the trees. In IPT, this consists of a large-scale map of the route the patient has traversed to arrive at his or her current interpersonal circumstances, and a detailed blueprint of the specific interpersonal and psychological difficulties with which he or she is struggling at the moment. The therapist can consider the patient's attachment style as the 'topography' of the map – a feature which inevitably dictates the general route to be taken, though there are many alternative paths along the way. The more detailed features – the trees – are the patient's current interpersonal relationships. These trees are either felled or nurtured by the patient's interpersonal communications.

There are several reasons that attachment must be examined during the assessment phase of IPT. First and foremost, the assessment should lead to a determination about whether the patient's attachment style renders him or her a suitable IPT candidate. Second, the patient's attachment style is closely correlated with his or her prognosis in therapy, allowing the therapist to make a reasonable prediction about how therapy will proceed and finish. Third, specific techniques follow directly from the patient's attachment style.

Table 4.1 *Assessment of Attachment*

The patient's attachment style should be assessed to determine:
• Suitability for IPT.
• Likely prognosis in therapy.
• Interventions to be used in therapy.

The assessment of attachment style

In assessing a patient's attachment style, there are three main issues:

1 The content of the patient's description of relationships.
2 The quality of the patient's narrative.
3 The patient–therapist relationship.

THE CONTENT OF THE PATIENT'S DESCRIPTION OF RELATIONSHIPS

The initial assessment of the patient's attachment style should begin with an evaluation of their past and current relationships. Simply asking open-ended questions about the patient's relationships is a good way to start. More specific inquiries can be directed towards determining what the patient does and communicates when distressed, ill, or otherwise seeking care. The patient should also be queried about his or her typical responses when asked to assist others.

This information is easy to obtain, requires little in the way of inference, and is an obvious way to evaluate the patient's attachment style. Both directive and open-ended questions can be used in the service of better understanding the ways in which patients function in relationships.

The primary source of information is the patient's *current relationships*. This should include both specific questions as well as questions which require slightly more insight on the part of the patient. For instance, the patient can be directly asked about any patterns that he or she has noticed in relationships. Typical ways of beginning and ending relationships can also be reviewed. The patient should also be asked about the ways in which he or she asks for help if it is needed, and the ways in which he or she communicates with others when feeling upset or angry.

Both intimate and family relationships should be explored in detail, and work relationships should also be covered. A good history of dating or sexual relationships is important, as the therapist can glean information about how the patient typically forms these types of relationships.

The information obtained should be both historical and current. Though IPT does not focus therapeutically on reworking past relationships, information about past relationships should still be obtained. Questions about the patient's interactions with primary care-givers, for instance, are an excellent way to begin to develop hypotheses about the patient's attachment style.

Table 4.2 *Typical Questions Used to Assess Attachment*

- 'How did your parent(s) react when you accomplished something, such as good marks in school?'
- 'How did your parent(s) react when you were hurt?'
- 'How did he or she react when you were angry?'
- 'How did you go about asking for help if you needed it?'
- 'Were there other people besides your parents who were primary care providers for you?'
- 'How do you and your siblings get along?'
- 'What were your relationships with your siblings like when you were growing up?'

The list of potential questions is endless – the point is to gather information directly from the patient in order to begin developing an idea about his or her attachment style. As attachment has everything to do with the ways in which relationships are formed and maintained, this information is crucial to develop an accurate interpersonal formulation, and to determine if the patient will do well with IPT.

Of equal importance in this narrative information is the patient's *perception* of his or her style of relating to others. The reported interactions and the patient's perception of his or her interpersonal behavior may be congruent, or they may be entirely different. Both situations obviously provide a lot of information about the patient. Patients whose perceptions match their reported interactions generally have much more insight, particularly of the type useful in IPT. In other words, they are able to recognize the way in which they are communicating, can appreciate that their communications have an impact on others, and realize the specific effects that their communications have on others. Patients whose reports do not match their self-perceptions generally lack this kind of insight, and the therapist will face greater problems with such patients because they require that therapy be started at a more basic level.

The following two case examples illustrate this point.

Case example 1: Congruent narrative and self-perception

Therapist: Tell me how you and your wife get along.
Patient: Up until this fight about my mother-in-law, we got along pretty well. When I get mad, she just withdraws and gives me the silent treatment. Last week things came to a head, and we had a huge fight about whether to put her mother in a nursing home or have her come live with us. I have to say though, from her perspective, I would have been angry too – when I get mad, I tend not to listen, and I tend to be pretty tenacious. She doesn't really have much choice but to keep quiet, I suppose.

Case example 2: Non-congruent narrative and self-perception

Therapist: Tell me how you and your wife get along.
Patient: We have been having this huge fight about my mother-in-law. I have been furious because she hasn't considered my needs at all, and wants to have her mother live with us instead of going to a nursing home.
Therapist: When you get mad, how do you react?
Patient: I just get mad. . . . you know . . . you'd be mad too if your wife did that to you.

There are many technical terms that can be used to describe factors which lead clinicians to consider patients to be good (or not so good) candidates for therapy. However, they all boil down to a simple question which is based more on intuition, experience and clinical judgment than anything else, and that question is:

Would you want to work with this patient?

With respect to the specific examples above, it doesn't take a rocket scientist (or an MD or a PhD) to figure out that patient 1 is obviously the best psychotherapy candidate. Technically speaking, he is already able, without prompting by the therapist, to recognize that his communications impact others. He is already acknowledging some responsibility for the problem, and appears to have at least an inkling of the way that his communication style may be a problem. Narrative and self-perceptions are congruent.

It is important to keep in mind that all of the patient's narrative information, though easily obtained, is generally not completely representative of the patient's style of interacting and his or her patterns of attachment. In any therapeutic situation, there is always some information that is withheld, misrepresented, or conflated by the patient. This occurs for any number of reasons, but some of the salient reasons for IPT are: (i) the patient may want to present him or herself to the therapist in the best possible light; (ii) the patient may be motivated to blame others for his or her problem rather than taking responsibility him or herself; (iii) the therapeutic bond and degree of trust in the therapist is not yet sufficient for the patient to be more revealing or open; (iv) the patient is looking to please the therapist and is reporting the 'right answer' that he or she thinks the therapist wants to hear; and (v) the therapist has not asked the right questions or shown enough interest for the patient to take a risk with self-disclosure. It is simply human nature that people withhold or distort personal information at times, and the therapeutic situation is no exception.

As a consequence, the therapist should always be mindful of the fact that it is both what is said, and how it is said, that forms the basis for the assessment of the patient. This is a reflection of patients' tendencies to withhold or distort information that they give to their therapists. This withholding may be conscious, but most often is a manifestation of the very difficulties which led to the patients' problems or led them to seek treatment.

Bowlby[1] (p. 425) summarizes this concept well:

'The fact is that much of the most relevant information refers to extremely painful or frightening events that the patient would much prefer to forget. Memories of being held always to be in the wrong, of having to care for a depressed mother instead of being cared for yourself, or the terror and anger you felt when father was violent or mother was uttering threats, of the guilt when you were told your behavior would make your parent ill, of the grief, despair and anger you felt after a loss, of the intensity of your unrequited yearning during a period of enforced separation. No one can look back on such events without feeling renewed anxiety, anger, guilt, or despair. No one, either, cares to believe that it was his very own parents, who at other times may have been kind and helpful, who on occasion behaved in some most distressing way. . . . Thus, we find defensive processes are as frequently aimed against recognizing or recalling real life events as ever they are against becoming aware of unconscious impulse or fantasy. Indeed, it is often only when the detailed course of some disturbed and distressing relationship has been recalled and recounted that the feeling aroused by it and the actions contemplated in reply come to mind.'

In addition to the information that can be directly obtained from the patient, there-fore, the therapist should also seek data which can be inferred from the patient's narra-tive and from the patient–therapist relationship. In those cases in which there is a significant other who is willing to come to several sessions of therapy, information can also be obtained from that person. All of these sources coalesce to form the foundation for the interpersonal formulation.

THE QUALITY OF THE PATIENT'S NARRATIVE

In addition to collecting information directly about the patient's relationships, infer-ences about the patient's attachment style can be drawn from the 'quality' of the patient's narrative. In simple terms, the quality of narrative is nothing more than the patient's ability to tell a good story.

In thinking about this, the therapist should consider what it is that makes a story compelling. Better yet, the therapist might think about those times when he or she has been affected by a story that a patient has told – those that have affected the therapist are usually prototypes for good narratives.

First, a good story should have a coherent plot. In other words, it should make sense. In therapy, it should come in context, rather than being told 'out of the blue.' The action should make sense, the story should make a point, and there should be a beginning and end to the story as well. In therapy, patients who tell really good stories often add an anticipatory ending – a look ahead to the way they want things to be when they finish treatment.

Second, a good story or compelling narrative should have some action. Something should be happening between the characters. Dialogue should be occurring, interper-sonal interactions should be described. The more descriptive the action the better, and lots of affect, both in the content of the story and in the telling, make for a good tale as well.

Third, there should be details which place the story in some kind of context. In ther-apy, stories should not be of the 'once upon a time' variety – they should specify the time when the event took place, and place it in a meaningful interpersonal context. For instance, a story about a conflict with a spouse should be located in real time and space.

Consider the two following examples:

Case example 3: A non-compelling narrative
Therapist: Tell me about your father's funeral.
Patient: I don't remember much about it really. It was a rainy day. . . . Most of my family had come, and we had a wake at the church afterwards. I don't really remem-ber talking to anyone. My father and I weren't very close.
Therapist: How did your father die?
Patient: He had cancer, prostate I believe. He was sick quite a long time.

Case example 4: A compelling narrative
Therapist: Tell me about your father's funeral.
Patient: There's not much to tell – it was a typical Irish affair . . . actually, it was the kind of wake that my father always wanted. He was a fun-loving man, and he had always talked about having a wake where everyone could come and remember the good times they had with him. He was an amazing man, really – even with the

> prostate cancer, which he suffered with for almost 2 years, he never lost his sense of humor. I remember visiting him in the hospital several days before he died. It seemed like we talked for ever, and I think that we both knew that the end was coming. It's hard to describe what it was like – on the one hand, I don't think that I've ever felt as close to him as at that moment, when we both just held each other and said 'I love you.' Yet I still feel so sad just thinking about it, because we'll never have any more time like that. As I was leaving, he said to me 'make sure your son knows how much you love him too.' I cried when I told that story during the eulogy. . . .

The ability to relate narrative in a meaningful way is important for several reasons. First, every form of psychotherapy requires that the patient produce some material for discussion. It may be dreams, it may be cognitions, it may be free associations or reports about desensitization exercises, but all therapies require that the patient have something to report. The more detail the better, as there is more material to be examined, and more information which can be used to understand the patient.

The ability to relate interpersonal narrative is essential in IPT. An integral part of the therapy involves having the patient produce narrative information – the patient will be asked time and again in IPT to reproduce in therapy specific interpersonal interactions, complete with dialogue, emotional content, and non-verbal information. The more information the patient is able to produce, and the more accurately it is produced, the better the patient will do in treatment.

Second, the ability to relate narrative in a compelling or meaningful way is intimately connected to the patient's ability to communicate his or her experiences to others. This in turn has a profound impact on the quality of the patient's social support network. Those patients who can describe their experiences in ways in which others are drawn in generally have much larger and more intimate social support networks than those patients who do not have that capability.

Third, the patient's innate ability to describe his or her experience is connected to his or her ability to deal with specific individual conflicts. Those patients who can convey their experiences, emotions, and need for support effectively will be able to resolve specific conflicts more effectively than patients who cannot.

Fourth, the patient's ability to tell a compelling story makes a difference because it more effectively engages the therapist. Being more human than not, therapists are influenced by exactly the same factors which affect others in the patient's interpersonal world. Therapists are drawn to listen to compelling stories – those patients who tell them are fun to work with, and therapists are more invested in such patients. This does, of course, subtly but profoundly affect outcome.

In short, the more compelling the story, the better the outcome is likely to be. The more securely attached the patient, the more likely the story is to be compelling, and the more likely the patient is to be able to meaningfully engage others and share his or her experiences. During the assessment, the therapist should directly ask the patient to tell some meaningful or interesting interpersonal stories.

THE PATIENT'S DESCRIPTIONS OF OTHER INDIVIDUALS

In addition to the quality of the narrative in general, the way in which the patient describes other people in his or her interpersonal world is telling with respect to attachment style. As with stories, the therapist should directly ask for descriptions of others with whom the patient interacts.

Those patients who are more securely attached are generally able to describe other people in 'three-dimensional' terms. In other words, they are able to portray other people as real, with good points and bad, altruistic and selfish motives, idiosyncrasies and strengths. This reflects their more accurate working model of relationships, or their relative lack of parataxic distortions. More securely attached people are able to 'call it like it is' more precisely.

Those patients with more anxious ambivalent attachments often portray others in more 'two-dimensional' terms. Because such patients are concerned or preoccupied with getting their attachments needs met, they are loathe to be critical of others who might provide them with care. Hence an idealized, or on occasion, a devalued description of others will be provided. Hypochondriacal patients are classic examples of this kind of attachment and corresponding descriptions, as they will completely idealize current and potential care providers while decrying those that have failed them before. None of the figures in an anxious ambivalently attached patient's world is complete – they have only good or only bad parts. Psychoanalytically speaking, splitting influences the way that such patients typically conceptualize others.

Patients with more avoidant styles of attachment, in contrast, will usually describe others in 'one-dimensional' terms. With these patients, there is literally no detail at all. There is literally nothing to hang one's hat on – no information, no details . . . nothing. This is a reflection of the avoidant patient's interpersonal world, in which relationships carry much less meaning than for others.

Consider the following three examples:

Case example 5: Secure attachment

Therapist: Tell me about your mother.
Patient: My mother . . . well, she and I get along pretty well now, though she certainly has her moments. When I was growing up, she was great. I remember when I was five and had the chicken pox, she took off from work and stayed home with me. We played games, read books . . . it was great. During my teen years . . . well, that was another story. She was a bit old fashioned, and she and I got into some pretty loud arguments about what I was going to wear and how late I could stay out. I guess all told she has been pretty supportive. Like with my kids – she is always willing to lend a hand to help watch them, and is great with them, but she still has a tendency to be critical of some of the ways that we have decided to raise them.

Case example 6: Anxious ambivalent attachment

Therapist: Tell me about your mother.
Patient: My mother . . . well she is just the greatest. She is always there to help, she's great with the kids . . . frankly, I don't think I could have asked for a better mother. I can't think of a single thing I'd change about her.
Therapist: I thought just a minute ago you had mentioned that you and she were having a big conflict about how you were raising your children.
Patient: Oh that . . . well, that hardly ever happens . . . it wasn't really that important.

Case example 7: Anxious avoidant attachment

Therapist: Tell me about your mother.
Patient: My mother . . . well, she's 56 years old.
Therapist: What is she like?
Patient: She's pretty nice, a good mom I guess.
Therapist: Any specific things about her come to mind?
Patient: No, not really. She was a good mom.

Though rather simplistic examples, the preceding do demonstrate the types of responses that patients with varying attachment styles may give to direct inquires about other people. In the first case, the securely attached patient is able to provide a well-rounded view of her mother – she has good and bad points, the patient is able to describe them, and the patient has integrated them into a coherent and meaningful whole person. Even better, she spontaneously produces narrative material that provides context and details for her description.

In the second case, the patient's description is idealized. When confronted by the therapist, she seems unable to integrate the two different aspects of her mother into a coherent whole. The threat of losing her mother and what limited support she provides leads the patient to idealize. In addition to hypochondriacal patients, this unfortunately happens on occasion with victims of abuse, who despite severe trauma will continue to idealize the perpetrator of the abuse and blame themselves.

In the third case, the avoidant patient is simply unable to provide much meaningful information at all. One can easily imagine that such a patient would be difficult to work with in therapy. This is not only because of the poor quality of information that she is providing, but also because she seems to have an inability to convey her inner experiences, feelings, and perceptions to others. In addition, such a patient will quickly become a burden to most therapists because she cannot effectively engage even the therapist.

There is clearly a great deal of overlap in attachment styles. All individuals have some combination of secure and insecure attachment traits. However, some are more secure than others, and it is these patients who will typically have a better prognosis in therapy.

THE PATIENT–THERAPIST RELATIONSHIP

The last part of the assessment of attachment and communication triad is that of the therapeutic relationship. As with the patient's report about relationships, and as with the quality of the patient's narrative, the patient–therapist relationship has far-reaching implications both about the patient's attachment style and his or her prognosis in therapy.

As the assessment phase proceeds, and for that matter, as all of therapy proceeds, the clinician should be acutely attuned to the therapeutic relationship. In particular, the therapist should be keenly aware of his or her reactions to the patient. This is crucial because both attachment and communication can be assessed in this way.

Attachment can be assessed because the relationship that the patient develops with the therapist is a reflection of the style of attachment that the patient manifests in relationships outside of therapy. The patient's interpersonal working model, or parataxic distortions, will be imposed upon the therapist. These may or may not be readily apparent. With a less securely attached patient, they will often come to the fore in the first session, as the patient's working model is so inaccurate that discrepancies are immediately evident. The raging borderline, the narcissist, and the antisocial all come to mind as examples of such patients. On the other hand, those patients with more secure styles of attachment do not impose such distorted attributes upon the therapist, or at least do not do so in such short order. They are cooperative, readily accept help, and are pleasant to work with.

Communication can be assessed because the patients' specific communications and metacommunications in therapy, as do all of their communications outside of therapy, elicit a characteristic response. In this case, they elicit a response from the therapist. Thus, the therapist should be keenly aware of his or her reflexive responses to the patient. Does the patient make the therapist feel helpless? Angry? Bored? Effective and helpful? Each reflexive response is indicative of the patient's specific communication style.

In order to make the assessment of attachment complete, the therapist should also conduct an assessment of the match between him or herself and the patient. The old adage to 'know thyself' cannot be overemphasized, for therapists – like patients – also have idiosyncratic styles of attachment and communication. Therapists who tend to be overly directive may have difficulty with avoidant patients, for example. Therapists who find it difficult to terminate treatment may encounter problems with patients with dependent attachment styles. Securely attached therapists, as patients, will more effectively utilize therapy.

ASSESSMENT OF ATTACHMENT AND COMMUNICATION: SUMMARY

The patient's attachment and communication style should be assessed in IPT using at least three different sources of information. First, the patient's direct report of relationships should be examined. Second, the quality of his or her narrative, particularly in response to direct inquiries to 'tell a story,' should be assessed. Third, the quality of the relationship between the patient and therapist should provide information. All of these come together to inform both the patient's suitability for IPT and his or her prognosis in therapy.

The patient's attachment style therefore has direct implications regarding his or her ability to develop a therapeutic alliance with the therapist and the likelihood that treatment will be beneficial. Unfortunately, in IPT as in all other psychotherapies, the old adage about the 'rich getting richer' holds true. Those patients with relatively secure attachment styles are usually able to form a working relationship with the therapist, and because of their relatively healthy relationships outside of therapy, are also more likely to be able to draw upon their social support system effectively. Individuals with more anxious ambivalent attachments can usually quickly form relationships with their clinicians, but often have a great deal of difficulty with the conclusion of treatment – a particular problem in time-limited therapy. Those with anxious avoidant styles of attachment may have difficulty trusting or relating to the therapist. Consequently, when working with anxious avoidant patients the therapist may need to spend several of the initial sessions in therapy working primarily on nothing more than developing a productive therapeutic alliance, waiting until a good alliance is established prior to moving into more formal IPT work.

In addition to evaluating therapeutic suitability, the therapist should use the assessment to forecast and plan for problems which may arise during the course of therapy. For example, since patients with anxious ambivalent attachment styles may have difficulty in ending relationships, the astute therapist may modify his or her approach by emphasizing the time-limited nature of the treatment, discussing the conclusion of treatment during the middle phases of therapy, and by beginning the conclusion process earlier. Significant others may also be included in sessions more frequently to ensure that dependency on the therapist does not become problematic. When working with avoidant patients, the therapist should plan to spend several sessions completing an assessment, taking great care to convey a sense of understanding and empathy to the client. Soliciting feedback from the patient about the intensity of treatment, particularly considering less frequent appointments, is another tactic which may improve the therapeutic alliance with these individuals.

TRADITIONAL PATIENT CHARACTERISTICS FOR TIME-LIMITED PSYCHOTHERAPY

In general, patients who have characteristics that render them good candidates for any of the time-limited therapies will be good candidates for IPT. There have been a number of authors who have described patient selection factors, and most stress that in short-term therapy, careful selection of patients is crucial to the success of the treatment.[2-5] The emphasis on these factors rests both on clinical experience and empirical data.

The empirical evidence regarding patient selection for short-term therapy suggests that there are several specific factors that have been associated with good outcome.[6-8] Although most of the research that has been conducted has investigated more psychodynamically oriented short-term treatments, the data nonetheless are useful in considering the suitability of patients for IPT.

The factors which are most commonly mentioned both in the clinical and empirical literature, and which are integral to the selection of patients for IPT, include:

1 Severity of illness.
2 Motivation.
3 The ability to form a therapeutic alliance.
4 Ego strength.
5 Psychological mindedness.

Severity of illness

The data on severity of illness as a predictor of outcome in short-term psychotherapy follow exactly the intuitive notion that the more severe the psychopathology, the less suitable patients are for treatment.[9,10] This includes not only psychiatric symptoms such as psychoses, but also more severe personality disorders.[11,12] High levels of symptomatic severity in disorders such as depression also portend poorer outcome in general.[13]

Motivation

The concept of motivation as it applies to time-limited therapy has been understood more as a desire to change as opposed to a simple desire to be rid of symptoms.[6]

Elements of such motivation include the patient's ability to recognize the psychological nature of the symptoms with which he or she is struggling, a willingness to participate actively in therapy, a willingness to explore new solutions to problems, and a willingness to extend oneself in pragmatic ways, such as sacrificing time to come to appointments and paying fees[14] – the latter being paramount, of course, for therapists as well as patients. The intuitive nature of these factors is obvious, particularly in IPT, as problem solving is a major component of the treatment. The empirical literature also supports the theoretical importance of motivation,[15] though several authors have suggested that motivation be assessed later in therapy as opposed to the initial session, as both the empirical evidence[16] and clinical experience indicate that later assessments of motivation may be more accurate.[2,17] This lends further credence to the contention that a thorough assessment is essential prior to selecting patients for IPT.

The ability to form a therapeutic alliance

The ability to form a therapeutic alliance includes many different facets of the therapeutic relationship, but in essence describes the patient's ability to work productively with the therapist. To do so, the patient must be able to position him or herself to seek and receive help, to report feelings honestly to the therapist, and to trust the therapist. In IPT, this is conceptualized in large part as the ability to attach securely to the therapist. The empirical evidence supports the importance of this factor, and as with motivation, the assessment of the therapeutic relationship, working alliance, or therapeutic bond appears to be more clearly correlated with outcome when measured several sessions into therapy.[18,19]

The quality of the therapeutic alliance has also been correlated with good outcome in IPT specifically. In the NIMH Treatment of Depression Collaborative Research Program (NIMH-TDCRP),[20] the quality of the therapeutic alliance was found to have a significant impact on outcome.[21] In particular, the patient's contributions to the alliance were found to carry great weight.[22] The patient's ability to engage in a productive therapeutic relationship was also found to have more impact upon the therapist's ability to competently conduct IPT than the severity of the patient's symptoms,[23] again emphasizing the importance of the therapeutic alliance.

Ego strength

Ego strength has a long tradition as an important factor in the success of psychotherapy. Ego strength as a general construct includes a host of factors, some of which are abstract, and others which serve as concrete representations of other underlying factors. Ego strength has been defined as the capacity to withstand internal or external stress, the ability to experience distressing material during the therapy process, and the ability to constructively integrate affect and experience.[24-26] Specific objective measures which may serve as markers of ego strength include the patient's intelligence, work history, and level of education.[3] Given the abstract nature of the construct, specific empirical literature is sparse, though several authors have found support for the concept as a positive predictive factor in general terms.[9,15] In IPT, it is certainly true that the ability to integrate affect with narrative material will serve the patient well.

Psychological mindedness

Psychological mindedness includes a number of elements such as a willingness to focus on one's internal processes, a capacity for introspection, and a curiosity about oneself with a willingness to explore one's own thoughts and feelings. Closely connected to this concept is the ability not only to be aware of one's own thoughts and feelings but also to be able to communicate them effectively to others.[24] This factor is crucial in any therapy, for if the patient is not able to describe his or her internal and external experiences, then therapy cannot proceed. Communicating one's experience is of course essential to IPT, both in terms of the therapeutic process itself and in terms of the patient's ability to effectively engage his or her social support network.

While the empirical data regarding the importance of psychological mindedness are mixed,[6] clinical experience with IPT clearly indicates that it is an important factor in outcome. The relative lack of empirical support may be due to the fact that different qualities of psychological mindedness may be important for different types of therapies. For instance, in IPT patients need to make connections between interpersonal events and symptoms, while in cognitive behavior therapy (CBT), the connections are between internal cognitions and symptoms. Dynamic therapies require yet again a different type of insight, and these propositions remain to be empirically tested.

Most of the factors common to all short-term psychotherapies are of the intuitively obvious type. In addition, most are at a fairly high level of abstraction, which largely accounts for the relative lack of empirical research and absolute conclusions that can be drawn from the literature. It is also important to note that diagnosis is not often cited as a primary basis for treatment selection. The best way to assess patients for IPT is to use these criteria generally, operating under the principle that 'you know it when you see it' – in other words, patient characteristics such as psychological mindedness and motivation can be recognized in therapy without much difficulty, even though they often elude more concrete description.

PATIENT CHARACTERISTICS SPECIFIC TO IPT

Characteristics specific to IPT which increase the likelihood that patients will benefit from IPT include:

1 A relatively secure attachment style.
2 The ability to relate a coherent narrative along with the ability to relate specific dialogue from their interpersonal interactions.
3 A specific interpersonal focus for distress.
4 A good social support system.

Secure attachment style

A secure attachment style is highly correlated with many of the other factors that are associated with good outcome in psychotherapy. Patients with more securely attached styles generally have more ego strength, are able to enter into therapy with a genuine desire to seek help, are able to trust their therapists to be of help, and can form more productive therapeutic alliances more quickly. They also generally have both the internal and external resources to do well in therapy: their ego strength leads them to be more able to take risks and to be motivated to change, and their social support systems are usually much better than those of patients who are less securely attached. A secure attachment style is likely the most important factor in determining which patients are most suitable for IPT.

Coherent narrative

In addition to being able to recognize interpersonal issues and connect them with symptoms and poor functioning, patients in IPT must be able to communicate their experiences in a coherent fashion. IPT in particular rests largely on communication analysis, which requires that the patient be able to relate, in detail, the communication which occurs in incidents outside of therapy. Being able to recreate dialogue, reflect on affect that is communicated, and to literally be able to tell a story is essential in IPT. In fact, specifically asking the patient to tell several stories about important interactions during the assessment phase will allow the therapist to make a reasonable judgment about this factor.

Specific interpersonal focus

Given the time-limited nature of IPT, patients who present with more focal problems will generally do better with the treatment. There is seldom enough time to deal with more general or historical issues as opposed to more focal and specific problems. Those patients who begin therapy having already made a connection between their symptoms and interpersonal issues are even better candidates for IPT, as they will need no convincing that IPT is a plausible and applicable treatment for them specifically. In essence, patients who present for treatment with complaints such as 'I just don't feel well, but I don't know why' are not good candidates; those who present with complaints such as 'I am in the midst of a divorce which is leading me to have trouble functioning and making me feel depressed,' are.

The concept of patient aptitude is also important to consider in IPT. Patients who frame their problems in interpersonal terms are likely to do better in IPT than those that do not. The patient's initial description of his or her problems is quite telling in this regard. For example, a woman who describes her postpartum depression as due to 'difficulties with conflicts with my husband and problems dealing with going back to work after the birth of my baby' – classic interpersonal disputes and role transitions – is likely to do well with IPT. In contrast, a woman who describes her problems as due to feelings that 'I don't measure up to other women as a mother, and I constantly worry that something bad may happen to my child' might do better with CBT, as her presentation is more consistent with distorted cognitive patterns. Research in this area is ongoing at present, but these distinctions have been found to be quite useful clinically.

Good social support

The better the social support, the more likely the patient is to improve with therapy. IPT in particular is focused on helping patients to utilize their social support systems to meet their attachment needs; hence, the more resources that are available, the more likely that patients will be able to get their attachment needs met. Good social support is highly correlated with attachment security, as securely attached patients generally have better social support systems. The therapist should also assess the intimacy of the relationships that patients have developed – those who are able to engage in deeper and more emotionally close relationships will do well in therapy, as they will have others with whom they can share their experiences and call on for support.

EMPIRICAL EVIDENCE FOR IPT

There are a number of studies which are relevant to the assessment of patients for IPT. First, there are a number of efficacy trials investigating the use of IPT with specific diagnoses. Second, there are several studies which have investigated the factors associated with a good response to IPT. The data from these studies should inform the clinician about what is likely to be helpful for a patient, but should by no means be the only or determining factor in making this decision. The empirical studies are all based on populations of patients – not specific individuals – and it is of course a unique individual with whom the therapist is working. In addition, all of the efficacy studies have limitations which restrict the conclusions that can be drawn about non-research use of IPT. Thus, while the empirical data should be a major factor in making decisions about treatment, final decisions about appropriateness should always also be based on clinical experience and should include a good measure of clinical judgment.

Efficacy studies have been conducted using IPT to treat a number of specific diagnoses. (For a more complete description of these and other studies, see Chapter 22.) IPT has been shown to be of benefit with a depression in general[13,27] as well as a number of other depressed populations including depressed geriatric patients,[28] depressed adolescents,[29] depressed patients who are HIV-positive,[30] and patients with dysthymic disorder.[31] IPT has also been used for perinatal depression, including postpartum[32] and antenatal depression.[33] In addition, it has been tested with patients with eating disorders,[34] and an open trial investigating the use of IPT with social phobia has also been published.[35]

Despite the variety of diagnoses which have been tested empirically, there are at present very few available data regarding the use of IPT in general clinical (i.e., non-research) settings, requiring that clinicians utilize their clinical judgment when faced with patients with comorbid diagnoses or personality pathology. There are, however, several studies which have investigated patient factors which have been linked with better outcome in IPT.

The presence of a personality disorder comorbid with depression has been associated with poorer outcome in terms of treatment for depression. In the NIMH Treatment of Depression Collaborative Treatment Program (NIMH-TDCRP), depressed patients with personality disorders had poorer outcome with respect to depressive symptoms and with respect to social functioning.[11] Although the empirical evidence is limited to this single study, the suggestion that personality disorders are likely to be associated with a more difficult course in therapy certainly has intuitive appeal.[36]

As a consequence, special attention should be paid to patients diagnosed with personality disorders, both because of the empirical data and because of the clinical experience that has accumulated with such patients. Those with cluster A disorders including paranoid, schizoid, and schizotypal personality disorders may be unable to form effective alliances with their therapists in short-term therapy, while those with severe cluster B disorders such as narcissistic, histrionic, border-line and antisocial personality disorders may require more intensive therapy than can be provided in an IPT format. However, many patients with depression or anxiety superimposed upon a personality disorder may benefit a great deal from short-term therapy with IPT which restricts its focus to the treatment of the depression or anxiety.

Additional data from the NIMH-TDCRP indicate that there are several other factors associated with a positive response to treatment with IPT.[37] These included a low level of social dysfunction at intake, as well as a high degree of interpersonal sensitivity. Patients who reported greater satisfaction with their relationships when they began treatment were also more likely to benefit from IPT as compared to the other treatments. The NIMH-TDCRP results can be summarized by stating that those patients without severe personality pathology, who have a relatively good social support system, and who have an awareness of the way in which they communicate in interpersonal relationships, typically fare well with IPT.

Several personality characteristics have also been found to be associated with outcome in IPT. Perfectionism has been shown to have a negative impact on outcome; Blatt et al.[38] noted that perfectionism began to impede therapeutic progress in the latter half of treatment, and have suggested that this may be due to the reaction of perfectionistic patients to an arbitrary, externally imposed termination date. In the NIMH-TDCRP, patients with more avoidant traits were found to fare better in CBT than in IPT, while patients with more obsessive traits had better outcomes when treated with IPT as compared to CBT.[39] Frank et al. found that, among women with recurrent depression who were treated with IPT, those with higher levels of self-reported panic and agoraphobic symptoms were less likely to respond to IPT.[40] Non-remitters were also found to have higher levels of somatic anxiety.[41]

Empirical data regarding biological predictors are limited, but studies investigating sleep parameters and their association with response to IPT have found that depressed patients with abnormal sleep electroencephalogram (EEG) profiles prior to treatment had significantly lower response rates than depressed patients with more normal sleep profiles.[42,43] More research regarding the predictive value of biological measures is clearly needed.

The empirical data regarding patient selection can be summarized as follows. First, good empirical data are available supporting the efficacy of IPT for a number of well-specified diagnoses, though the effectiveness data are quite limited. The presence of personality disorders, though obviously not a contraindication to IPT, may complicate its course and be associated with poorer outcomes. Social factors such as a good social support system have been associated with good outcome. At present, more data are needed regarding biological markers of response.

CONCLUSION

The selection of patients can best be understood to be on a spectrum, with highly suitable patients at one end, and those who may be less suitable at the other. While there are no absolute contraindications to IPT, there are clearly patients who might benefit more from treatments other than IPT. Clinical judgment should be used to weigh the patient's suitability for short-term treatment, the empirical evidence supporting efficacy of the various treatments available, and the clinical value of the treatment options.

In summary, the assessment process should assist the therapist to evaluate the patient's suitability for IPT, and it should be based on clinical experience, empirical data, and clinical judgment. An assessment of the patient's attachment style and communication patterns should be undertaken, as well as a thorough psychiatric assessment. The assessment should assist the therapist to anticipate and plan for potential problems in therapy, such as resistance or dependency, and should direct the therapist as to how to modify the therapeutic approach so that these problems are minimized. The assessment will often take several sessions to complete, given the number of tasks that need to be completed. It is only after the assessment, and the determination that the patient is suitable, that IPT should begin formally.

REFERENCES

1. Bowlby, J. 1977. The making and breaking of affectional bonds, II: some principles of psychotherapy. *British Journal of Psychiatry* **130**, 421–31.
2. Malan, D.H. 1976. *The Frontier of Brief Psychotherapy*. New York: Plenum.
3. Marmor, J. 1979. Short-term dynamic psychotherapy. *American Journal of Psychiatry* **136**, 149–55.
4. Schneider, W.J., Pinkerton, R.S. 1986. Short-term psychotherapy and graduate training in psychology. *Professional Psychology: Research and Practice* **17**, 574–9.
5. Sifneos, P. 1972. *Short-term Psychotherapy and Emotional Crisis*. Cambridge: Harvard University Press.
6. Lambert, M.J., Anderson, E.M. 1996. Assessment for the time-limited psychotherapies. In: Dickstein, L.J., Riba, M.B., Oldham, J.M. (eds), *American Psychiatric Press Review of Psychiatry*. Volume 15. Washington, DC: American Psychiatric Press, 23–42.
7. Barber, J.P., Crits-Cristoph, P. 1991. Comparison of the brief dynamic psychotherapies. In: Crits-Cristoph, P., Barber, J.P. (eds), *Handbook of Short-term Dynamic Psychotherapy*. New York: Basic Books, 323–56.
8. Demos, V.C., Prout, M.F. 1993. A comparison of seven approaches to brief psychotherapy. *International Journal of Short-Term Psychotherapy* **8**, 3–22.
9. Luborsky, L., Crits-Cristoph, P., Mintz, J. 1988. *Who Will Benefit from Psychotherapy?* New York: Basic Books.
10. Hoglend, P. 1993. Suitability for brief dynamic psychotherapy: psychodynamic variables as predictors of outcome. *Acta Psychiatrica Scandinavica* **88**, 104–10.
11. Shea, M.T., Pilkonis, P.A., Beckham, E., *et al*. 1990. Personality disorders and treatment outcome in the NIMH Treatment of Depression Collaborative Treatment Program. *American Journal of Psychiatry* **147**, 711–18.

12. Shea, M.T. 1992. Some characteristics of the Axis II criteria sets and their implications for assessment of personality disorders. *Journal of Personality Disorders* **6**, 377–81.
13. Elkin, I., Shea, M.T., Watkins, J.T., *et al*. 1989. National Institute of Mental Health Treatment of Depression Collaborative Research Program: general effectiveness of treatments. *Archives of General Psychiatry* **46**, 971–82.
14. Sifneos, P.E. 1987. *Short-term Dynamic Psycotherapy*. New York: Plenum.
15. Orlinsky, D.E., Grawe, K., Parks, B.K. 1994. Process and outcome in psychotherapy noch einmal. In: Bergin, A.E., Garfield, S.L. (eds), *Handbook of Psychotherapy and Behavioral Change*. 4th edition. New York: Wiley.
16. O'Malley, S., Suh, C.D., Strupp, H.H. 1983. The Vanderbilt psychotherapy process scale: a report on the scale development and a process-outcome study. *Journal of Consulting and Clinical Psychology* **51**, 581–6.
17. Garfield, S.L. 1989. *The Practice of Brief Psychotherapy*. New York: Pergamon.
18. Strupp, H.H. 1981. Toward the refinement of time-limited dynamic psychotherapy. In: Budman, S.H. (ed.), *Forms of Brief Therapy*. New York: Guilford, 219–25.
19. Binder, J.L., Henry, W.P., Strupp, H.H. 1987. An appraisal of selection criteria for dynamic psychotherapies and implications for setting time limits. *Journal of Psychiatry* **50**, 154–66.
20. Elkin, I., Parloff, M.B., Hadley, S.W., Autry, J.H. 1985. NIMH Treatment of Depression Collaborative Treatment Program: background and research plan. *Archives of General Psychiatry* **42**, 305–16.
21. Krupnick, J.L., Sotsky, S.M., Simmens, S., *et al*. 1996. The role of the therapeutic alliance in psychotherapy and pharmacotherapy outcome: findings in the National Institute of Mental Health Treatment of Depression. *Journal of Consulting and Clinical Psychology* **64**, 532–9.
22. Zuroff, D.C., Blatt, S.J., Sotsky, S.M., *et al*. 2000. Relation of therapeutic alliance and perfectionism to outcome in brief outpatient treatment of depression. *Journal of Consulting and Clinical Psychology* **68**, 114–24.
23. Foley, S.H., O'Malley, S., Rounsaville, B., Prusoff, B.A., Weissman, M.M. 1987. The relationship of patient difficulty to therapist performance in interpersonal psychotherapy of depression. *Journal of Affective Disorders* **12**, 207–17.
24. Bauer, P.B., Kobos, J.C. 1987. *Brief Therapy: Short-Term Dynamic Intervention*. London: Jason Aronson.
25. Malan, D.H., Osimo, F. 1992. *Psychodynamics, Training, and Outcome in Brief Psychotherapy*. Boston: Butterworth-Heinemann.
26. Davanloo, H. 1980. *Short-Term Dynamic Psychotherapy*. Northvale, NJ: Aronson.
27. Weissman, M.M., Prusoff, B.A., DiMascio, A. 1979. The efficacy of drugs and psychotherapy in the treatment of acute depressive episodes. *American Journal of Psychiatry* **136**, 555–8.
28. Reynolds, C.F., Frank, E., Perel, J.M. 1992. Combined pharmacotherapy and psychotherapy in the acute and continuation treatment of elderly patients with recurrent major depression: a preliminary report. *American Journal of Psychiatry* **149**, 1687–92.
29. Mufson, L., Fairbanks, J. 1996. Interpersonal psychotherapy for depressed adolescents: a one-year naturalistic follow-up study. *Journal of the American Academy of Child and Adolescent Psychiatry* **35**, 1145–55.
30. Markowitz, J.M., Klerman, G.L., Perry, S.W. 1993. Interpersonal psychotherapy for depressed HIV-seropositive patients. In: Klerman, G.L., Weissman, M.M. (eds), *New Applications of Interpersonal Psychotherapy*. Washington, DC: American Psychiatric Press, 199–224.
31. Markowitz, J. 1998. *Interpersonal Psychotherapy for Dysthymic Disorder*. Washington, DC: American Psychiatric Press.

32. O'Hara, M.W., Stuart, S., Gorman, L., Wenzel, A. 2000. Efficacy of interpersonal psychotherapy for postpartum depression. *Archives of General Psychiatry* **57**, 1039–45.
33. Spinelli, M.G., Weissman, M.M. 1997. The clinical application of interpersonal psychotherapy for depression during pregnancy. *Primary Psychiatry* **4**, 50–7.
34. Fairburn, C.G., Jones, R., Peveler, R.C. 1991. Three psychological treatments for bulimia nervosa: a comparative trial. *Archives of General Psychiatry* **48**, 463–9.
35. Lipsitz, J.D., Markowitz, J.C., Cherry, S., Fyer, A.J. 1999. Open trial of interpersonal psychotherapy for the treatment of social phobia. *American Journal of Psychiatry* **156**, 1814–16.
36. Shea, M.T., Widiger, T.A., Klein, M.H. 1992. Comorbidity of personality disorders and depression: implications for treatment. *Journal of Consulting and Clinical Psychology* **60**, 857–68.
37. Sotsky, S.M., Glass, D.R., Shea, M.T., *et al.* 1991. Patient predictors of response to psychotherapy and pharmacotherapy: findings in the NIMH Treatment of Depression Collaborative Research Program. *American Journal of Psychiatry* **148**, 997–1008.
38. Blatt, S.J., Zuroff, D.C., Bondi, C.M., Sanislow, C.A., Pilkonis, P.A. 1998. When and how perfectionism impedes the brief treatment of depression: further analyses of the National Institute of Mental Health Treatment of Depression Collaborative Research Program. *Journal of Consulting and Clinical Psychology* **66**, 423–8.
39. Barber, J.P., Muenz, L.R. 1996. The role of avoidance and obsessiveness in matching patients to cognitive and interpersonal psychotherapy: empirical findings from the Treatment for Depression Collaborative Research Program. *Journal of Consulting and Clinical Psychology* **64**, 951–8.
40. Frank, E., Shear, M.K., Rucci, P., *et al.* 2000. Influence of panic-agoraphobic spectrum symptoms on treatment response in patients with recurrent major depression. *American Journal of Psychiatry* **157**, 1101–7.
41. Feske, U., Frank, E., Kupfer, D.J., Shear, M.K., Weaver, E. 1998. Anxiety as a predictor of response to interpersonal psychotherapy for recurrent major depression: an exploratory investigation. *Depression and Anxiety* **8**, 135–41.
42. Thase, M.E., Buysse, D.J., Frank, E., Cherry, C.R. 1997. Which depressed patients will respond to interpersonal psychotherapy? The role of abnormal EEG sleep profiles. *American Journal of Psychiatry* **154**, 502–9.
43. Buysse, D.J., Tu, X.M., Cherry, C.R., *et al.* 1999. Pretreatment REM sleep and subjective sleep quality distinguish depressed psychotherapy remitters and nonremitters. *Biological Psychiatry* **45**, 205–13.

5

Negotiating the Treatment Contract

INTRODUCTION

Interpersonal Psychotherapy, like all other psychotherapies, requires the collaborative establishment of a set of 'rules' for its conduct. The contract in IPT is for the benefit of both the patient and the therapist. For the patient, it establishes expectations for the treatment along with the obligations of both the patient and therapist in the conduct of IPT. For the therapist, the IPT treatment contract provides a practical and theoretical guide to treatment, particularly with patients whose individual attributes increase the likelihood that problematic psychodynamic processes will emerge during the therapy. Since both the patient and therapist have important contributions to make to the contract, it should be a collaboratively negotiated 'treatment agreement' between patient and therapist, rather than being rigidly dictated by the therapist.

WHY IS A CONTRACT NECESSARY IN IPT?

Unlike human relationships outside of a clinical setting, the therapeutic relationship is constrained by ethical and practical concerns (although one might well argue that it would be desirable if all relationships were bound by similar ethical concerns). The concept of clinical 'boundaries' is one of the best examples of this. In addition to the practical necessity of agreeing to a specific time and place to meet for therapy, therapeutic relationships nearly always have limits to such issues as contact with the therapist out of hours, the establishment of a workable arrangement for payment for services, and so on. Ideally, these are established clearly and a priori rather than emerging as problems later in the therapy. Setting these boundaries both preserves the integrity of the therapeutic relationship and serves to protect the patient and therapist from exploitation. As a part of the process of negotiating the treatment contract, the patient and therapist should establish the boundaries of the therapeutic relationship.

Despite the emphasis throughout this book upon the need for flexibility and clinical judgment on the part of the therapist, IPT remains a highly structured and focal intervention. Establishing a therapeutic contract that both 'sets the scene' and limits the scope of therapeutic intervention will help the therapist to ensure that the patient will obtain the greatest benefit from treatment.

Like all of the components of IPT, the treatment agreement involves a collaborative process between the patient and therapist. While the agreement may need to be literally 'set in stone' in some circumstances, the ability to revisit and renegotiate the treatment contract should remain throughout the treatment course. Clinical judgment should naturally guide this process.

The negotiation of the treatment contract is in essence an interpersonal process between patient and therapist. As a consequence, the contract should be negotiated after the therapist has had the opportunity to assess the patient's clinical presentation, attachment style, and social and financial situation. The therapist should have a fairly well-developed feel for the nature of the therapeutic relationship after a thorough assessment has been completed.

The contract should also include mutually negotiated therapeutic goals. If the patient and therapist enter a treatment contract with a shared view of the clinical goals, the likelihood of the treatment being successful in alleviating the patient's psychological symptoms is greatly increased. As a result, the therapist should help the patient to articulate his or her specific goals for treatment with IPT – that is, the specific outcomes in the nominated interpersonal problem area – as clearly as possible. The patient's attachment style also guides this process to some extent: those patients with more secure attachment styles are much more likely to tolerate the therapist 'taking the lead' in setting goals, while those with more insecure styles of attachment will likely feel alienated or rejected if the therapist is too directive in setting the agenda.

THE CONTRACT IN IPT

The core components of the treatment contract in IPT include the following.

Table 5.1 *The Core Components of the IPT Contract*

• The number, frequency and duration of sessions.
• The agreed clinical foci.
• The expectations of the patient and therapist.
• Contingency planning.
• Treatment boundaries.

Depending upon the therapist's clinical judgment, the contract in IPT can be either a written or a verbal agreement. The provision of a written description of the conduct of IPT and a description of the patient's role in treatment is extremely helpful in formalizing the contract with some patients (a patient information sheet is included in Appendix A). The use of tools such as this should be determined to a large degree by the individual patient with whom the clinician is working, rather than being applied dogmatically to all patients. Patients who are more securely attached are likely to do quite well in therapy without the need for a written agreement, while those patients with evidence of insecure attachment and more problematic interpersonal styles may benefit from a clearly written description of the conduct of IPT and the specific goals and expectations of their roles in the treatment.

Whether written or verbal, the contract in IPT should specifically address:

- *The number, frequency and duration of sessions*: this should be determined primarily on the basis of the severity of the patient's problems and his or her attachment style. Sessions may also vary with the style and availability of the therapist, but in general will be on the order of eight to twenty sessions, each of 50 minutes' duration. Issues of cost and payment should also be clarified.
- *The agreed clinical foci*: this should include the problem areas and relationship issues which have been identified by the patient and therapist, and may also include limitations on discussion of more psychodynamic issues or explorations of the patient's early experiences.
- *The expectations of the patient and therapist*: the patient is expected to take responsibility for both utilizing the sessions as well as working between sessions on problems in his or her social environment and interpersonal relationships. Patients frequently have the incorrect assumption that the bulk of change in IPT will take place in the sessions rather than in the context of their interpersonal functioning outside of sessions. The 'bottom line' in IPT is changing the patient's functioning in his or her social environment; hence 'work' must occur between sessions.
- *Contingency planning*: this includes matters such as missed sessions, lateness, or illness. In general, if the therapist is late or misses a session, the time should be made good at a later time. If the patient misses sessions or is late for reasons that are, after discussion between patient and therapist, considered unreasonable, then the time is usually considered lost. The therapist should frame the lateness or absence as an overt interpersonal behavior, rather than examining the psychodynamic underpinnings of such behavior directly with the patient. The therapist can also use this information about the patient's behavior to further develop his or her hypotheses about the patient's interpersonal relationships and attachment style. The therapist can then draw attention to other circumstances in which the patient has been late or not met obligations with others in his or her social network, as opposed to discussing such issues within the therapeutic relationship.
- *Treatment boundaries*: 'boundaries' in clinical practice are perhaps best defined as the ethical and practical constraints that distinguish the therapeutic relationship from other non-professional relationships. Relevant 'boundary' issues include the degree of therapist self-disclosure, clinical and non-clinical contact out of hours, appropriate arrangements for emergencies out of hours, and expectations regarding substance use and aggressive or inappropriate behavior. While many would argue that these are implicit in any therapeutic relationship, it is frequently worthwhile discussing these formally with the patient and negotiating common ground between the patient and therapist.

'VIOLATIONS' OF THE CONTRACT

'Violations' or breaches of contract may occur, even with explicit contracts. These may range from simple matters such as lateness or delayed fee payments to more significant problems such as inappropriate behavior in sessions or inappropriate contact outside of therapy. While all of these problems can be viewed as having psychodynamic and transferential significance, the focus of the IPT therapist's responses to such occurrences is to address them as interpersonal behaviors in the 'here-and-now' rather than as unconsciously determined behaviors.

Contract or boundary violations, conceptualized as conscious interpersonal behaviors, often provide valuable information about the patient's experience of the therapeutic relationship, as well as his or her behavior in relationships outside of therapy. In some cases the behavior may have a simple explanation such as logistical difficulties (time off work, child care, etc.) or financial limitations, which are best dealt with by the therapist pragmatically. In others, they reflect the patient's attachment style and corresponding difficulties with communication, and may also reflect personality difficulties and psychological defenses. It is the therapist's task to analyze this information, integrate it into a coherent understanding of the patient as a whole, and use it to help the patient improve his or her communications with others outside of therapy.

Boundary violations in IPT should generally be dealt with using a three-step process. First, the therapist should state directly to the patient that a boundary violation has occurred. A brief discussion should follow to ensure that the patient recognizes this, and that there is continuing agreement on the limits to be set. Second, the therapist should clearly communicate his or her expectations to the patient. In other words, the therapist should direct the patient to the specific kind of behavior that the therapist wants instead of the patient's disruptive behavior. Third, the therapist should direct the discussion towards problems that similar behaviors may have caused the patient in relationships outside of therapy.

For example, if a patient has been calling the therapist too frequently between sessions, the therapist should directly point out to the patient that they had agreed that calls would be limited. Next, the therapist should direct the patient to new behavior – calling the emergency room after hours, or having the patient call at a specific time during the week as opposed to the random out of hours calls. The therapist should at this point establish that the patient understands both the inappropriate behavior and the way it should be modified.

After this, the therapist can then use the information gleaned from the contract violation to begin asking questions about the patient's relationships outside of therapy. For instance, the therapist might ask the patient how he or she typically asks others for help when distressed. What happens when he or she calls other people frequently? Has he or she ever received negative feedback from others about being too persistent? How has the patient dealt with this?

In IPT, most boundary violations can be dealt with very directly in this way. All provide important information to the therapist about potential problems that the patient may be having in his or her social relationships. Rather than using boundary violations to focus more on the patient–therapist relationship, in IPT the discussion should be quickly turned to similar problems outside of therapy.

Regardless of the nature of the boundary violation (with the exception of aggression against the therapist or others), any intervention in the area of 'contractual violations' should be designed to be therapeutic and for the benefit of the patient.

Practical reasons for contract violations

Many patients have quite legitimate practical reasons for missing appointments, payments, or for not fulfilling other parts of the treatment contract. As an advocate for the patient, it is certainly within the purview of the therapist to actively assist the patient to seek out and utilize resources in the community that might be available. Referrals for assistance with payments for treatment, housing resources, childcare resources and the like can be provided by the therapist. Though this is clearly not the primary goal of IPT, if the patient is unable to come to treatment for these types of practical reasons, then treatment will obviously not be successful. The patient is fully responsible for utilizing the resources, but the therapist can direct the patient to them, rather than interpreting the patient's inability to find and use such resources as resistance to therapy.

In some cases, the contract violations arise as a result of a misunderstanding by the patient, which may merely reflect his or her problems in communication. Reframing the boundary violation as a consequence of poor communication between patient and therapist may therefore reinforce the need for clear communication in other relationships as well, and examples from other relationships can be discussed in therapy. When the problem arises as a consequence of unrealistic or unreasonable expectations on the part of the patient, this too can be addressed as a process that may be typical of the patient's other relationships.

What does a contract violation imply about the patient's social relationships?

It is axiomatic in IPT that whatever occurs in the therapeutic relationship parallels processes in other relationships. The therapeutic relationship is a real relationship influenced by the same factors that affect all of the patient's relationships. The patient's attachment style and experience of other relationships will affect the way in which he or she experiences the constraints of the therapeutic contract. If problems emerge in the therapeutic relationship, they therefore shed light on these factors, and on the relationships that the patient is involved in outside of therapy. The patient's experience of, and reaction to, the therapeutic contract is therefore extremely valuable information about his or her interpersonal relationships.

What does a contract violation imply about the therapeutic relationship?

In some cases, the patient's boundary violations or reactions to the therapist may be so extreme or difficult to manage that the therapeutic relationship must be directly addressed. The preservation of the therapeutic relationship must be the primary consideration in IPT, as without it, therapy cannot proceed. If the therapeutic relationship is threatened, the therapist may choose to renegotiate the therapeutic contract with the patient. Doing so may have additional therapeutic benefits for the patient as he or she may experience this process as a new way of behaving and communicating that may generalize to other relationships. If this fails, the therapist should strongly consider moving to another form of therapy in which the patient–therapist relationship is more directly addressed.

Is the patient aware of the effects of his or her behavior?

In many circumstances, the patient may be unaware of the nature and implications of his or her interpersonal behaviors. Such 'blind spots' or communication problems experienced by the patient may only be apparent to the therapist when they are examined against the background of the therapeutic contract. Using this information, the therapist can then begin to examine other situations in which the patient's lack of insight about the consequences of his or her communication may be problematic. The therapist can address this by hypothesizing that others are likely to respond to the patient in the same way that the therapist has, and that situations that provoke or elicit such a response from others occur in the patient's relationships. Discussing these kinds of interactions and reflecting on the likely responses from others, informed by the therapist's experience with the patient in a similar interaction, is a potent way to help the patient develop insight into his or her communications and what follows in their wake.

In summary, the therapist's actions should always reinforce the contract by implication, and by explicit reminder if needed. Interventions regarding the contract should first and foremost be pragmatic: a gentle reminder of the contract agreement, and then discussion of the patient's social relationships in which similar communication problems are likely to be occurring.

Case example: Barry

Barry was a 21-year-old man in a stable relationship who had been referred by his local physician for management of depression. Barry described experiencing difficulties in his relationship with his girlfriend and had suffered periods of dysphoria leading to vague suicidal ideation. Barry's local doctor had started antidepressant medication, which had provided some benefit in relieving his symptoms.

Following an evaluation for therapy, Barry and his therapist negotiated a treatment contract and agreed to meet for twelve sessions of IPT. They discussed a reasonable fee structure, the process for rescheduling appointments, and the possibility of decreasing the frequency of the latter sessions of treatment. After completing the interpersonal inventory, Barry selected an interpersonal dispute with his girlfriend and an interpersonal dispute with his mother as interpersonal areas upon which to focus the treatment.

Barry arrived 10 minutes late for session 4, citing work restrictions. The therapist conducted a shortened 40-minute session and highlighted the need for Barry to try to make full use of the time set aside for treatment. Barry arrived on time for session 5, but cancelled session 6, 2 hours prior to its scheduled time. The therapist decided that the session would not be made up as Barry had not provided 24-hour notice prior to cancellation as they had initially agreed he would do. The therapist discussed this series of events with Barry, and reiterated the need for Barry to make an effort to be on time, as to do otherwise was limiting the benefit he was getting from therapy.

The therapist noted that she was feeling frustrated with Barry's behavior and was irritated that Barry did not seem to be valuing her time or professional efforts. Being an astute therapist, however, she recognized that her reactions were a reflection of the ways in which Barry was likely to be interacting with others. Putting aside her frustration and annoyance, the therapist reminded herself that any course of action she took should be fundamentally therapeutic and of benefit to the patient. Rather than feeling compelled to act reflexively to Barry, the therapist realized that her reactions were important 'diagnostic' information, and could be used to address problems in Barry's relationships outside of therapy.

Barry arrived 10 minutes late for session 7, prompting the therapist to address the therapeutic contract right at the beginning of the session. She planned to move from there to a discussion about other relationships in which Barry had difficulty in maintaining his commitments.

Therapist: Barry, over the last several sessions you have had problems either keeping the appointments or being here on time. I wanted to remind you that we had agreed that we would meet for 50-minute sessions, and when you are late we aren't able to meet for that long. While you might still get a lot of benefit from the time that is left in the session, I don't think that you are getting the full benefit of treatment by being late. It's almost like taking half of a dose of medicine – you might feel somewhat better, but the effect isn't as great as the full dose.
Barry: I can see your point . . . I have just had trouble getting everything organized to get here on time.
Therapist: We had also agreed that you would call at least 24 hours ahead of time if you had to miss an appointment, and I wanted to remind you of that as well.
Barry: I'll try my best, but the time I missed I had a real emergency at work.
Therapist: I appreciate that things come up, but I do want to make sure that we are clear on our expectations of each other. Barry, since this has happened several times during our work together, I wonder if this is a problem in other relationships you have. What are your thoughts about that?
Barry: Well, my girlfriend is always getting on me about being late. She says that is one of her main complaints with me – that if I'm late, it means that I don't take things seriously enough.
Therapist: What's your reaction to that?
Barry: I have tried to convince her that my being late has nothing to do with her – it's just a bad habit that I've gotten into. I wish she wouldn't take it so personally.
Therapist: It sounds like your being late is being understood by her in a way that you aren't intending.
Barry: That's right. But I haven't been able to convince her otherwise.

Barry agreed that some of his behavior was frustrating, and then began to explore ways in which he might be able to more effectively manage his behavior, recognizing that it was a problem for others, and was not communicating what he intended.

CONCLUSION

The contract is an essential part of the initial phase of IPT. Establishing a clear and consistent contract is crucial because it is a referent to which both therapist and patient can return when therapeutic boundaries are threatened. Since addressing the therapeutic relationship is discouraged in IPT, the contract carries even greater weight because it allows boundary problems to be addressed without recourse to discussions of transference.

The Interpersonal Inventory

INTRODUCTION

The Interpersonal Inventory[1] is, in essence, a register of the key contemporary relationships in the patient's life. It is a unique feature of IPT in that it structures the process of history gathering and formulation of interpersonal problem areas as well as providing a reference point for conducting IPT. Although the Interpersonal Inventory is typically compiled during the first two to three sessions of IPT, it is best considered a 'work in progress' as most therapists and patients find that their perspectives of relationships and the problems associated with them change during the course of IPT.

IPT is a focused intervention which requires that the patient and therapist maximize the use of the limited time available to achieve meaningful change in problematic relationships. The Interpersonal Inventory functions as the main structural component of this process by focusing the patient and therapist specifically on:

1 Contemporary relationships.
2 The history of the patient's current problems.
3 Information that is relevant to the process of resolving the interpersonal problem, e.g., communication styles or patterns of interaction.
4 Setting appropriate treatment goals by examining the patient's expectations regarding his or her relationships and ensuring that they are realistic.

While the Interpersonal Inventory can be compiled in a more formal fashion, it is in essence a thorough and extended social history with a significant difference – the emphasis of the Interpersonal Inventory (as befits the 'here-and-now' focus of IPT) is on current relationships that are potentially relevant to the patient's current psychological distress.

Introducing this focal and structured method of collecting interpersonal data at the beginning of the treatment establishes the manner in which the patient and therapist will approach the therapy, as well as giving a clear guide as to what direction it will follow.

Table 6.1 *The Interpersonal Inventory*

- Includes all significant contemporary relationships, including recent losses.
- Contains specific details of the history of problematic relationships as well as the history of particular problem areas.
- Contains details about social support.
- Includes current communication problems.
- Includes current problems with expectations in relationships.
- Facilitates the planning of treatment interventions.
- Evolves and changes during the course of IPT and serves as a monitor for treatment progress.
- Provides a reference point for 'regrouping' and for 'reorienting' therapy.

FEATURES OF THE INTERPERSONAL INVENTORY

Among the features of the Interpersonal Inventory are the following:

- *It includes all 'significant' contemporary relationships including recent losses.* The Interpersonal Inventory should focus primarily on the patient's significant relationships in the 'here and now.' While not an exhaustive history of every relationship, it should refer to all relationships in which the patient has a significant attachment. By implication, this literally pushes the patient both to focus on current relationships and to work on changing them, as opposed to speaking more about past history.
- *It contains specific details of the history of problematic relationships as well as the history of particular problem areas.* The history obtained from the patient should be more a reflection of his or her experience of problems rather than an exhaustive attempt at uncovering the 'truth.' The therapist must ensure, however, that the information gathered is as complete as possible, as some patients are prone to leave out details that might implicate them as being responsible for the problem. Past history is relevant as far as it illuminates the patient's actions in the present, and the extent to which past history is collected must be determined using clinical judgment.
- *It contains details about social support.* In addition to particular problematic relationships, the therapist should collect information about the patient's social support in general. One of the primary goals of IPT is to help the patient more effectively utilize his or her social support; thus, an accurate appraisal of the available resources is crucial. This information will also help the therapist to understand more about the patient's attachment style and ability to enlist the support of others.
- *It includes current communication problems.* The Interpersonal Inventory should note the patient's attempts to deal with his or her particular problems as well as his or her associated affective response to those problems. The therapist's inquiries regarding the history of disputes or transitions should also contain examples of problematic communication and interactions with the involved significant other, as these frequently lead directly to specific IPT interventions.

- *It facilitates the planning of treatment interventions.* The issues highlighted in the Interpersonal Inventory will not only help the therapist and patient understand the relationship problems at hand, but will also provide a guide as to which particular interventions are likely to be of help. For example, if a patient has problems with an interpersonal dispute, and during the development of the inventory describes what appears to be poor communication within the involved relationship, the therapist might anticipate that the best techniques to approach the problem are likely to be those focused on improving communication. Techniques such as communication analysis and role playing would be well-suited to this purpose. From these initial points of intervention the progress of the interpersonal work will follow logically.
- *It evolves and changes during the course of IPT and serves as a monitor for treatment progress.* The Interpersonal Inventory is best considered an evolving story or 'work in progress' by the patient and therapist. The Interpersonal Inventory as it initially unfolds is often incomplete or distorted by the patient – sometimes by intent – as the patient wishes to avoid portraying him or herself in a negative light, and sometimes because the patient is either unable to organize the information fully or because he or she may be avoiding difficult issues. However, as the course of treatment progresses, the patient's perceptions change, more information typically emerges, and the patient's situation changes as a result.

At the conclusion of acute treatment, the patient and therapist should refer to the initial conceptualization of the Interpersonal Inventory and compare it to its current state in order to review the progress that has been made, as well as to discuss the work that remains to be done in the future. The reorganization and reintegration of this material in ways that the patient can better understand, and particularly in ways which lead the patient to appreciate his or her contribution to the problem and the ways in which he or she can work to resolve it, is an important part of the therapy.

The nature of the attachment that forms between the patient and therapist will influence the way in which IPT progresses. The process of developing the Interpersonal Inventory is no exception to this rule. A patient who forms an insecure attachment to the therapist will be less likely to divulge sensitive or highly distressing information to the therapist, thus distorting the way in which the inventory is compiled. It is therefore imperative while conducting the Interpersonal Inventory, as during any part of IPT, that the therapist recognize the nature of the patient's attachment and remain vigilant for information or issues that may not have been disclosed at a time when the therapeutic relationship was tenuous.

- *IPT provides a reference point for 'regrouping' and for 'reorienting' therapy.* IPT is not immune to psychodynamic processes such as transference and resistance. When these processes become problematic, the patient and therapist may find themselves confused or disoriented about which direction the treatment should progress. In these circumstances it is useful to refer to the Interpersonal Inventory for 'regrouping' and for 'reorienting' the treatment. When temptation to address the therapeutic relationship directly strikes, both patient and therapist can literally return to the specific problem areas that were illuminated in the inventory. The Interpersonal Inventory can metaphorically be considered to be a beacon or lighthouse that can illuminate the path of the therapeutic process when intratherapy processes threaten to displace the interpersonal focus of IPT (Figure 6.1). As such, it can help the therapist to navigate a clear path rather than straying into the Scylla of transference and the Charybdis of resistance (unless of course the therapist has been trained as an argonaut or analyst).

The Interpersonal Inventory need not be a formal document, and is often a series of notes in the patient's file (Figure 6.2). Some therapists prefer to have the Interpersonal Inventory as a separate structured form in the patient's file and prepare it as a key document in IPT (Figure 6.3). The inventory can also be collected in a fashion similar to a genogram, but should also include information about significant others outside of the patient's family. In order to promote the collaborative nature of IPT, the patient may be given a copy of the document for his or her own use. An Interpersonal Inventory form is included in Appendix C.

USING THE INTERPERSONAL INVENTORY DURING THE COURSE OF IPT

Initial phase

In the initial sessions of IPT, the Interpersonal Inventory is used to orient the therapy. The Interpersonal Inventory also has conceptual utility, as the patient's descriptions of relationships will provide a wealth of information about their attachment style and communication tendencies. Inconsistencies in the patient's accounts of events, or the lack of detail about an interpersonal problem, may be informative about a patient's perceptions or expectations about a relationship. The patient's report of his or her communication style or attempts at problem solving are also informative. Moreover, the Interpersonal Inventory may highlight problematic processes that are consistent across a number of relationships which are only apparent when these are scrutinized as a whole. In other words, the Interpersonal Inventory should provide a good view of both the forest and the trees.

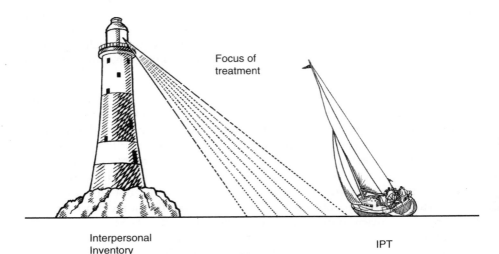

Interpersonal
Inventory

IPT

Figure 6.1 *The Interpersonal Inventory as a Guide for Treatment.*

Interpersonal Inventory

Bill (Husband)
- Married 6 years (together 9)
- Wanted a baby
- Used to communicate well

- Talked about it before she got pregnant
- Seemed committed

Problems
- Wont talk
(NB. She reports very hostile interactions)
- Won't contribute

- Gets angry when confronted
- Seems to hide in work

Expectations
- Wants him to keep his word (to be a father)
- 'Equal time'
- Less hostile in communicating

Communication – Seems to not communicate point clearly

Problem solving – Previously present

Figure 6.2 *The Interpersonal Inventory.*

Interpersonal Inventory

Patient Name: Jeffrey Snout
Date of Birth: 9–11-71
Other Clinicians:
Insurance Details: Blue Cross – "HMO Buster" Top
Date of First Consultation: 3–23-00
Contracted Number of Sessions: 12

Name of Other: Jemima
Relationship: Girlfriend
Patient's Account of Problem:
- Together for 2 years – work in same firm
- She wants to move in he said no – symptoms
- 'Won't talk' – says she does not do conflict well
- Communicates OK
- They initially travelled, got on well
- His expectations 'Fun and friends' – Hers???

Areas Requiring Further Clarification: Communication? Roleplay; Problem solving

Agreed Problem Area: Disputes   Role   Grief and   Interpersonal
                                    Transition   Loss   Sensitivity

Special Issues:

Figure 6.3 *The Interpersonal Inventory – Structured.*

When compiling the Interpersonal Inventory, questions to be addressed include:

- How does the patient engage social support?
- How does the patient resolve interpersonal problems?
- How does the patient deal with loss?
- How does the patient deal with attachment disruptions?
- How does the patient care for others?

The answers to these questions will help to identify the patient's strengths and vulnerabilities, and should guide the course of IPT so that specific interpersonal problems can be addressed.

Middle phase

As described previously, the Interpersonal Inventory serves as a reference point for the conduct of treatment. It is therefore quite useful at this stage of treatment for reorienting the focus of treatment when diversions such as transference and resistance threaten.

Conclusion of acute treatment and maintenance treatment phases

The Interpersonal Inventory serves as a measure of the patient's progress through treatment. At the conclusion of treatment, it is often helpful to review the original inventory with the patient to sum up the changes that have occurred over the course of therapy. This includes not only the resolution of identified problems, but also any changes in the patient's conceptualization of relationships and problems. For instance, at the conclusion of therapy the patient may see an interpersonal dispute less as an irreconcilable conflict and more as a problem with communication. Emphasizing areas in which the patient has gained insight into his or her contribution to the problems that were discussed is very helpful, as is a review of the steps that the patient took to solve them.

The Interpersonal Inventory also serves as a guide to the discussion of potential future problems. If the initial version of the inventory indicates that a particular interpersonal problem arose consistently or was present for a long time – for instance, a pattern of complicated grieving or dysfunctional response to loss – this should suggest a focus for the future when additional losses may lead to exacerbations of the patient's psychological symptoms.

The Interpersonal Inventory assumes great significance with maintenance IPT. The focus of maintenance treatment is usually upon ongoing work in one or two problem areas. The Interpersonal Inventory serves to preserve the interpersonal focus of maintenance treatment and to optimize the use of the time available.

Case example: Lana

Lana was a 34-year-old married woman who was receiving IPT in combination with antidepressant medication for an episode of depression. She presented for help with a conflict with her husband which she described as one of the main contributors to the development of her illness. In the initial sessions of IPT, Lana appeared well engaged in the therapy, participated in the process of discussing her interpersonal dispute, and seemed to be motivated to address her interpersonal problems.

During a session in the middle stage of IPT, Lana asked the therapist to advise her as to whether she should disclose some previous indiscretions to her husband. The therapist suggested that rather than telling Lana what to do, it would ultimately be more helpful for her to decide, though he was very willing to spend time discussing the options and the pros and cons of each. He also stated to Lana that his role in IPT was to assist her to determine what the best decision was for her, rather than to make the decision for her. Though not directly communicated to Lana, the therapist also felt that this position was more ethical, and was certainly more consistent with the approach to treatment used in IPT.

Lana became very angry as a result of the therapist's refusal to tell her what to do, but did not directly communicate this to the therapist. Instead, she began to withdraw from the therapeutic relationship by becoming increasingly silent and withholding. Recognizing that this was likely to be what happened in her relationships outside of therapy, the therapist planned to move the discussion to situations when this occurred with Lana's husband, and to explore the ways in which she dealt with her anger with others. However, the therapist also recognized that Lana's reaction to him were causing the therapy to deviate from the established focus on Lana's conflict with her husband, as the problematic patient–therapist interaction was standing in the way of progress.

At the beginning of the following session the therapist chose to directly address the conflict between himself and Lana. Rather than explore the implications of the conflict within the therapeutic relationship, however, he then immediately shifted the discussion to similar conflicts Lana had experienced with her husband.

'Lana, over the last few weeks you seem to have been quite angry with me and obviously very frustrated with the treatment – we seem to have come to an impasse when I didn't respond like you wanted to your request for advice about how to approach your husband. I have been wondering how this problem might inform us both more about the problems you came here to solve. If we go back to the Interpersonal Inventory, we determined that the main problem was a 'dispute' with your husband. At the time, we compiled the inventory we agreed that some of your expectations of your husband, and the way you communicated these to him, were a problem that we should tackle. I wonder if your expectations of me, and the ways you have communicated your frustration to me for not meeting them, might help us to better understand how this occurs with him. What happens, for instance, when he doesn't live up to your expectations?'

Lana began describing an incident in which she felt her husband had been unresponsive to her requests, and went on to relate how she had 'shut him out' as a way of communicating her frustration with him. The treatment was effectively refocused on the dispute with her husband thereafter.

CONCLUSION

The Interpersonal Inventory is a critical element of IPT. It is, in some ways, the hallmark of the treatment as it orients both patient and therapist to the specific interpersonal problems that are to be addressed in therapy. Further, the inventory helps to maintain the therapeutic focus throughout treatment, and aids in resisting the temptation to stray from an interpersonal focus. The inventory is also a helpful tool when reviewing the patient's progress during therapy and when planning for problems that may arise in the future.

REFERENCE

1. Klerman, G.L., Weissman, M.M., Rounsaville, B.J., Chevron, E.S. 1984. *Interpersonal Psychotherapy of Depression*. New York: Basic Books.

The Interpersonal Formulation

INTRODUCTION

The ability to develop an accurate and concise psychological formulation of a patient's problems is an invaluable skill for all clinicians. A valid formulation synthesizes information about an individual's biological and psychological make-up, attachment style, personality, and social context, creating a plausible hypothesis explaining his or her psychological symptoms. The formulation should lead to:

- An enhanced understanding of the patient's experience.
- A plausible hypothesis explaining the origin of the patient's symptoms.
- A guide to the therapeutic stance to be taken in treatment.
- A guide to the use of specific therapeutic techniques.
- An accurate assessment of prognosis.

In essence, the 'formulation' of a 'case' is nothing more than a theoretically grounded working understanding of the unique individual with whom the clinician forms a relationship in therapy. In many respects, stripping away the jargon inherent in the terms 'formulation' and 'case' is extremely helpful. Both terms can be dehumanizing: the first, 'case,' because it lumps a unique individual into a reified category of illness or pathology; the latter, 'formulation,' because it presumes that the therapist can more accurately understand and synthesize the patient's experience than can the patient him or herself. It cannot be emphasized enough that *working to understand the unique individual who is seeking help* is the most important therapeutic task in IPT. The formulation is not a definitive interpretation of the patient's problem by an omniscient therapist.

In IPT, however, the formulation also serves a purpose which need not involve this kind of dehumanizing approach. In fact, if applied properly, the development of a formulation of the patient's problems, and the presentation of the formulation to the patient, should enhance the therapeutic alliance and convey the therapist's genuine attempts to understand the patient. Because the theoretical orientation of IPT is based on attachment and communication theory, the formulation is an approximate under- standing of the patient's experience from that perspective. As such, it bridges the gap between a general theory of human behavior and the patient's specific and unique problems.

In summary, the formulation is nothing more than an hypothesis (informed in IPT by attachment and communication theory) which addresses the following questions:

1   How did the patient come to be the way he or she is?
2   What factors are maintaining the problem?
3   What can be done about it?

The Interpersonal Formulation is not a diagnosis to be presented to the patient – rather it is a 'hypothesis,' arrived at collaboratively by the patient and therapist, which describes how the patient's distress has developed. The formulation emphasizes both the interpersonal factors involved in the origin and context of the problem, as well as how IPT will help the patient overcome his or her symptoms. It is therefore a pivotal part of IPT, as the successful collaboration between patient and therapist to provide a valid formulation 'sets the scene' for the conduct of treatment.

The Interpersonal Formulation should provide the patient and therapist with:

1   A plausible *hypothesis* explaining the patient's problems and their onset, clinical manifestation, and course.
2   A *validation* of the patient's experience and a way of understanding his or her problems.
3   A *mutually determined focus* for intervention based on the four problem areas.
4   A *plausible rationale for treatment* with IPT and for the use of specific IPT techniques.

THE BIOPSYCHOSOCIAL MODEL

The biopsychosocial model of mental illness[1] asserts that biological, psychological, and social factors coalesce within an individual to produce a unique diathesis or response to stress. When faced with a sufficient interpersonal crisis, vulnerable individuals are likely to have psychological difficulties. The biopsychosocial model therefore frames psycho- logical difficulties as the response of a unique and multifaceted individual to a unique stressor rather than as categorical illnesses.

The utility of the biopsychosocial model in current clinical practice has become increasingly evident as movement towards a dimensional view of mental health has continued. This dimensional view of biopsychosocial functioning incorporates 'good' mental health as well as illness states, acknowledging both strengths and symptoms rather than simply identifying pathological syndromes. As a consequence, the biopsy- chosocial model offers both the patient and therapist a 'user-friendly' way of under- standing the complex and multiple determinants of psychological symptoms and interpersonal distress.

While the medical model of mental health requires that an individual's problems be categorized as syndromal diagnoses, the biopsychosocial model emphasizes the whole person and his or her suffering rather than focusing exclusively on an illness. This by no means diminishes the importance of diagnoses, but rather emphasizes the person who is suffering. This is much more congruent with the aim in IPT that the therapist should work to understand the patient in the context of his or her unique personal and social circumstances, and that the patient begin to appreciate the influence of these factors as well. The true value of the biopsychosocial model is that it conceptualizes illness as being determined by many factors, none of which alone can explain the patient's distress, its manifestation, or its course.

The biopsychosocial model as it is applied to the Interpersonal Formulation in IPT thus acknowledges:

- *Biological factors* such as genetic vulnerabilities, physical illness, substance abuse, medication side-effects, and injuries to the central nervous system.
- *Psychological factors* such as attachment style, temperament, psychological defense mechanisms, cognitive style, intelligence, personality, psychological development, and ego strength.
- *Social factors* such as losses, available social supports, financial resources, culture, family functioning, and work environment.

THE ELEMENTS OF THE IPT FORMULATION

The Interpersonal Formulation is built upon the foundation of the biopsychosocial model. In addition, as befits the theoretical basis for IPT, there is a strong emphasis on both attachment and communication theory. The hypotheses regarding the patient's current functioning are not static or fixed; rather, they should be continually modified by the collaborative efforts of the patient and clinician as therapy continues. The formulation will evolve and change emphasis over time as the patient and therapist come to better understand the patient's unique circumstances.

Biological contributions to distress

GENETIC FACTORS

Documented or suspected illnesses or symptoms in family members are of clear significance. A common oversight is to take at face value a negative family history. The therapist should not merely inquire about diagnoses or treatments, but should also ask about the presence of abnormal symptoms or behaviors suggestive of illness in family members.

DRUG AND ALCOHOL USE

These may not be reported by the patient, as recreational drug and alcohol use is common in many societies. Heavy use may not be reported by the patient for fear of reprisals, or because of denial. The therapist needs to help the patient understand the subtle effects of even moderate psychoactive substance use, which may disturb psychological health and interpersonal functioning in ways which may not be apparent to the patient. Both the contribution of these factors and the interpersonal determinants of drug and alcohol use should be included in the interpersonal formulation.

MEDICAL ILLNESS

A comprehensive medical history must be obtained during the evaluation phase of treatment. Some illnesses will be readily acknowledged by the patient, though they may not be recognized as being connected to psychological difficulties. Some disease processes, particularly those involving the central nervous system, may not be apparent to the patient. Questions which review neurological problems in depth should be asked, and they should be framed in language that is understandable to the patient, such as asking about 'fits, faints, or funny turns' when asking about seizure activity. Similarly, viral infections and physiological changes such as menarche or menstrual hormonal fluctuations may be significant biological factors that are not recognized by the patient as relevant to psychological symptoms.

EFFECTS OF MEDICAL TREATMENTS

Many medications have psychological sequelae and may be relevant to the Interpersonal Formulation. The use of medications that in many cases may be lifesaving often presents a dilemma, as the medications are necessary but cannot be stopped despite unwanted psychological side effects. Corticosteroids, for instance, often fall into this category of medication. The formulation should not only acknowledge the effects of medical treatments, but should also include the patient's response to his or her medical illness and its interpersonal significance. Examples are medications which produce sexual side effects, such as some agents used to control hypertension or to treat depression. The use of these medications may lead to intrinsic psychological disturbances in the patient, and may also lead to significant interpersonal difficulties in marital or other intimate relationships. The issue of compliance with psychotropic medications that create these kinds of problems should also be addressed – an antidepressant medication which causes fatigue and sexual dysfunction is apt to have both physical and interpersonal consequences which may affect compliance.

Psychological contributions to distress

ATTACHMENT STYLE

The patient's attachment style is usually evident in the way in which the patient has functioned in both previous and current relationships. A patient who describes long-standing difficulties in meeting his or her attachment needs will likely relate a childhood history replete with a lack of affection or closeness within his or her family of origin, as well as difficulties functioning with peers at school. Relationships in early adulthood may be described as being short-lived or unsatisfactory. Work histories that are chaotic or lacking in a central theme are also commonly reported by patients with more insecure attachment styles. Maladaptive responses to losses, such as the death of relatives or loss of friendships, are also characteristic of insecurely attached patients.

The therapist's experience of the patient in therapy should also help him or her to understand how the patient's attachment style has contributed to the current problems. The therapist may find it difficult to 'connect' with the patient, or may find that the patient frequently challenges the therapist. Other factors communicating ambivalence or anxiety in attachment may arise in boundary issues such as lateness or problematic transference.

TEMPERAMENT

Temperament can be considered to be the genetically and biologically determined manner in which an individual responds to his or her environment. Many authors have described specific features of temperament; one of the more operationally useful in IPT is the description proposed by Cloninger.[2] According to Cloninger's theory, individuals can be described along three axes which define temperament. Those who are 'harm avoidant' respond to their environment and interpersonal relationships with vigilance and reserve. Those who are 'stimulus craving' tend to approach these in an impulsive and at times chaotic manner. Those who are 'reward-dependent' tend to seek approval from others and are highly vulnerable to rejection. The therapist can evaluate the patient's temperament in a manner similar to that used to examine the patient's attachment and defense mechanisms.

COGNITIVE STYLE

The patient may display problematic cognitive processes such as generalizations or selective abstraction, particularly when discussing his or her relationships. Statements such as 'this always happens to me,' or 'he only stays because of the children,' may be very informative, as the patient's cognitions about his or her relationships are often the most strongly held. The therapist should attempt to establish if this type of thinking pattern pervades other interpersonal aspects of the patient's life. Methods of dealing therapeutically with these unrealistic expectations or cognitive sets is described in subsequent chapters, but the primary focus in IPT is to deal with the interpersonal aspects and ramifications of such cognitions.

PSYCHOLOGICAL COPING MECHANISMS

The way in which a person deals with intrapsychic stress is a key determinant of mental health. Valliant[3] has argued that psychological defense mechanisms can be broadly categorized as 'mature' and adaptive, or as 'immature' and maladaptive. Individuals who respond to psychological and interpersonal distress with psychological defenses such as 'somatization' or 'acting out' are more prone to develop illness and interpersonal distress, as their ability to deal with internal and external stress is likely to be compromised. The therapist can develop an impression of the patient's coping mechanisms by considering how the patient describes his or her attempts to deal with current interpersonal problems. Questions such as 'What happens to you when you get angry?' or 'What happens to you when you get distressed?' can provide additional details.

Consider for example a patient who is dealing with an impending divorce. He may describe frequent physical symptoms or a preoccupation with his health. He may describe behavior such as physical aggression or hazardous substance use. While discussing the breakdown of his marriage, he may exhibit a lack of affect, or perhaps may endow his estranged wife with all manner of personal faults that seem more his own. In this situation the therapist can infer that the patient probably relies on more 'immature' or 'neurotic' coping mechanisms such as 'projection,' 'acting out,' and 'isolation of affect.' This not only helps the therapist to understand how the patient has come to be in his or her current situation, but also how he or she is likely to deal with the challenges of IPT, and the type of obstacles that he or she is likely to present to the therapist during the treatment.

Social contributions to distress

In this section of the Interpersonal Formulation the therapist needs to highlight the ways in which the patient's current interpersonal difficulties, as encapsulated in the four problem areas, have contributed to the development of psychological symptoms. The ways in which the patient's current interpersonal functioning has been affected by his or her symptoms should also be explored. The therapist should not only place the patient's psychological distress in an interpersonal context, but should also establish a temporal relationship between the onset of the symptoms and the development of the interpersonal problems.

In addition, the patient's current social milieu should be assessed. The absence of support, or of people who can provide secure attachment relationships for the patient, has a profound effect on the patient's current distress. Conversely, those patients who have extensive social support systems will be less vulnerable to psychological difficulties when faced with crises.

PRESENTATION OF FORMULATION TO THE PATIENT

Once the therapist has completed a full clinical assessment, he or she should present to the patient a formulation of the patient's psychological problems using a biopsychosocial model which incorporates the key elements described above. The Interpersonal Formulation should also include the core problem areas of IPT which are relevant to the patient. It is not the therapist's objective to depict one or all of the four problem areas as the only cause of difficulty for the patient, but rather to use the Interpersonal Formulation to place the patient's problems in a social and interpersonal context. Doing so will emphasize to the patient that intervening in these areas is likely to help achieve symptom relief. The process of integrating the biological, psychological, and social components into the Interpersonal Formulation is depicted in Figure 7.1.

The therapist should present the Interpersonal Formulation to the patient in a collaborative fashion, posing the hypotheses as tentative and asking for the patient's feedback. The formulation must be meaningful to the patient, and validate not only his or her suffering but also any concerns about his or her perception of the significance of the various factors that have interacted to create the crisis. Some patients will attribute their psychiatric symptoms entirely to their family histories or physical health problems rather than to their interpersonal problems. Similarly, patients who see only the inter-

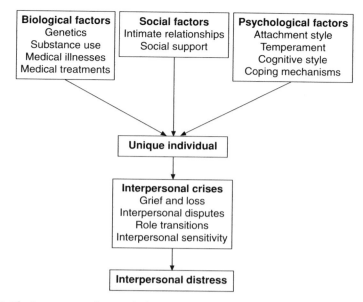

Figure 7.1 *The Interpersonal Formulation. Based upon the biopsychosocial model, biological, psychological and social factors combine with an interpersonal crisis to cause interpersonal distress in vulnerable individuals.*

personal contributions to their situation will also benefit from considering other aspects of their make-up that have helped create their situation.

Case example: Penny

Penny, a 32-year-old legal secretary, was referred to a psychiatrist for assessment of an episode of depression that followed the birth of her daughter three months earlier. She complained of irritability, poor concentration, self reproach, loss of interest in her usual activities, and excessive tearfulness. She recognized that these symptoms were a marked departure from her usual self, and had resulted in an ongoing conflict with her husband since the birth of her baby.

Penny told her psychiatrist that she and her husband had discussed the arrangements for the arrival of the baby, and had agreed that she would take maternity leave for a year while her husband, Brad, would continue to work full-time. According to Penny, Brad was also supposed to contribute to the running of the household and had agreed to take care of the baby on weekends in order to give Penny some 'time to herself.' Penny had also discussed care-taking arrangements with her mother, who had agreed to offer one day a week to look after the baby in order for Penny to keep up with things at work, despite the fact that she was officially on maternity leave.

After the arrival of the baby, Penny found that she had less time to spend with her husband as the demands of childcare left her tired. In order to keep up with the house payments, Brad had started working longer hours to offset the drop in income created by Penny's maternity leave. Penny found also that her mother was increasingly unreliable in fulfilling her child care agreement.

Penny described being physically well throughout her pregnancy. She stated that during the pregnancy she felt 'terrific,' but since the birth had experienced a major 'let down' which she felt was hormonal. She reported having intermittent mood swings during the latter half of her menstrual cycles, though she had not sought any treatment for this previously. The decision to have a child was, according to Penny, based largely on her age. She stated that she had determined that if she were going to have children, it had to be now, as it would be much more risky if she were any older.

Penny was the only child of her parents' marriage. She said that her mother had suffered from depression throughout Penny's childhood, apparently with postpartum onset. Penny's relationship with her mother during adolescence was described as conflicted, and she reported feeling closer to her father during that time. She described her mother currently as helpful at times but unreliable in general. In contrast, she stated that since she had been married, she had little contact with her father.

Penny said that throughout her schooling she excelled academically, although she did not want to pursue tertiary studies. She stated that as a student she was always noted for her impeccable bookwork as well as her dedication to her chosen sport of swimming. She said that her working life was highly satisfying as she was a valued member of the team at her legal firm. She pointedly mentioned that the partners always asked her to assist with their cases. She enjoyed work, and stated that she missed the social support she received there.

Penny had been married for 8 years. She described being happy in her married life, although she felt that the lack of time she and her husband had together, as well as her inability to regularly see her friends and colleagues, was 'taking its toll.' Her description of her relationship with her husband was telling, as Penny said they had got married because, 'they worked well together.' She reported that her husband had complained on occasion that their relationship lacked intimacy, and was frequently dissatisfied with their sexual relationship, but Penny stated that she was quite satisfied with both of these aspects of her marriage.

Penny described herself as a perfectionist and told the psychiatrist that her self-esteem was related to her ability to achieve things. She reported being 'in control' of her life prior to the arrival of her baby, but the lack of structure and continual demands of motherhood coupled with the lack of definite goals was difficult. She reported some difficulties in breast-feeding her child in the first few weeks, which she found made her feel, 'even less in control of things.'

The factors contributing to the Interpersonal Formulation of Penny's interpersonal distress and the development of her postpartum depression included:

1   Biological factors:
- History of depression in her mother.
- Predisposition to hormonally influenced mood swings.

2   Psychological factors:
- Insecure avoidant or self-reliant attachment traits.
- Obsessive-compulsive personality traits.
- Reward dependent temperament.

3   Social factors:
- Poor support from family.
- Fair support from husband.
- Good support from work colleagues.

4 Interpersonal crises:
- *Role transition* into motherhood – adjusting to the physical and psychological demands of motherhood, as well as the loss of the benefits of full time work.
- *Interpersonal dispute* with her mother – unmet expectations of child care and support as well as difficulty communicating her needs.
- *Interpersonal dispute* with her husband – unmet expectations between Penny and her husband.

The Interpersonal Formulation for Penny is depicted in Figure 7.2.

This conceptualization of Penny's distress and depression was compatible with several treatment options:

1 *Cognitive behavioral therapy*: Penny described a degree of perfectionism and in her history highlighted a number of thoughts that seemed to reflect dysfunctional cognitive schema. Her need for perfectionism and her tendency to 'all or nothing thinking' would provide material for focal cognitive interventions.

2 *Self-psychology*: Penny described a distant relationship with her mother, and there was evidence that this was re-emerging as a significant issue in the context of her own motherhood. Self-psychology would offer Penny a therapeutic relationship that offered opportunities for 'mirroring or idealizing' transference. This would potentially improve Penny's symptoms and functioning, but would be primarily focused on facilitating the evolution of her 'disorganized selfhood.' Despite the fact that Penny does not show evidence of severe personality disturbance, there would likely be benefits to this approach, although its long-term nature may be problematic, particularly considering the logistical limitations imposed by her new parenting responsibilities.

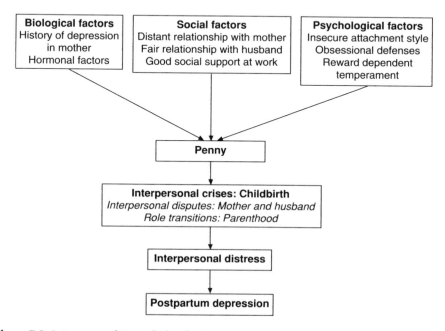

Figure 7.2 *Interpersonal Formulation for Penny.*

3 *Family therapy*: Penny and her extended family system appeared to be in crisis largely because of the introduction of a baby as a new member in the family system, with clear changes in the relationship between Penny and her husband and mother. There would potentially be benefit in bringing the family into therapy in order to deal with the difficulties that the family system encountered since Penny's transition into parenthood.

4 *Interpersonal psychotherapy*: while there are clearly numerous determinants to Penny's distress, the most pressing issues for Penny in her current situation were the changes in her relationship with her husband and the difficulties she was experiencing with her mother, framed within the transition to her new role of mother. IPT offers Penny a framework for understanding her distress, as well as a method for helping Penny develop solutions to her interpersonal problems, with the ultimate aim of symptom relief. The time-limited and focal nature of the treatment is well-suited to her need to resume functioning as quickly as possible, so as to develop a healthy attachment to her child. In addition, IPT may have more intuitive appeal as the concepts of role transition and interpersonal conflict are directly relevant to her experience.

Presentation of the formulation to Penny

Once the therapist and patient have collaborated to develop an Interpersonal Formulation this must be communicated to the patient in a plausible and understandable manner. Typically, it is verbally communicated to the patient, but a written formulation can also be presented for discussion. The verbal presentation allows the patient to have further input into the formulation rather than the therapist seemingly 'imposing' his or her interpretation upon the patient. Providing the patient with a written formulation may serve a formal and symbolic function and allow the patient time to reflect upon what has been presented.

In this case, the therapist offered Penny the following Interpersonal Formulation:

'Penny, I believe that you have developed an episode of major depression, which is why you have been experiencing all of the symptoms that you have mentioned. Depression is a complex illness that is influenced by a number of things. There seem to be physical factors that are important in your case, such as the fact that your mother has suffered from depression. This suggests that there is likely to be a genetic component to the depression. In addition, the fact that you have had mood swings that correspond to your menstrual periods suggests that there may be hormonal factors at work as well.

There also appear to be factors within your psychological make-up which are contributing to your problems. It seems that you have usually been able to deal with life very successfully by working hard and being a high achiever, and that feeling in control of your life has been very important to you. No doubt that sense of control has been changed with the arrival of your daughter – babies are experts at keeping their parents on an irregular and unpredictable schedule.

In going through this life transition to parenthood, it seems that other relationships have also been affected. You were quite clear that your relationship with your husband, which was very good before the baby, has been affected by the new responsibilities that you both face. It sounds like your relationship with your mother has also become more of a problem since your daughter was born.

All of these factors are important, and it seems to me that you became depressed after the birth of your daughter because of a combination of all of these things. The transition to becoming a mother has clearly brought about major changes in your life – both good and not so good – and has challenged your ability to cope with things as you normally have in the past.

In working out a plan to provide some help, I believe that it will help a great deal to work on the transition you are going through, and on the relationship conflicts you described with your husband and mother. IPT would seem to be a natural fit, as the primary focus of treatment is to help people resolve interpersonal conflicts and adjust to major life changes like having a child. Using IPT as a treatment will also allow us to get a handle on your symptoms without needing to use antidepressant medication, since you're concerned about the effect that medication might have on your baby.

How does that sound to you?'

The discussion of the formulation need not be technical, as it should be framed in terms that are readily understandable to the patient. Further, it is extremely helpful to emphasize the patient's strengths. In this case, Penny had a number of coping strengths; the magnitude of the transition to parenthood was simply too great for her to deal with at the moment given her typical coping style and interpersonal resources. One can imagine, for instance, that had she had a better relationship with her mother, she may have weathered the postpartum period with fewer problems, or if she had been less obsessional and less driven to be controlling, she may have been able to adjust more suitably to her new situation. Framing the patient's difficulties as a temporary reaction to a difficult situation both reinforces his or her ability to cope with stress and implies that the difficulty is time-limited and will be overcome.

The discussion about the formulation should always be collaborative. The therapist should always ask the patient for feedback, be receptive to it, and be willing to incorporate the feedback and the new information that will develop in therapy into the continually evolving formulation.

CONCLUSION

The Interpersonal Formulation in IPT is the result of a collaborative process in which the patient and therapist arrive at an understanding regarding the genesis of the current problems the patient is experiencing. The formulation is the product of an integration of the biological, psychological, and social factors that create a vulnerability to psychological distress, and the interpersonal factors that precipitate it at a given point in the patient's life. This process ultimately validates the patient's experiences and links these factors to his or her interpersonal distress. The formulation also provides the rationale for the use of IPT as a therapeutic intervention, as well as providing information to the therapist about which specific IPT techniques are likely to be most beneficial for the patient.

REFERENCES

1. Engel, G.L. 1980. The clinical application of biopsychosocial models. *American Journal of Psychiatry* **137**, 535–44.
2. Cloninger, C.R. 1987. Systematic method for clinical description and classification of personality variants. *Archives of General Psychiatry* **44**, 573.
3. Valliant, G. 1977. *Adaptation to Life*. Boston: Little and Brown.

Section 3

IPT Techniques

INTRODUCTION

IPT relies on a number of specific techniques, all of which are important to the success of the therapy. *More important that any technique, however, is the establishment of a productive therapeutic alliance.* Warmth, empathy, genuineness, and unconditional positive regard, though not sufficient for change in IPT, are all necessary for change in IPT. Specific techniques are of no effect if the patient is not engaged in the therapy. Without a productive alliance, the patient will simply discontinue therapy, an obstacle which no amount of technical expertise can overcome.

The primary goal of the IPT therapist is to understand the patient. If the patient does not perceive that the therapist is truly committed to doing this, the patient will not disclose information as readily, will not feel valued as an individual, and will not develop a meaningful relationship with the therapist. Working to understand the patient should always take precedence over any technical interventions.

All IPT interventions should be therapeutic. Though this seems obvious, the ultimate guide to the value of an intervention is the degree to which it will help the patient.

Techniques should not be used simply to follow a manualized protocol – the benefit to the patient should guide the interventions used in treatment.

The techniques section of this book can metaphorically be considered as a 'tool box,' with the wrenches, hammers, and saws contained within it corresponding to the various IPT techniques. While it is customary to use specific tools for specific jobs, from time to time a handyman may need to use different tools for jobs that appear similar, an assortment of tools for a complicated job, or may need to bang away with a variety of large hammers to correct a particularly stubborn problem. More frequently, smaller and more delicate tools are needed to solve a problem without creating additional damage. IPT techniques – like the tools in the box – are there to help patients resolve different kinds of interpersonal distress. It is a poor handyman who hammers away as if every patient is a nail.

The following sections contain descriptions of IPT techniques. They should always be used following the principles above.

8

Clarification

INTRODUCTION

Clarification is one of the most frequently used techniques in IPT. It is the 'heart and soul' of the initial sessions of IPT but may be used at any time during the course of IPT. Clarification in essence is nothing more than:

- Asking *good* questions so that the therapist can better understand the patient's experience.
- Asking *very good* questions so that the patient can understand his or her own experiences better.
- Asking *extraordinarily good* questions so that the patient is motivated to change his or her behavior.

Clarification is a 'non-specific' psychotherapeutic technique, and its use is not unique to IPT. As in other therapies, clarification facilitates the IPT therapist's understanding of the patient, the patient's understanding of him or herself, and increases the therapeutic alliance. The process of collaboratively exploring a particular aspect of a patient's interpersonal experience is therapeutic in a number of ways:

1 It provides the therapist an opportunity to validate the patient's experiences and distress.
2 It provides an opportunity for the patient to explore and reflect upon his or her interpersonal experiences within a supportive and constructive therapeutic relationship.

3   It helps the patient to more clearly communicate his or her experiences to others, as practice in doing so occurs under the therapist's guidance.
4   It helps to consolidate the therapeutic alliance by emphasizing that the patient and therapist are involved in the collaborative process of exploring the patient's experiences.

Despite the apparent simplicity of clarification, asking questions is a real art. It requires that the therapist take a genuine interest in the patient, and that the therapist be able to convey this interest to the patient. Patients who are less securely attached are apt to be particularly vigilant for therapists who are less than genuine, so that clinicians may need to work very diligently and creatively to use clarification to foster a productive therapeutic relationship with such patients. The primary goal of clarification, therefore, should be to understand the patient and to foster the development of the therapeutic alliance.

CLARIFICATION IN IPT

Clarification as a technique is best considered an integration of:

1   *Directive questioning*: the therapist should gently guide the patient towards pertinent interpersonal issues during the clarification process. The focus on interpersonal issues is an aspect of clarification that is characteristic of IPT.
2   *Empathic listening*: the therapist should validate the patient's experiences and concerns regarding his or her interpersonal problems.
3   *Reflective listening*: the therapist should work to ensure that he or she is correctly understanding the patient, often using statements such as, 'so what you've said is. . .' to check his or her comprehension of the issue at hand.
4   *Encouragement of spontaneous discourse by the patient*: the therapist should use verbal and non-verbal cues to encourage elaboration by the patient.

The aims of clarification in IPT are to:

- Facilitate the therapist's understanding of the patient's experience.
- Develop a therapeutic alliance.
- Direct the treatment.

CLARIFICATION AND THE PATIENT'S ATTACHMENT STYLE

During the process of clarification, the therapist can gain valuable insight into a patient's attachment style by evaluating the way in which he or she responds to open-ended questions about relationships. Such inferences may help the therapist understand the patient's experience of interpersonal problems, as well as helping to anticipate potential problems in the therapeutic relationship. It should also guide the therapist in determining to what degree close or open-ended questions should be used, and the degree to which the questions should be directive. More securely attached patients can generally tolerate more directiveness on the part of the therapist, while those that are less securely attached may need more empathy and reflection from the therapist in order to sustain a good alliance, particularly early in therapy.

THE ART OF CLARIFICATION

The use of clarification requires a balance between encouraging spontaneous narrative by the patient and using more directive questions in order to keep the discussion on focus. The therapist should be prepared to allow some degree of drift, as it may lead to the disclosure of new material which is relevant to the problem area under discussion.

The artful use of clarification can be compared to a damper on a fireplace. More directive questions can be used to 'open the damper' and generate a more intense fire, while less directive and more empathically driven questions can be used to 'close the damper' so the fire doesn't get out of control. Enough heat is needed to keep the patient motivated to change; too much and the patient will (psychologically) spontaneously combust. More securely attached patients can generally tolerate more intrapsychic heat than those less securely attached. The therapist's job is to keep the fire burning at the most efficient level by directing the interview in this way.

In more 'expressive' and psychodynamically based treatments, the therapist often encourages the patient to produce narrative that is free-flowing and at times may be circumstantial or discursive. While this may be useful for uncovering latent or unconscious psychological content, it is outside of the scope of IPT.

Why is such associative discourse discouraged in IPT? First, it distracts from the focus on symptom resolution. Second, the intrinsic time-limit in IPT requires a more specific focus for discussion than is used in less structured treatments. Allowing an open-ended focus over a longer time period is likely to move the treatment to a transference based therapy. Finally, and most importantly, focusing the therapy, and particularly using more directive clarifications, allows that therapist to encourage the patient to make changes in his or her communication and to resolve the problems with which he or she is faced outside of therapy.

USING CLARIFICATION TO BEGIN SESSIONS

Mindful of the need in IPT to maintain an interpersonal focus and to direct the patient's attention to the specific problem at hand, the therapist should typically begin sessions by avoiding general non-directive statements such as:

'How are things since we last spoke?'

More appropriate and directive questions would include those that draw the patient's attention to the interpersonal problem last discussed, and which clearly convey to the patient the expectation that work is to be done on these issues between sessions. Such directive questions might include those such as:

'Over the last few weeks we have been discussing the problem you are having with your spouse. Can you update me as to how this has been progressing?'

The latter statement establishes a focus for the discussion of interpersonal problems, directs the patient's attention to the specific problem at hand, leads naturally into a continuing discussion of the problem in the current session, and reinforces the therapist's expectation that the patient will work on the problem between sessions.

POTENTIAL DIFFICULTIES WITH CLARIFICATION

The patient who continually 'wanders off subject'

The therapist must be constantly attentive to the direction of the discussion. If the patient begins to wander off topic, then redirection or gentle confrontation may be helpful. The therapist should highlight the need to remain on interpersonal topics, and it may be necessary to review the Interpersonal Inventory with the patient to emphasize the specific problem areas that were determined to be therapeutic foci. The use of more closed-ended questions may be helpful to redirect the discussion to interpersonal areas, with a return to more open-ended questions once the focus of discussion is firmly refocused upon the interpersonal problem.

The therapist who continually 'wanders off subject'

There are occasions when even the most experienced IPT therapist finds him or herself roaming into IPT 'no-man's-land.' Many times this is because the patient's psychodynamic processes are too intriguing, and the therapist falls prey to the temptation to ask about dreams or the patient's fantasies about the therapist simply because it is so fascinating. This is particularly difficult for therapists who come from a more psychodynamic background, because there are times during which the therapist may feel that he or she has to 'hold back' and not follow transferential leads that might be used in less-structured approaches. Recognizing this temptation when it occurs is the best way to prevent drift, and if the patient begins to share a fascinating dream, the therapist can simply ask him or her how the meaning in the dream is communicated to significant others.

Patients who are vague at times or who have trouble organizing their thoughts well tend to engender digression in the therapy. When a therapist finds himself or herself following a divergent lead, it is best to 'regroup' by consulting the Interpersonal Inventory. Returning to the original problem areas allows the therapist and patient to refocus the discussion. It may also be useful to examine the 'confusion' as an interpersonal communication, and to discuss the ways in which it might cause problems in the patient's extra-therapy relationships. For instance, the therapist might comment:

'There have been a few times now when our discussion has led us to areas that seem to be a little "off the track." This seems to have made us both a bit confused about where we are heading in working with your problems. Do you find that this happens when you are discussing this problem with others? How does it seem to affect your relationships with other people?'

Case example: Henry

Henry was a 36-year-old legal assistant who presented with worsening anxiety in the context of a marital problem. Henry had received some benefit from treatment with cognitive therapy, although his ongoing relationship difficulties had continued to result in symptoms.

Henry complained to the therapist that his wife, 'did not understand him,' and that he 'didn't want to be in the marriage anymore.' After an evaluation, Henry and the therapist agreed to twelve sessions of IPT with a specific focus upon the dispute between Henry and his wife.

Henry gave an account of his relationship with his wife that implied a great degree of indifference about its survival. They had been together only six months before getting married; his wife had suggested marriage, with which Henry 'went along.' The therapist asked if Henry recalled any of his thoughts at the time of his wife's suggestion of marriage, to which Henry replied, 'I don't really know, and I haven't really given it much thought.' His other relationships seemed to be equally 'unimportant' to Henry.

While compiling the Interpersonal Inventory, the therapist attempted to clarify the dispute between Henry and his wife further:

Therapist: Henry, tell me more about your wife.
Henry: Well, um, there isn't really much to say.
Therapist: Well, perhaps you could tell me about the early days.
Henry: Not a lot to say really – we met, she proposed, I didn't think too much about it, we got married.
Therapist: Tell me more about your meeting.
Henry: Like what?
Therapist: Well, like how you felt about her then and now.
Henry: Much the same really.

Based on Henry's responses and the pattern of relationships he described, the therapist hypothesized that Henry's style of attachment was insecure and avoidant. Further, Henry's tendency to be dismissive of relationships was a potential threat to the therapeutic relationship. It soon became apparent that the therapist needed to do two things, and to do them skillfully. First, the therapist needed to direct the therapy so that more specific information about Henry's interactions with his wife could be obtained. At the same time, the therapist needed to make sure that the therapeutic alliance was strengthened so that Henry wouldn't literally dismiss the therapist. Thus, an artful mix of directive questions, empathy, warmth, and a genuine effort to understand Henry was required.

Therapist: Let me slow down the pace a bit – I really want to understand as best I can what your experience with your wife has been like for you.
Henry: It's hard to describe really, but it has been quite frustrating.
Therapist: It sounds like it has been – it's hard for me to imagine what it must be like for you. Could you tell me more about your experience?
Henry: Nothing I do seems to make any difference to her. She doesn't seem to appreciate that I have feelings too, even though I may not be quite so direct about it as she is. I really hate it when she says that I never communicate my feelings. I think that she just doesn't listen.

> **Therapist:** That does sound frustrating. If we could, I would like to focus a bit more on one or two specific interactions you have had with her, so that I can understand the details a bit better.
> **Henry:** Uh huh.
> **Therapist:** Tell me about the last time you and she had a disagreement.
> **Henry:** OK.
> **Therapist:** Where were you?
> **Henry:** At home.
> **Therapist:** What was it that you were both doing at the time?
> **Henry:** I was watching a ball game and she was talking at me.
> **Therapist:** 'Talking at you' – that's an interesting way to describe it. Can you remember some specific things she said?
> **Henry:** Yeah, she said, 'You are always doing something else except talking to me!'
> **Therapist:** How did you respond to that?
> **Henry:** I said, 'Well, I'm talking to you now, aren't I?'
> **Therapist:** What did she say then?
> **Henry:** Well, I think she said, 'Can you turn the damn Roosters game off and commit to the conversation?'
> **Therapist:** OK, and how did you respond?
> **Henry:** I didn't really respond, I just kept watching the game – they were playing the Eels after all.

The therapist continued to clarify the specific aspects of Henry's interpersonal dispute with his wife. He remained mindful of Henry's attachment style, and continued to artfully use both open and directive questions to elucidate Henry's interpersonal experiences.

CONCLUSION

Clarification is much more than merely asking the patient questions. Clarification involves a delicate balance between directive queries and encouragement of narrative, which will vary depending on the patient's attachment style. Clarification is a fundamental method for establishing and maintaining an interpersonal focus in IPT. The art of using clarification is to develop an understanding of the patient's interpersonal experiences which helps the patient develop insight and which motivates him or her to change.

9

Communication Analysis

INTRODUCTION

The basic premise of IPT is that individuals have difficulties because they are faced with an overwhelming stressor in the context of insufficient social support, both in their intimate relationships and in their general social network. Though the lack of sufficient social support is often due in part to deficits within patients' support systems, it is also frequently due in part to poor communication. This is largely because patients are not communicating their needs clearly, nor in a way to which their social support system can productively respond. As a direct consequence of these maladaptive styles of communication, patients do not get their attachment needs or their needs for emotional and physical support met adequately.

THE GOALS OF COMMUNICATION ANALYSIS

In essence, *communication analysis is simply a formal means of investigating the hypothesis that the patient's difficulties are being caused, perpetuated, or exacerbated by poor communication.* The goals for communication analysis are to:

- Help the patient identify his or her communication patterns.
- Help the patient recognize his or her contribution to the communication problem.
- Motivate the patient to communicate more effectively.

To do this, the therapist should work sequentially with the patient through the following steps:

1 Collect information about the patient's interpersonal relationships and the communication which occurs within them.
2 Develop hypotheses about the cause of the communication problem.
3 Present the hypotheses to the patient as feedback about his or her communication.
4 Solicit responses from the patient about the therapist's critiques.
5 Revise the hypotheses if needed.
6 Problem solve to develop and practice new ways of communicating.

A strong therapeutic alliance must undergird this process, as the patient must be able to tolerate feedback from the therapist for it to have any impact, and for it to lead eventually to change. The specific ways of giving feedback must also be selected, carefully considering the patient's attachment style and insight.

SOURCES OF COMMUNICATION

The obvious requirement for communication analysis is that there must be communication to analyze. In IPT, the therapist relies on four potential sources of information:

1 The patient's description of his or her communications, both generally and specifically.
2 The quality of the patient's narrative to the therapist.
3 The patient's in-session communication with the therapist.
4 The reports of significant others in the patient's social network.

Each of these provides extremely important information, and can literally be thought of as providing different glimpses of the proverbial 'communication elephant.' Thus, communication analysis must be preceded by an extensive social history, a detailed description of the patient's relationships, and his or her expectations of others. Moreover, the therapist should also explore the patient's perceptions of the expectations that others have of him or her. The rule rather than the exception is that interpersonal difficulties are caused not only by poor communication but by expectations that are unrealistic or non-reciprocal.

Most patients are able to provide a fairly accurate accounting of their expectations of others, although this will be colored to some degree by the patient's ability to relate narrative, and his or her insight. Unfortunately, a patient who has difficulty in communicating directly to others in his or her social network will usually also have difficulty communicating directly to the therapist. Further, patients who misunderstand the communication or intent of others will often report a biased view of the communication they have with others. Such patients may attribute malevolent or uncaring motives to others when their attachment needs are not met, despite the fact that the significant other may be communicating clearly and may be invested in the relationship. The therapist should therefore explore the possibility that the problems in communication arise from any or all of the following:

- The patient is not communicating his or her needs clearly.
- The patient is not communicating his or her needs in a way to which his or her social support system can respond.
- Individuals in the patient's social support system are not communicating clearly to the patient.
- Individuals in the patient's social support system are not communicating in a way to which the patient can productively respond.

The patient's description of his or her communications

During the initial history and the development of the Interpersonal Inventory, the patient will undoubtedly spontaneously provide the therapist with a great deal of information about his or her communication patterns. This may involve direct descriptions of communication by more insightful patients, or it may come in the form of general complaints by the patient such as, 'my husband never understands me,' or 'my wife never listens to me.' Inferences that communication in such relationships has gone awry are not difficult for the therapist to make in the latter cases.

The IPT therapist should make direct inquiries about communication during the evaluation as well as in subsequent sessions. Direct queries on the part of the therapist might include such questions as:

- 'What kinds of patterns do you see in your relationships?'
- 'What kinds of patterns do you see in your communications with others?'
- 'What kinds of things do you have difficulty talking to others about?'
- 'What is it like for you to express anger or displeasure to others?'
- 'How do you respond when others get angry with you?'
- 'What kinds of relationships do you have trouble with?'
- 'What do you do when you are under stress?'
- 'How do you communicate your needs to others when under stress?'
- 'How do you typically respond to others when they ask you for help?'
- 'What feedback have you gotten from others about your relationships?'
- 'How well do you think others understand you?'

The patient's responses to these questions should lead the therapist to develop hypotheses about the specific communication difficulties that the patient is having. This information is particularly useful in judging a patient's insight and his or her ability to be empathic and to understand others' points of view. For instance, if a patient recognizes when responding to these questions that he or she is contributing to the communication difficulties, and if he or she can understand the kinds of responses that are being elicited, therapy will be much less difficult than with a patient who blames others for all of his or her problems.

The direct report provided by a patient is colored by a number of factors that the therapist should take into consideration. These include the patient's insight, motivation, ability to disclose personal information, and ability to be empathic. The patient's attachment style also dramatically affects his or her presentation. Patients who are more securely attached are more trusting early in therapy, more able to readily disclose information, and are generally more understanding of other's points of view.

Another piece of information to which the therapist should be attentive is the degree to which the patient tends to generalize descriptions of his or her communications. Patterns which are described in absolutes, such as 'my boss *never* recognizes my accomplishments,' or 'my spouse *always* criticizes me,' signify much more entrenched and less insightful ways of understanding one's communications and relationships. When met with such generalizations, the therapist should move to the use of Interpersonal Incidents as described in the next chapter.

In general, the concept that the 'rich get richer' applies in the area of communication analysis as in other areas of therapy. Patients with better communication skills are better able to describe the relationship problems they are having, they are better able to listen and to understand other's reactions to them, they are more insightful, and more accepting of feedback from the therapist. In contrast, those patients whose communication skills are poor manifest that communication style in therapy, making it more difficult for the therapist to understand the problem, to give feedback about it, and to assist the patient to develop insight. Consider the following examples from the evaluation phase of treatment with two patients with marital conflicts.

Case example 1

Therapist: Tell me how you react when others are critical of you.

Patient: In general, I don't like it. I tend to take criticisms very personally. . . . Even though I know that the other person may be trying to give me some feedback I can use, I often see it as critical. And then when I feel criticized, I withdraw from the other person. I remember one time when I was getting dressed for work several days ago, and my wife said, 'that tie doesn't look quite right with that shirt.' Intellectually, I knew that she was just trying to help, but it felt like she was criticizing my competence and trying to put me down. And I was mad because she was probably right about the tie, so I felt even worse.

Therapist: What did you do after your wife's comment about the tie?

Patient: I reacted like I usually do – I just kind of looked at the floor and pouted. She's to the point that she's pretty fed up with that, so she started to leave. But as she was going downstairs, I walked into the hall after her and said, 'I know you were just trying to help, but I can't stand it when you criticize me.' We talked about it for a few minutes, but then we both had to leave for work.

Case example 2

Therapist: Tell me how you react when others are critical of you.

Patient: Boy, that's a good question. My wife criticizes me all the time for no reason. She has a real bad habit of losing her temper – you just can't reason with her.

Therapist: Tell me about a specific time when you felt she was critical of you.

Patient: Happens all the time . . . last week, yesterday, next week for sure. There's no changing her.

Therapist: What do you do when you feel she's being critical?

Patient: I react like anyone would – I tell her to cut it out. In a reasonable way, of course. . . . I don't yell and scream like she does. . . .

As a means of making concepts such as insight and empathy more concrete, the reader may simply want to consider which of these two patients he or she would prefer to work with. The first patient recognizes his communication pattern of withdrawal under fire, has insight into his own reactions as well as insight into his wife's motives and, even better, has already attempted to address the conflict directly with his wife. In contrast, the second patient has externalized the problem, presents his wife as completely at fault, and has no motivation to change his own behavior, much less of an ability to recognize how he might be contributing to the communication problem.

The first patient has provided a very good description of the way in which communication occurs in his relationship. The therapist can use this information directly to give feedback to the patient, and to help him modify his communication patterns. While the therapist must draw some inferences about the way in which the second patient is communicating, hypothesizing that he has difficulty communicating directly, tends to be critical, and tends to generalize is quite reasonable and is supported by the patient's presentation.

The quality of the patient's narrative

In addition to the information provided by the patient in response to the therapist's direct questions about communication, the quality of the patient's report also reflects the patient's communication style. The patient's ability to produce a coherent narrative, for example, is a clear reflection of the way in which he or she communicates outside of therapy. If the patient is unable to present a clear picture of the problem to an empathic therapist who is *trained* to help the patient tell his or her story, it is certain that the patient gets bogged down when trying to communicate in his or her social environment. The therapist should attempt to answer the following questions about the patient's narrative:

- How coherent is the patient's report of communication patterns?
- To what degree does the patient spontaneously produce examples of communication problems?
- How compelling is the narrative? In other words, how well does the patient engage the therapist in the narrative?
- How well are emotions conveyed by the patient?
- How specific is the information presented? Is it nothing more than a generalization, or can the patient describe specific interactions?

The patient's in-session communication with the therapist

The patient's communication with the therapist during the session is another extremely important piece of information. In IPT, since the patient–therapist relationship is typically not directly addressed, this information usually being gathered by the therapist experientially rather than by direct inquiry. A slightly different way of understanding this source of information is to think of it as derived from the process which occurs during the therapy. In other words, how does the patient 'work' with the therapist, and within that framework, how does the patient specifically communicate to the therapist?

For instance, when the therapist is negotiating the contract with the patient, how capable is he or she of participating in the process? Does the patient simply passively accept the therapist's suggestions, does he or she immediately complain that there won't be enough sessions, or is he or she able to productively engage in the discussion, give input, and compromise? When discussing homework, does the patient have the capacity to work productively with the therapist, to offer his or her own suggestions, or does he or she resist suggestions passively or even aggressively? All of the interactions in therapy are potential sources of this kind of information.

One of the basic premises of IPT is that the patient behaves and communicates consistently across relationships, including the therapeutic relationship. Simply put, *people just can't help but be themselves*. Thus, the information gleaned from the therapeutic relationship has direct implications about the patient's relationships outside of therapy. Questions about those relationships should be directly informed by the therapist's experience with the patient in session.

Reports from the patient's significant others

Some of the best sources of information about the patient's communications are the patient's significant others. While it may not always be possible, in IPT it is strongly encouraged that the therapist meet with the patient's partner or spouse during the therapy. This serves as a means of providing psycho-educational information about the treatment to the partner, serves to demystify therapy, and also helps to enlist the partner in the recovery of the patient. Most important, however, is the opportunity it gives the therapist to observe the couple's communication 'in vivo' and to obtain information from an outside observer.

This can best be illustrated by noting the experience that most therapists have had when meeting the spouse of a patient two or three sessions into a course of individual therapy. The patient may have described his or her spouse in great detail, but when the therapist has the opportunity to meet the spouse in person, rarely does the description do justice to the reality. A patients may describe a spouse who is distant and uncaring, only to have the therapist find after meeting the spouse that he or she is quite reasonable and not at all like the patient's description. Conversely, a patient may describe his or her spouse in glowing terms, with the therapist only later discovering upon meeting the spouse that the description is completely inaccurate, and that the spouse is in reality a wolf dressed in the sheep's clothing of the patient's over-idealized description.

Communication analysis is based on the premise that communication problems are directly involved in the patient's symptoms and interpersonal difficulties. However, an important caveat to this approach is that the therapist must be mindful of the individuals who are the recipients of the patient's communications, because it is likely (if not certain) that those individuals also have limitations in their ability to communicate. If so, improvement in the patient's communication skills may still be met with rejection or misunderstanding by others.

In addition, the motivations of others with whom the patient is communicating may be very different from those of the patient. For instance, a patient may be attempting to get his or her attachment needs met in a romantic relationship in which the partner has little or no investment. More direct communications on the part of the patient may continue to be met with responses that are negative.

This being the case, it is nearly always helpful for the therapist to meet with the significant others who are involved in the patient's social support system, and particularly those that are involved in marital or intimate relationships. This is even more desirable in situations in which an interpersonal dispute is at issue. Doing so allows the therapist to:

- Observe the communication in the relationship '*in vivo*.'
- Obtain information from the significant other about his or her perception of the problem.
- More accurately gauge the investment of the significant other in the relationship.
- Provide psycho-educational information to the significant other.
- 'Demystify' the therapy experience for the significant other.
- Assign communication homework to the couple.
- Gauge how effectively the patient has implemented the changes in communication which have been discussed in therapy.

THE PROCESS OF COMMUNICATION ANALYSIS

Much time has been spent on the methods of collecting information about the patient's communications for two reasons. First, the evaluation process which occurs while this is happening is crucial to the therapy, as it informs the therapist not only about the patient's suitability and prognosis for therapy, but also directs the interventions that the therapist will subsequently use. The second reason is that the remainder of the communication analysis process is quite simple technically – *it is nothing more than developing a hypothesis about what is causing the patient's communication difficulties, and reflecting that hypothesis back to the patient in a way in which he or she can accept the feedback and use it to make changes.* However, while the technical aspects are straightforward, the art of giving useful feedback is much more complicated, as the therapist must be able to modify his or her style to account for the idiosyncrasies of a given patient.

The feedback to be given is simply a synthesis of all of the information gathered from the patient about his or her communications, applied to a specific situation. Data from the patient's direct report of communications, the therapist's impressions of the patient's narrative, the therapeutic alliance, and information from others (if available) should all be included. These should all be integrated and summarized for the patient, presented in the context of a specific interpersonal relationship. For instance, in the first case described above, the therapist might comment on the marital dispute as follows:

> 'Based on what you have told me about your relationship with your wife, it appears to me that you are quite sensitive to her comments, and have a tendency to take what she says very personally. Once that happens, your typical reaction seems to be to withdraw. My impression is that when you pull away emotionally or shut down communication in that way, you would like your wife to recognize what you are doing and would like for her to approach you to make amends. What are your thoughts about that?'

Rather than viewing the formulation of the patient's communication difficulties as set in stone, the therapist should always see it as a work in progress. It is a true hypothesis, which should take into account additional information as it is developed. IPT continually revolves around the gathering of more and more detailed information about relationships and communications; thus, the hypotheses that are developed by the therapist should be under constant revision.

Further, presentation of the formulation of the patient's communication difficulties is not a one-off occurrence. It is a continuing process in which a tentative hypothesis is offered, the patient responds to it, and more information is collected. This forms the basis for yet another, more precise hypothesis, which is then discussed again. Wrapped into this process is discussion about how the patient's communication could be modified and the problem alleviated.

Giving feedback to the patient

Once the therapist has gathered information from some or all of the sources noted above, and has developed a preliminary hypothesis about the patient's specific communication difficulties, the interactive process of giving feedback to the patient should begin. The most crucial aspect in this process is the therapeutic alliance.

In Kiesler and Watkins's terms,[1] the patient–therapist relationship must have a high degree of *inclusion* in order for the therapist's feedback to the patient to make a difference. In other words, the therapeutic relationship has to be important to both patient and therapist. The patient must attach importance to the therapist's feedback – it has to have an impact on the patient. If the relationship is tenuous, or if the feedback is given prematurely, the therapist's comments to the patient will be easily dismissed.

The ideal outcome of the feedback process is that the patient respond to the therapist's comments by literally replying, 'You really think so?' The emphasis is on the 'you' – the therapist – who is valued and whose opinion has meaning for the patient. The degree of importance, respect, and recognition of expertise that the patient attributes to the therapist – i.e., the quality of the therapeutic *relationship* – will be the primary factor which determines how the feedback is received. The therapist should establish this kind of relationship with the patient by conveying warmth, empathy, genuineness, and unconditional positive regard[2] – all of the factors which, though not sufficient for change in IPT, are necessary for change in IPT.

The therapist must also modify his or her style to accommodate the attachment style of the patient. More securely attached patients are able to tolerate more direct feedback, and their security allows them to tolerate feedback earlier in therapy. In contrast, those patients with ambivalent attachment styles should be encouraged to develop their own ideas about the problems in their communications, rather than having the therapist give them a lot of direct feedback. Less directive interventions are usually warranted so that passive resistance or dependency does not become a major issue. Those patients who are more avoidant in attachment style require more time to develop a strong therapeutic alliance, so feedback may need to be delayed until such time as the alliance allows the patient to tolerate it.

An important part of the process of giving feedback to the patient is having the patient respond verbally to the therapist's ideas. This means that the conceptualization developed by the therapist is not framed as a definitive 'interpretation' of the patient's problems, in which the therapist provides the patient with the 'correct' understanding which the patient must accept in order to gain insight. Instead, the therapist should literally offer his or her conceptualizations as hypotheses – concepts that offer a reasonable explanation but which are open to further investigation and exploration.

The therapist should couch such feedback to the patient in a way which reflects this. Statements such as, 'The information you've given me about your relationships seems to suggest . . .' or 'I wonder if you are having pro blems with . . .' should be used, rather than more definitive statements. And each should be followed by an invitation to the patient to respond: 'What do you think?'

The more ownership the patient has of the conceptualization, the better. Thus, patients should be asked to develop their own ideas about their communication problems. Questions such as, 'What do you think are the major patterns in your communications?' or 'How do you see all of these things coming together?' may be very helpful. Input into the conceptualization from the patient should be strongly encouraged.

It should also be clear that in IPT, communication analysis does not necessarily require an understanding of the psychological or historical factors involved in the communication problem. While it is of great benefit if the patient does appreciate the historical precedents to the problem, it is not necessary. *What is required in IPT is that the patient recognizes his or her current communication patterns, appreciates the kinds of responses that he or she elicits from others, and makes changes in his or her communication to resolve the problem.*

The implications of this statement are profound. What this means, in essence, is that even though patients who are less insightful, less motivated, and less securely attached are more difficult to work with in therapy, they are still amenable to treatment because the IPT approach does not require deep psychological insight. It simply requires that the patient recognize that there is a communication problem and that by changing his or her communication, it can be improved or resolved. In fact, it is even possible that the patient can still see the problem as being external (i.e., the fault of another person), but can recognize that changing his or her communications will cause others to respond differently and will resolve the problem. Thus, even very difficult patients are amenable to the IPT approach to therapy.

This is not to say that insight and intrapsychic change should not be encouraged in IPT – it is always better that this happen than not. However, IPT can be used with patients who appear to lack the capacity for insight, who are not psychologically minded, or who for other reasons are poor candidates for more insight-oriented therapies.

Perhaps the best example of this is the work in IPT that can be done with patients with somatization disorders. In general, such patients are very poor candidates for therapy, as they have maladaptive attachment styles, very poor insight, a distrust of the medical system, and are poorly motivated to seek treatment. Moreover, they are often hostile towards caregivers, and most importantly, are quite fixed in their beliefs that their problems are physical rather than psychological. They are not exactly the optimal candidates for therapy.

Nonetheless, even if such patients continue to blame their problems on a medical care system that simply does not respond to their needs, they can often come to recognize that changing their communications leads to better provision of care. The goal in IPT is to help such patients to recognize that changing their communications will result in a more effective response to their attachment needs.

For instance, a patient who frequently visits the emergency room for physical complaints may recognize during therapy that this is not an effective way to get his or her physical problems addressed. Emergency rooms are very busy, so the patient will have to wait; the patient is likely to see a different physician at every visit, and is clearly not going to get the personal attention that the patient desires. On the other hand, scheduling regular appointments with a family physician who knows the patient well and is able to give more personal attention is likely to get his or her attachment needs met more effectively.

Somatizing patients may not develop any understanding of the dynamic processes that drive their care-seeking behavior. They may continue to externalize the problem, blaming the medical system or even individual emergency physicians who 'don't give patients the time they deserve.' But most will grudgingly agree that they are more satisfied seeing a doctor who knows them well rather than sitting for hours in an emergency room. They are able to recognize that changing their communication results in better care.

Case example: Fred

Fred was a 32-year-old male who sought treatment for complaints of marital dissatisfaction. He described that frequent fights with his wife Sandra were causing him to have trouble sleeping, were making him more irritable, and had also affected his work. He also stated that he was 'fed up,' and was particularly upset about the fact that Sandra had not been willing to go to therapy with him. He denied any previous history of psychological treatment, and also denied any problems with substance abuse.

Through the first two sessions, Fred described that his attempts to be more intimate with his wife had all been met with rejection. He reported that she, 'never wants to talk, and consistently rejects any attempts I make to be affectionate.' He felt that the relationship may have been coming to an end, but was willing to give it one last try.

In the third session, the therapist asked Fred to describe his relationship with his wife in detail:

Therapist: Fred, tell me more about your wife.
Fred: Well, when I first met her, I thought she was the greatest thing since sliced bread. We had such a close relationship. Over the last several years, things have gotten really bad. I don't think that she really cares about me any more.
Therapist: What kinds of patterns do you see in your relationship with her?
Fred: Patterns? I hadn't really thought about that. . . . I guess the main one I would say is that I don't get enough affection from her. Yeah, that's pretty consistent.
Therapist: What about patterns in your communication with her?
Fred: She thinks that I am too demanding – I don't agree though – but it's been a consistent complaint of hers. She grew up in a home where there was hardly any physical affection, and I think that has affected her a lot.
Therapist: How do you ask her for affection or let her know that you want to be closer?
Fred: Usually I feel much closer to her when we are, you know, when we get together – you know, sleep together.
Therapist: It sounds like your sexual relationship is very important to you.
Fred: That's right! And she hasn't been willing to do anything at all recently – she says that she doesn't feel close to me and won't even consider sex.
Therapist: How have you responded to that?
Fred: I figure that if she really cared about me, she'd know how important the sexual part of our relationship is. After all, as long as we've been married, she ought to know me by now.
Therapist: So how do you tell her that you are upset about it?
Fred: I tell her that if she really loved me she'd take better care of me and pay attention to what I need.

Therapist: How is that said exactly – I mean, tone of voice for instance.

Fred: I just say it to her in a very matter of fact way – I hardly ever get angry – so she should certainly be aware of how I feel. It would sure be helpful if you could see her so that you could talk some sense into her!

The therapist was able to draw several tentative conclusions from this interaction and other information provided by Fred. The direct report that Fred gave indicated that communication was occurring, but that Fred was making several assumptions about what his wife understood. He was making the assumption that she should understand his needs without communicating them when he stated that, 'she should know how important the sexual part of our relationship is.' He also seemed to assume that she would behave in a particular way, 'if she loved me.' Assumptions that others can literally 'read the mind' of the patient and will respond appropriately to his or her needs are quite common in marital disputes.

The narrative that Fred produced was fairly coherent, but notable for what appeared to be a dichotomous presentation of his wife. His description of her when they met was glowing, but he described their current relationship in very negative terms. There did not appear to be any balance in Fred's description of her. A more two-dimensional picture was emerging, with Fred's wife being either idealized or devalued. Further, the whole narrative was literally framed by Fred's complaints that his wife was not 'caring for him.' Rather than a dispute over a particular issue, Fred's problems seem to be related primarily to a general sense that his needs were not being met.

Fred's insight also appeared to be quite limited. His report indicated that his wife was to blame for his problems, and he presented his own communications in the best possible light: 'I just say it to her in a very matter of fact way – I hardly ever get angry – so she should certainly be aware of how I feel.' Based on the other parts of Fred's report, the therapist strongly suspected that this was not the case, and that Fred's communications to his wife were neither clear nor presented in a 'matter of fact' way. More likely there was a lot of emotion being communicated by both Fred and his wife.

On the other hand, Fred did appear to have the potential for insight. His response to the therapist's question about patterns in his relationship was met positively, and seemed to get him thinking. The therapist was encouraged that this might be a fruitful area with which to continue.

Fred's in-session communication to the therapist, and the way in which he was forming a therapeutic relationship, was also informative. Though there were not overt signs of dependency, the therapist did note Fred's statement that, 'It would sure be helpful if you (the therapist) could see her so that you could talk some sense into her!' This struck the therapist as more information supporting the hypothesis that Fred had some dependent personality traits as well as some anxious ambivalent attachment traits, and that these were being manifest in his attempts to get his wife (and the therapist) to 'care for him.'

When evaluating the ways in which feedback might most effectively be given to Fred, the therapist considered three options. First, he could give Fred direct feedback. This might be in the following form:

'It sounds from what you have told me that you and your wife are clearly having some trouble communicating, and that you don't feel that she is responding to you the way you would like. I wonder if some of the things you feel that you are communicating clearly might not be quite so clear to her. For instance, you seem to be assuming that she will know what you want, both in terms of emotional closeness and sexual response, but it doesn't sound as if that has been communicated to her clearly. She may be operating under a completely different set of assumptions than you have been. What are your thoughts about that?'

This option might be quite reasonable for a patient who was relatively securely attached, and who had already developed a solid alliance with the therapist. Both would be required for the patient to be able to tolerate this kind of direct feedback. If the patient were able to use it productively, it would probably be the most direct and helpful way to work on the problem. In Fred's case, however, the therapist judged that Fred was neither able to tolerate such feedback at this point in therapy, nor would he be able to use it – he would likely experience it as critical and as an empathic failure on the part of the therapist.

Option number two was to gently persist with similar questions about Fred's interactions with his wife, with the goal of helping him to appreciate how his communication style and expectations of his wife were leading to problems. The therapist would begin to move to questions that pushed Fred to think about things in more depth, and which would (hopefully) stimulate some insight. This might be in the following form:

'Fred, it's clear that you don't feel your needs are being met by your wife, and that you have been trying to communicate this to her, but she doesn't seem to respond to you as you would like her too. I would like to try to understand better how this happens, and to figure out why this seems to keep happening. What are your thoughts about why the two of you aren't connecting on this?'

Such an approach would likely be much more tolerable to Fred, as the therapist would carefully convey empathy, and not 'blame' Fred for the communication problems. Asking for Fred to take the lead, rather than giving him direct feedback to which he could respond, would also be more compatible with his insecure attachment style. The therapist would also be particularly careful to frame his statements as attempts to 'understand' Fred. This process, however, requires much slower pacing than the direct feedback approach.

Option three, which the therapist elected to follow, was to have Fred invite his wife to therapy for a session. Despite Fred's initial protestations to the contrary, when he asked his wife directly she came quite willingly to therapy. The therapist used this opportunity to collect information from her about Fred's style of communication, and to observe their communication directly. It became clear quite quickly that Fred's wife was invested in the relationship, but was beginning to get fed up with what she perceived to be his unreasonable demands. She felt that he was not at all clear about what he wanted, and tended to pout when he didn't get his way.

Therapist: Thanks for coming in today.
Sandra: You're welcome. I told Fred that I'd be glad to come in for therapy – I even suggested that we see someone together, but he said he didn't want to do that.
Fred: I did not – I said that I wanted to work on my problems, but I never said that you couldn't come!
Sandra: Well, that's not what I remember.

Therapist: At any rate, now that you're here, I would like to do two things. First, I would like to get some feedback from you, Sandra, about your perception of the communication that's occurring between you and Fred. Second, it sounds like we need to do some planning about how to proceed with therapy after this session.

Sandra: My perception is that Fred and I have had a pretty good relationship for the most part, but that recently it has gotten worse. I can even put my finger on when I think that things started to go badly – I had a miscarriage about six months ago, and we haven't really been close since then. Fred just kind of stopped talking after that. I'm not even sure that he knows how I feel about it – he sure hasn't asked.

Fred (to the therapist): Oh, I forgot to tell you about that – that was really difficult for both of us.

Therapist: That does sound like a pretty important piece of information. What was that experience like for both of you?

Both Fred and Sandra began to share their experiences with the therapist, and in the process of doing so, began to feel that they were at least being heard by their partner. At the end of the session, the therapist raised the possibility that he could meet with Fred and Sandra for two or three more sessions before returning to individual work with Fred. Both agreed to this, and time was spent both on the grief issues surrounding the miscarriage as well as the communication difficulties the couple was having. Fred continued in individual therapy for several sessions thereafter, and at the end of treatment felt that the conflict was largely resolved. He was also able to appreciate that he needed to be more active and clear in communicating with Sandra.

In summary, the case is an illustration of the value in obtaining information about communication from a variety of sources. It also illustrates the classic IPT paradigm in which an acute psychosocial stressor leads to interpersonal problems in a vulnerable individual. In this case, Fred's insecure attachment traits and communication style led him to be vulnerable to the loss experience of the miscarriage.

CONCLUSION

Communication analysis is an extremely important part of IPT, as it is aimed directly at one of the root causes of patient's distress – namely that his or her attachment needs are not being met sufficiently. Helping the patient to recognize patterns in communication, understand ways in which his or her communication is not effective, and then helping the patient to change his or her communication is the essence of the technique.

REFERENCES

1. Kiesler, D.J., Watkins, L.M. 1989. Interpersonal complimentarity and the therapeutic alliance: a study of the relationship in psychotherapy. *Psychotherapy* **26**, 183–94.
2. Rogers, C.R. 1957. The necessary and sufficient conditions of therapeutic personality change. *Journal of Consulting Psychology* **21**, 95–103.

Interpersonal Incidents

INTRODUCTION

One of the explicit and overriding goals of IPT is helping patients to improve their inter-personal communication. The therapeutic aim, given the patient's underlying attach-ment style, is to help the patient more closely meet his or her attachments needs by communicating them more effectively to others. In IPT, one of the most powerful means to bring this about is to collect information about Interpersonal Incidents. The technique allows for a more thorough understanding of the communication that is occurring, and is also helpful in assisting the patient to begin to appreciate the ways in which he or she is not communicating effectively with others. Interpersonal Incidents are frequently used as a form of communication analysis.

In essence, an Interpersonal Incident is an episode in which communication occurs between the patient and significant others. An 'Interpersonal Incident' is a description by the patient of a *specific* interaction with his or her attachment figures or social contacts – it is not a description of a general pattern of interaction. For instance, if an identified dispute is a conflict between spouses, the therapist might ask the patient to 'describe the last time you and your spouse got into a fight,' or to 'describe one of the more recent big fights you had with your spouse.' The therapist should direct the patient to describe in detail the communication which occurred in each of the specific incidents, taking care to recreate the dialogue as accurately as possible. The patient should also be directed to describe his or her affective responses as well as both verbal and non-verbal responses, and to describe observations of his or her spouse's non-verbal behavior.

The purpose of discussing an Interpersonal Incident is four-fold:

1   To collect information regarding the miscommunication that is occurring between the parties.

2   To provide insight to the patient about the unrealistic view that the problem is insoluble.
3   To help the patient recognize his or her style of communication and its consequences.
4   To motivate the patient to change his or her communication.

CLARIFYING INTERPERSONAL INCIDENTS

In psychotherapy, patients will often describe interactions with significant others in very general terms, leaving the therapist with little information about the specific communication which has occurred. For instance, a patient may say that her husband, 'never listens to her.' This statement strongly implies that the patient believes two things:

1   The problem is pervasive – her husband literally never listens to her, and there are no exceptions.
2   The situation is permanent and unchangeable – i.e., her husband not only doesn't listen to her now, but will continue to ignore her in the future.

Given these beliefs, it is no surprise that such a patient feels a sense of hopelessness. If her statement and the implications are in fact true – if in fact her husband never listens to her and never will – the only options left to the patient are to put up with the relationship and continue to suffer, or to end the relationship. No middle ground, compromise, or improvement in the communication is possible.

A general statement like this, which conveys to the therapist the hopelessness of the patient and her frustration with a primary relationship, cannot be allowed to stand in therapy. Irrespective of the approach taken, the therapist must work on the patient's sense of frustration and helplessness, or the relationship problem will continue, along with the psychological distress the patient is suffering. Externalized attributions of problems by the patient must be challenged by the therapist.

There are several different ways of approaching a patient who makes a general statement like this in therapy. First, the therapist might choose to challenge the veracity of the patient's statement. For instance, the therapist might ask if it is really true that her husband always ignores her all of the time and under all circumstances. Exceptions would be sought – perhaps there were times in the past that were different. A cognitive therapist might challenge the distorted and absolute thinking of a patient who made a statement like this, perhaps assigning homework with the specific intent of determining whether her husband did in fact always ignore her.

In contrast to an approach which questions the accuracy of the patient's cognitions, the IPT therapist is interested in the way in which the patient communicates his or her attachment needs. IPT is directed at the patient's communications, and is concerned with the ways in which the communication between the patient and her significant other is maladaptive. In other words, rather than addressing any internal processes, the IPT therapist is concerned with examining the interpersonal communication which is occurring in the relationship.

The hypothesis under which an Interpersonal Incident is analyzed is that the 'problem' presented by the patient is the result of poor communication. In other words, something is going 'wrong' in the communication between the patient and her husband.

IPT does not presuppose blame; rather, it is assumed that the communication in the system is maladaptive. In fact, in a situation in which there is a clear-cut dispute between two individuals, it is preferable to meet with both in therapy to observe the communication *in vivo*. Unfortunately, it is often not possible to do so – in marital disputes one partner may not be willing to attend the sessions; in conflicts at work only one party may attend; and there are a variety of situations in which only one of the people involved in the conflict is willing or able to come to therapy. The principle in IPT in such a situation is to work with the person who does come, with the hope that as that individual changes his or her communication, the system as a whole will change as well.

Thus, the hypothesis is that the patient (and her husband) are not communicating in such as way that the patient's attachment needs are being met. (It is, of course, quite possible that her husband's interpersonal and emotional needs are not being met either.) The IPT therapist works from the position that both parties are not communicating effectively, and that both likely have unmet needs. It is also likely that both are assuming that their communication is being understood and that they are understanding the other person as well, when in fact this is almost certainly not the case.

A general statement such as 'my husband never listens to me,' also conveys a great deal about the patient's reluctance to address her own behavior and her possible contributions to the problem. In other words, such unqualified statements are at one level an attempt by the patient to influence the therapist, so that he or she will come to share the same absolutist view as the patient – i.e., that 'blame' for the problem is external to the patient. Such a statement literally 'elicits' a response from the therapist in which he or she is drawn to sympathize with the patient and to say something like 'if I had a husband like that, I'd feel frustrated too.' Thus, the patient's statement is in part an attempt to pull in the therapist as an accomplice in blaming her husband for the problem.

Consider, for example, the differences in presentation below. In the first example, the patient makes a general statement about her husband which indicates a complete externalization of the problem – it is all her husband's fault. The first patient is literally attempting to elicit a response from the therapist which confirms her world view and which absolves her from responsibility for change. Conversely, in the second example, the patient indicates some degree of insight, an openness to change, and enlists the therapist to help to create that change.

Case example 1: General statement

Patient: It's all my husband's fault – he never listens to me!

(Note that blame is placed on the husband with no acknowledgment by the patient of any responsibility for the communication problem. Insight is very limited. The therapist can respond by accepting the patient's statement as fact, by challenging it, or by asking for more information about the situation.)

Therapist: Tell me more.

Patient: Well, he has a bad habit of always ignoring people, and as soon as he thinks anyone is being critical, he simply walks away. He'll never change.

(The patient attempts to elicit a sympathetic response from the therapist, hoping to gain an accomplice in blaming her husband. An IPT therapist would move here into an Interpersonal Incident to get more information about the communication that is occurring and to begin to challenge the absolute statement of the patient.)

Case example 2: Specific statement

Patient: My husband and I have been having some problems lately in talking about things. I feel very frustrated.

(Note the absence of absolute conditions, the framing of the problem as mutual and systemic, and the inclusion of a description of feeling state by the patient. The patient moves to enlist the therapist as an expert in helping her solve the problem.)

Therapist: Tell me more.

Patient: Well, over the last several months when we try to talk about the finances, both of us end up getting really frustrated. He has a tendency to withdraw when he thinks that I am getting critical, but he doesn't seem to understand how worried I am about our money right now.

(The patient recognizes her husband's response to her communication, has some insight into her contribution to the problem, and also understands that there is a mutual communication problem. This patient will be much easier to work with as she is open to change, as opposed to the patient in the first example.)

General statements such as 'my husband never listens to me,' though containing a grain of truth, almost always represent only one (very biased) side of the story. What is more likely is that while the patient's husband may indeed be insensitive, some of his non-responsiveness is due to the communication style of the patient. She may, though intending otherwise, come across as critical or uncaring, or may simply be trying to communicate at a time when it will not be well received. She may also be unwittingly ignoring important communications from her husband.

The general statement does not contain any of this information. More detail must be obtained. Therefore, when eliciting Interpersonal Incidents, the therapist's goal is to have the patient recreate, in as much detail as possible, a specific interaction between herself and her husband. This should not be a *typical* interaction, which will allow the patient to continue making general statements – it must be a *specific* incident. As this is not usually what patients spontaneously talk about, the therapist must direct the patient to produce this material. The goal is to use this 'step-by-step' (or perhaps better put, 'blow-by-blow') report to understand the way in which the patient conveys her attachment needs, acting on the hypothesis that she is communicating in such a way that she is being misunderstood and is therefore not being responded to as she would like.

Case example: Maude

Maude was a 42-year-old woman who sought treatment for a marital problem. She had been married for 11 years, and had two children aged five and seven. She reported that things in her marriage with Harold had been deteriorating over the last 2 years, culminating with his decision to quit his job and become a day trader in stocks. She reported that she was very concerned about their finances, and that he had not been willing to talk to her in detail about them. By her report he got very defensive when she questioned him about their financial situation. She reported that she felt that the family was essentially living off of her salary while Harold was 'gambling' with the family's future.

Her initial description of the conflict was a classic general statement about the relationship:

> **Therapist:** Tell me about your relationship with your husband.
> **Maude:** He never seems to listen to me. I am getting very worried about the finances, and he will never talk about it. He just gets defensive. To be honest, I came to therapy in part to try and decide if it would be better if the children and I left him.

A grid can be used to display graphically the process which occurs while exploring Interpersonal Incidents (Figure 10.1). The patient's communications can be divided into general statements and specific statements, and the emotional descriptions of events can also be either general or specific. The process with Maude began with her general statement about her husband, 'he never listens to me.' If this were true, and if the situation is as she describes, her concerns are quite warranted, and it is quite understandable that she would think about a divorce as a way of escaping the situation. Before accepting this as fact, however, the therapist should move into a specific Interpersonal Incident to determine if her general statement is accurate.

The next step in the process is to ask the patient to connect her affective responses to the general statement. In essence, the therapist should ask the patient to describe how she feels about the situation in general. The goal is to connect symptoms with the interpersonal problem, and to help the patient become more affectively engaged in the process – it is important because it is causing distress (Figure 10.2). In this case, Maude described feeling very hopeless, frustrated, and angry.

	Specific incident	**General statement**
Content		My husband never listens to me
Affect		

Figure 10.1 *Interpersonal Incidents: General Statement.*

	Specific incident	**General statement**
Content		My husband never listens to me
Affect		I feel depressed, frustrated and angry

Figure 10.2 *Interpersonal Incidents: General Affect.*

After obtaining information about the emotional content of the conflict and connecting it to the interpersonal communication problem, the therapist should specifically ask the patient to describe an Interpersonal Incident. This can be done by asking the patient to describe either a recent conflict, or to describe an incident that is a good example of the conflict problems – the patient should not, however, describe the 'typical' pattern of interaction, as this will perpetuate the presentation of the general statement of the problem. The therapist must direct the patient to present a *specific* interaction so that the specific communication can be examined in detail. Directives such as 'Tell me about the last time you and your husband got into conflict,' or 'Tell me about one of the big conflicts you have had recently,' are good ways for the therapist to do this.

Once the patient begins to describe the interaction in detail, the therapist must then direct the patient to produce, as closely as possible, the exact dialogue that occurred. In addition to the spoken communication, the patient should also be directed to describe the non-verbal communication, and should also describe the emotional content of the communication in detail. At this point, the goal of the therapist is to recreate, in as much detail as possible, an exact description of the episode of conflict.

The therapist should ask not only about the verbal interactions that occur, but also the non-verbal communications, such as using silence in a hostile fashion, slamming doors, or leaving the situation in the middle of an interaction. This should include a detailed description of what the patient said to begin the interaction, how her husband responded, what she understood him to say, how she responded in turn, and so forth until the end of the interaction. Special note should be made of the end of the interaction, as many conflicts may carry over to the next day, or may be brought up again in subsequent disagreements.

When asking Maude about this, the following dialogue ensued:

Therapist: Tell me about the last time that you and Harold had a disagreement about the finances.

Maude: Oh, we fight about it all the time.

Therapist: It would be most helpful if you could tell me about a specific time – perhaps one that has happened recently or is clear in your mind. I'd like to know about the specific details as much as possible.

Maude: Well, the last time that comes to mind is a fight we had last Tuesday after dinner. We were eating late, and had put the kids to bed.

Therapist: What happened?

Maude: I asked him how his day was, and then we got into a fight.

Therapist: Tell me more about what exactly was said.

Maude: I think I said something like 'I suppose you have been making loads of money again today.'

Therapist: That's the way it started?

Maude: Yes, and then he said 'Don't start that up again.'

Therapist: What did you say next?

Maude: I said 'We've got to talk about this sometime, so quit trying to avoid it.'

Therapist: What happened next?

Maude: He got up and left.

In contrast to Maude's initial report, the additional information suggested that there was more to the story. Asking about a specific incident allowed the therapist to

	Specific incident	General statement
Content	Tuesday evening we had a fight after dinner	My husband never listens to me
Affect		I feel depressed, frustrated and hopeless

Figure 10.3 *Interpersonal Incidents: Specific Incident.*

more clearly examine the communication that was occurring, and to draw more accurate conclusions about what was causing the conflict and what might be done to resolve it (Figure 10.3).

The next task in the process is to connect emotional responses to the dialogue. In addition to the spoken words, the emotional content of the communications should be examined. Asking questions about what was affectively conveyed, how the patient felt about specific statements, and even the way in which she perceived her husband to be responding emotionally are crucial (Figure 10.4).

The following interaction occurred as the specific incident was discussed further:

Therapist: Tell me about your emotional reactions during that specific interaction.
Maude: I was furious. You know, I guess I was really quite mad going into the discussion – it had been building up for a long time, and I really wanted to let him know how angry I was with him.
Therapist: What was the tone of voice that you used when you made the statement about him making loads of money.
Maude: I was furious. I'm sure there was an edge to my voice, though I don't usually yell. In fact, I know that there was – I really want him to know how angry I am.
Therapist: How well do you think he understood what you were feeling?
Maude: I am quite sure he knew I was angry – no doubt about that.

	Specific incident	General statement
Content	Tuesday evening we had a fight after dinner	My husband never listens to me
Affect	I feel angry and hopeless	I feel depressed, frustrated and hopeless

Figure 10.4 *Interpersonal Incidents: Specific Affect.*

> **Therapist:** How do you think he was reacting emotionally as this particular conversation was occurring?
>
> **Maude** (pausing): I don't really know. That's a good question. I guess he must have been pretty frustrated too – I hadn't really thought about it.

At this point, the therapist has clarified the emotional aspects of the interaction in more detail. As the therapist asks questions about the emotional reactions Maude had, questions about her husband's reactions and motivations are introduced. The purpose in doing this is not only to collect more information, but also to generate some insight on the part of the patient. The idea is to move the patient from a feeling of anger, sadness, or hopelessness to a feeling of being misunderstood. This allows the patient to reframe the situation as one which she can do something about – if she is being misunderstood, then a change in communication may help resolve the problem.

In addition, questions about Harold's reactions and motivations are designed to help Maude reframe the situation as a problem within the relationship rather than externalizing it entirely to Harold. If she is able to understand his position, or if she becomes motivated to find out more about how he is reacting, communication will be improved.

The interaction continued:

> **Therapist:** It sounds like both of you may have had pretty strong feelings. I suspect that neither of you really got across what you were intending. You were clearly trying to let Harold know how angry you were, but I wonder if he really understood that you wanted to talk about it. His reaction – walking away I mean – would sure suggest that he didn't understand what you wanted.
>
> **Maude:** True enough, though I still think that he should know what is important to me. Now that I think about it, maybe it is a little much to ask for him to read my mind.
>
> **Therapist:** What do you think he was trying to communicate to you?
>
> **Maude:** Probably that he was angry too – and I think he is probably getting tired of having me pester him about the finances. Still, I don't know what to do – we've got to talk about it, and I am really worried that we are getting into a really deep hole.

At this point, the therapist elected to move on to some problem solving. Maude seemed to appreciate that her communication wasn't getting her what she wanted, and also was beginning to realize that her husband was communicating something too, although it wasn't entirely clear to her what that was (Figure 10.5). The problem solving

	Specific incident	**General statement**
Content	Tuesday evening we had a fight after dinner	My husband never listens to me
Affect	I felt misunderstood	I feel depressed, frustrated and hopeless

Figure 10.5 *Interpersonal Incidents: Introducing the Possibility of Change.*

was focused on two issues: first, to assist Maude to find some different ways to address her concerns so that she could get the response from Harold that she wanted, and second, to have her collect more information about what Harold was trying to communicate.

> **Therapist:** Let's try and do some brainstorming about how you might communicate more clearly – so that Harold can really understand what is bothering you in detail.
> **Maude:** Well, I suppose I could ask him directly to spend some time talking – the last several months I have been so angry I have just made snide remarks to get his attention. Still, it's such a hot topic for us that I don't know if that will work.
> **Therapist:** It may not work, but the results won't be any worse than what is happening now.
> **Maude:** That's certainly true – we don't seem to be getting anywhere now.
> **Therapist:** How could you find out more about what he is really feeling?
> **Maude:** I guess I'll just have to ask him.
> **Therapist:** When would be a good time to ask him about it, and to have the conversation?
> **Maude:** Tuesday evenings are the best – we have dinner late, and the kids are in bed – I hope we haven't set a precedent with our last fight!
> **Therapist:** Tuesday it is then. You'll have to let me know next week how it went.
> **Maude:** I'm a bit more optimistic now – he's not such a bad guy, you know.

At the end of the interaction, Maude had a different picture of the interaction between herself and her husband. Rather than viewing the problem as intractable, Maude now saw some hope that things could be different. By changing her communication, it was possible that she could get her needs met more effectively. Further, it was possible that her husband would do likewise in response if she were able to take an interest in what he was feeling and thinking instead of being critical. Finally, Maude and the therapist developed a plan of action designed to specifically address the problem, also giving her a sense of hope that things would improve.

The interaction can be depicted graphically – Maude's general statement began with an absolute that her husband never listened to her. The associated affect was that she felt depressed, frustrated, and hopeless. When discussing the specific Interpersonal Incident, she initially described feeling angry and hopeless. As the interaction was

	Specific incident	**General statement**
Content	Tuesday evening we had a fight after dinner because I started the conversation being critical	My husband never listens to me if I am critical of him
Affect	I felt misunderstood	I feel hopeful that things can change

Figure 10.6 *Interpersonal Incidents: Affective Shift.*

discussed in detail, her views changed as she began to see that she could change her communication and perhaps bring about different results. Her affect shifted to more of a feeling of hopefulness, and the hope that she felt about the specific interaction was then generalized, so that the absolute statement, 'he never listens to me' was transformed into a qualified, 'he doesn't listen to me when I approach him critically.' The affect in general was also shifted (Figure 10.6).

Over the next week, Maude attempted some of the communication changes that she and the therapist had discussed. Though she and her husband continued to have some conflict, Maude felt that the continued problem solving and refinement of her communication was quite helpful. Maude and the therapist continued to review additional Interpersonal Incidents to explore what was working, and what was not working, in the couple's communication. After about eight sessions, Harold – seeing the changes that were occurring with Maude – relented and came in for several sessions. He also reported that he felt the marriage had improved.

CONCLUSION

Communication analysis is simply a formal means of investigating the hypothesis that the patient's difficulties are being caused, perpetuated, or exacerbated by poor communication in a general sense. In contrast, the technique of examining Interpersonal Incidents expands upon this concept by focusing on particular key interactions in a patient's life. It is particularly useful in dealing with disputes and issues of interpersonal sensitivity, and in helping patients with less secure attachments to understand how their style of communicating may be contributing to the relationship problem.

Table 10.1 *Interpersonal Incidents*

The therapeutic goals are to:

- Collect information regarding the miscommunication that is occurring between the parties.
- Provide insight to the patient about the unrealistic view that the problem is insoluble.
- Help the patient recognize his or her style of communication and its consequences.
- Motivate the patient to change his or her communication.

The therapist's tasks are to:

- Actively investigate specific interpersonal incidents.
- Help the patient identify problematic communication.
- Assist in problem solving so that communication can be improved.

11

Use of Affect

INTRODUCTION

As in any form of psychotherapy, recognition of the patient's affective state is crucial in IPT. The more affectively engaged the patient is in therapy, the more likely it is that change will occur.

In IPT, there are several goals regarding affect:

1   To assist the patient to recognize his or her immediate affect.
2   To assist the patient to communicate his or her affect more effectively to others.
3   To facilitate the patient's recognition of affect that may have been suppressed, or that the patient may find painful to acknowledge.

CONTENT AND PROCESS AFFECT

The most obvious technique that the therapist can use to reach these goals is to give direct feedback to the patient regarding how he or she perceives the patient's affective state. This must be done, of course, in the context of a relationship in which the patient can tolerate this feedback, and also make use of it. This requires a high degree of inclusion in the treatment relationship and reflects the importance of the therapeutic alliance. If these conditions are met, remarking to the patient that he or she appears sad, angry, pleased, or demonstrates other affective states may be of great help.

A variation of this technique with particular relevance to IPT rests on the therapist's observation of 'process' and 'content' affect. *Process affect* is the affect that the patient displays during the conduct of therapy, i.e., the affect that he or she displays in session

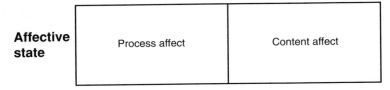

Figure 11.1 *'Content Affect' versus 'Process Affect.'*

with the therapist while discussing important issues. *Content affect*, on the other hand, is the affect that the patient reports having experienced in the past, in interactions outside of the therapeutic relationship (Figure 11.1).

These two types of affect may be congruent, or they may be dissimilar. For instance, when describing the death of a spouse a year previously, a patient may describe the following:

> 'When my husband died, I was an emotional wreck. I was really depressed, I couldn't eat for several days, and I slept terribly for a month.'

The *content affect*, or the emotional state reported at the time of the death, would be described as sad, upset, and depressed.

When describing the experience in therapy, however, the same patient may display a *process affect* very different from the *content affect* described in the past. For instance, the therapist may note that the patient describes the event in therapy in a very flat or monotonous voice, or is telling the story as if reporting that it happened to someone else. In a case like this, the *process affect* would be described as neutral or flat.

The converse might also occur. The woman might describe the death of her spouse in the following way:

> 'When my husband died, I was the one who kept the family together. I took care of all of the arrangements – I was so busy I never had the chance to cry. I mostly remember feeling numb.'

The *content affect* in this case would be described as flat or neutral at best.

When describing the experience in therapy, the patient might be upset, sad, or even tearful, and the *process affect* would be sad or depressed (Figure 11.2).

When working with content and process affect, it is extremely important for the therapist to be aware of incongruities in the patient's presentation. In other words, when process and content affect are dissimilar, it signals the therapist that the topic under discussion should be explored further. It also signals that the therapist, when the patient is able to tolerate the feedback, should point out the incongruity to the patient. This will assist the patient to become aware of emotions that he or she may be suppressing, or that he or she may be aware of but is finding difficult to acknowledge.

Case example: Joe

Joe was a 45-year-old man who came to therapy following the death of his father, which he identified as the primary issue leading to his depression. His father had died a year previously, and Joe had resisted coming to therapy until his wife had finally strongly suggested that he do so. Though he reported being able to function both at

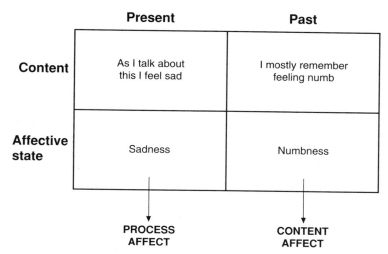

Figure 11.2 *Content and process affect.*

home and work, he reluctantly admitted that his productivity had gone down; he was having trouble concentrating, sleeping, and his libido was greatly decreased. Though he was reluctant to come to treatment, he was able to admit that, 'my wife was right, I should have come to therapy a long time ago.'

After completing the Interpersonal Inventory, both Joe and his therapist agreed that the primary problem area was grief and loss, and that work needed to be done regarding the death of Joe's father. In the third session, the therapist asked Joe to recount the circumstances surrounding his father's death, to which Joe replied:

> 'My father died quite suddenly of a heart attack ... he had been in good health, and no one expected it. My mother found him outside in the yard where he had been gardening, and he was already gone. My mother must have felt really guilty somehow, because she insisted that they do everything they could to save him, even though he had probably been dead for several hours. When they brought him to the hospital, they tried to do CPR and stuck him full of tubes and lines. ... When I finally got to the hospital they wouldn't let me in to see him. It was several hours later that I got in, and by then, he had wires and tubes stuck everywhere – it didn't even look like my dad.
>
> I don't remember feeling anything when I saw him, just thinking, "this isn't really him – I just need to get this mess cleaned up." So I started throwing all the needles and tubes and stuff away until a nurse came in and told me to stop.
>
> I didn't feel anything at the funeral either – I was too busy trying to help my mom, and I had to take care of all the funeral arrangements. I haven't even been to the cemetery since he was buried. ...'

During this report, the therapist noted that Joe's affect when relating the story was extremely sad and tearful. His voice was quivering, and he clearly had a great deal of difficulty in recounting the story without breaking down. Using the discrepancy in process and content affect, the therapist remarked:

> 'As you're telling the story, I can really begin to understand what that must have been like for you. It's clearly difficult to talk about – you even look sad and tearful as you're

speaking. There is clearly a lot of emotion you're experiencing now that you weren't in touch with at the time your father died. My experience has been that it is really helpful for a lot of people to talk about experiences like yours – when someone so important has died, it's important to have time to grieve, even if it is a while after the actual death.'

'Tell me some more about your experience.'

The content and affect incongruity was a clear signal to the therapist that the grief experience was at the core of Joe's difficulties. Furthermore, work needed to be done in helping Joe to express his emotional reaction to his father's death – both his reactions to the immediate circumstances surrounding it, and his current feelings. The therapist's open-ended query to 'Tell me more about your experience' was designed to get that process started.

Subsequent sessions, consistent with the IPT goals of helping patients to better communicate their needs and to build a more effective social support network, focused on a discussion about friends and family with whom Joe could talk to further about his experience and feelings about his father's death. He was able to quite readily share his feelings with his wife, who was very supportive. He also approached a friend at work who had also lost his father recently, and felt very supported in that relationship as well. Towards the end of therapy, he made a decision to speak with his mother, whom he had largely avoided, about his anger that she had not let his father 'die in peace' in the hospital. Though this issue was not resolved when therapy was concluded, he did feel that he had made some progress with her, and had at least 'opened the door' to developing a better relationship with her.

In addition to being an extremely useful technique when dealing with grief and loss issues, the use of content and process affect is also very helpful in dealing with interpersonal disputes. The technique is particularly effective when combined with the use of interpersonal incidents.

Many patients who report interpersonal disputes will do so in a dispassionate way. In other words, a patient will 'present the case' to the therapist in a logical and unemotional way, largely because one of the purposes in relating the conflict to the therapist is to externalize the blame for the problem. The goal is to convince the therapist that the patient him or herself is not to blame – rather it is the 'other person' with whom he or she is in conflict. A patient will often modify the way in which the dispute is presented so as to convince the therapist of the correctness of the patient's point of view. In order to do this more effectively and dispassionately, *patients will often report the emotional content of an Interpersonal Incident with a neutral process affect, despite reporting a very angry or hostile content affect.* Stories of conflicts which are fraught with content affect, such as yelling and screaming, are often initially reported by the patient with neutral and unemotional process affect.

When there is a clear discrepancy between the reported content affect in a conflict-laden Interpersonal Incident and the process affect that is apparent in therapy (typically lack of strong affect), it is a signal to the therapist to delve more into the conflict. The discrepancy should also point out the need for the therapist to reflect to the patient the difference in content and process affect. The purpose in doing this is two-fold: (i) it leads the patient to become more affectively engaged in the process of therapy, and as a consequence more likely to be motivated to change; and (ii) it gives the therapist a much more accurate report of the emotions that were expressed in the Interpersonal Incident, allowing both therapist and patient to understand more fully how the patient's communication in that incident was not effective.

Case example: Debbie

Debbie was a 32-year-old woman who reported difficulty in her relationship with her husband. Though she denied specific symptoms of depression and did not meet diagnostic criteria for any major psychiatric disorder, both she and her therapist felt that she would benefit a great deal from IPT with a focus on her relationship with her husband. While he was perfectly happy to have her come to therapy, she reported that he had no interest in attending sessions himself.

Early in therapy, Debbie related an incident which she felt characterized the communication between herself and her husband. The conflict involved the care of their 1-year-old son: several days before the session, her husband had called her at her workplace late in the afternoon to tell her that he had 'forgotten' he had a meeting that evening, and would be unable to pick up their son from daycare. After a brief phone call which concluded with her hanging up on him, she cancelled her last meeting of the day in order to be able to pick up her son herself. She reported that she felt her meeting was at least as important as that of her husband, and that she was furious about his refusal to keep his commitment to pick up their son. The following therapeutic dialogue ensued:

Therapist: Tell me more about the incident between yourself and your husband.
Debbie: I was in the midst of an important meeting when the secretary interrupted me to tell me I had an important call. At first, I was afraid that something serious might have happened to my son at daycare – calls like that always worry me. When I got on the line and found out it was my husband, I felt relieved at first. Then he told me that he had a late meeting that he had forgotten about, and wouldn't be able to pick up Jason from daycare. My first reaction, of course, was to make sure that Jason was alright – that someone would pick him up. Then I thought 'he (husband) always does this – he never follows through on things or keeps up his commitments.' I felt really angry at him (spoken with virtually no process emotion), but then I thought things through logically, and decided that if I didn't pick up Jason myself, no one would.
Therapist: How did the phone call end?
Debbie: Oh – I hung up on him . . . slammed down the phone I think. My husband is always doing things like that, you know. (Again spoken completely dispassionately, almost matter-of-factly.)

It was clear to the therapist that there was much more to the story – Debbie's process affect was quite neutral and objective, and she was communicating to the therapist that she was behaving logically and rationally. The fault, as she presented it, was entirely with her husband. However, there was a clear discrepancy between Debbie's content and process affect, as the content of her story revealed a great deal of anger that Debbie was not displaying in therapy. Slamming down the phone, for instance, was likely a very forceful communication of anger or hurt, but that affect was not apparent in Debbie's report in therapy. The therapist felt that helping Debbie to recognize the incongruity between her content and process affect would help her to better understand how she was communicating, and how her communications might be misunderstood by her husband. Further, the therapist believed that it would help her to become more engaged in therapy and increase her motivation to change. The therapist intervened in the following way:

Therapist: It sounds like there was quite a bit of conflict between the two of you even during that brief phone call. I noticed, however, that as you were relating the story, it was almost as if you were telling the story about someone else. I didn't get much of an idea about how you were really feeling. It would help me to understand better what that was like for you if you could tell me more about how you are feeling about that incident right now as we're talking about it.
Debbie: Well ... actually I am pretty angry about it. I don't like to think about that though, because I'm afraid that if I think about how angry I am, I won't be able to control it. One time that actually happened . . . .

Debbie went on to relate an incident during which she felt she had got really angry at her husband, and as she did so, she became much more affectively engaged in telling the story. With an emerging recognition of her feelings, Debbie and the therapist were able to examine how she was (or was not) accurately communicating her feelings to her husband, and they were able to explore ways that she might be able to communicate more directly and effectively.

CONCLUSION

The recognition of incongruity between content and process affect is extremely important in IPT. Recognizing these discrepancies will help both patient and therapist understand the ways in which the patient is communicating, and will also draw the patient more into the therapeutic process – the more affectively engaged the patient is, the more likely that change will occur. The technique is particularly helpful when dealing with grief and loss and interpersonal disputes.

Table 11.1 *Use of Affect in IPT*

The therapeutic goals are to achieve:
• Recognition of difficult affect and emotions.
• More accurate representation of communication.
• Increased engagement in the therapeutic process.
• Increased motivation for change.
The therapist's tasks are to:
• Recognize discrepancies between content and process affect.
• Identify these differences for the patient.
• Facilitate discussion of affect.

12

Role Playing

INTRODUCTION

Role playing is a technique in which the patient and therapist create an *in vitro* interaction in therapy to reinforce behavioral change outside of therapy. While role playing, the patient's communication style and his or her mode of affective interaction can be examined in detail. In addition, the patient can often gain a better understanding of the experience of others involved in the patient's social relationships.

Role playing is best used to depict key past or future interactions between patients and their significant others such as conflicts or situations involving interpersonal sensitivities. In both situations, role playing allows more effective communications to be discussed, modeled, and practiced. Role playing is not a mandatory intervention in IPT; it is best used with selected patients and with selected problems. It tends to be most effective when the therapeutic relationship is such that the patient is feeling supported and can tolerate a degree of confrontation by the therapist. Patients with more secure styles of attachment are more likely to benefit from role playing.

The goals of role playing in IPT are to:

- Help the patient develop new insights into his or her interpersonal behavior.
- Allow the therapist to model new modes of interpersonal behavior and communication.
- Allow the patient to practice new interpersonal communication skills.
- Help the patient to gain new perspectives on the reactions of significant others to the patient's communications.

THERAPEUTIC USES OF ROLE PLAYING

Role playing is helpful in achieving a variety of clinical ends in IPT. In essence it is useful in at least four ways:

1   *As a tool for gathering information*: the therapist, while observing the patient playing him or herself, can collect a great deal of information about the patient's style of communication. Problematic interactions can also be re-enacted, and examined for specific instances of miscommunication.
2   *As a tool for implementing changes*: the therapist can give the patient direct constructive feedback about his or her communications, which can then be incorporated into new ways to communicate more effectively.
3   *As a means of practicing and reinforcing communication*: new styles of communication can be practiced before extending them to the patient's social relationships.
4   *As a means of developing insight into a patient's interpersonal behavior*: as the patient observes him or herself interacting in a role playing situation, he or she can reflect upon what is really being communicated, and how clearly the communication is occurring. Role playing literally requires that the patient enlist his or her 'observing ego' as the communication occurs, and requires that the patient stop and think about what is being said.

TYPES OF ROLE PLAY

Role playing may be structured so that the patient plays him or herself or plays a significant other, with the therapist taking the complimentary role. In each of these formats, the emphasis of the role playing differs.

The patient as self

Having the patient play himself or herself in a role playing exercise is useful in at least two situations. During the initial phases of IPT, when the goal is to better understand the nature of the patient's interpersonal problems, role playing can provide very useful information about the way in which the patient 'really' communicates, as opposed to simply relying on the patient's self-report. The patient's particular style of communicating with, interacting with, and approaching others is often more readily apparent during role playing. Affect is also often more apparent while role playing. Role playing often reveals discrepancies between a patient's report of his or her communications and that which are actually occurring.

In later sessions, role playing may be an ideal medium for the rehearsal of new communication skills. Behavioral changes such as anger or anxiety management can be practiced. Specific situations, such as confrontations or interviews, can also be practiced.

In either situation, role playing is enhanced if the therapist is able to give the patient direct feedback about his or her specific communications. Doing so requires a solid therapeutic alliance, as this feedback can be threatening to some patients, particularly those with less secure attachment styles. Nonetheless, in such instances where the therapist judges that it will be helpful, interrupting the role play periodically to give direct feedback can be quite helpful.

An example in which direct feedback can be productively used is a role play of a job interview. As the patient plays him or herself, the therapist can intermittently step out of the interviewer role to give direct feedback to the patient about verbal communication, such as being too soft-spoken or too passive. Non-verbal communication can also be addressed, and is often even more important in such situations. The therapist might reflect, for instance, that maintaining more direct eye contact, or giving a more firm handshake, might better impress prospective employers.

The patient as other

Having the patient depict a significant other while role playing can provide the therapist with a unique window into the patient's experience of that person and the interpersonal problem in which they are engaged. Patients frequently become more affectively charged as they engage in role playing and more accurately convey the types of behavior exhibited by others – this is often quite enlightening for the therapist.

The patient may also alter his or her impressions of the significant other when depicting that person during a role-playing exercise. For instance, a patient may describe the other person to the therapist as unreasonable, but when depicting the other in the context of a role play, may recognize that some of the other person's responses may be provoked by the patient.

There is risk in having some patients play a significant other. If the patient is somewhat passive-aggressive, he or she may be bent on 'proving' to the therapist that the other, not the patient, is completely to blame for the interpersonal problem. The patient may then portray the other as completely unreasonable in an attempt to convince the therapist that this is the case. The patient may, by dramatically portraying a hostile significant other, make it nearly impossible for the therapist (playing the role of the patient) to respond. Therapeutic judgment should rule the day – if an aggressive, hostile, or histrionic patient is hell-bent on proving to the therapist that the other is at fault, the therapist should beat a hasty retreat and move on to other techniques.

The therapist as patient

Playing the patient role affords the therapist the opportunity to demonstrate different styles of communication for the patient. The therapist may model communication techniques such as reflective listening by paraphrasing what was said by the other person. Techniques such as assertiveness, non-confrontational feedback and appropriate handling of aggression may also be modeled by the therapist, and then reinforced by switching the roles so that the patient plays him or herself and can practice the techniques that have been demonstrated.

A portrayal of the patient which emphasizes his or her relative strengths in interpersonal interactions may be greatly reassuring for the patient, and a significant therapeutic intervention, particularly when interpersonal sensitivity is an issue. Positive reinforcement is nearly always therapeutic if honestly delivered. The therapist should, however, generally avoid depicting negative aspects of a patient's behavior, such as poor communication or maladaptive non-verbal communication, because it risks appearing insensitive at best, and derisive at worst. It is much better for the therapist to give such feedback directly to the patient outside of the role play, or to give such feedback to the patient when he or she is playing him or herself.

There is certainly good reason, however, for the therapist to model for the patient new and more positive ways of communicating. This can be done either subtly without calling direct attention to the new communications, or can be done after bringing the patient's attention to the new communication that is being demonstrated. The therapist should use his or her judgment to determine which is most suitable at any given moment in therapy.

The therapist as other

In this mode, the therapist depicts another significant individual. In the early stages of IPT this may be useful to gain insight into the patient's typical style of communication beyond what is obtainable through the patient's self-report; later in therapy it is useful as a means of having the patient practice new communication skills. New situations which the patient might encounter, particularly if interpersonal sensitivity is at issue, can also be enacted. In all of these situations, the therapist can intermittently stop the role play to give direct feedback to the patient about his or her specific communications.

POTENTIAL DIFFICULTIES USING ROLE PLAYING

The patient is reluctant or unable to role play

As role playing is an active and potentially anxiety-provoking process, some patients may be reluctant to participate in it, or may find it difficult or unpleasant. In these circumstances the therapist may choose to postpone the role play and move to a less confrontative intervention. The therapist should also consider the possibility that the therapeutic alliance is not sufficient for the patient to feel comfortable role playing, and if that is the case, should both delay the intervention and work on fostering the alliance.

The therapist may also explore the possibility that the patient's reluctance to partici-pate in the role-playing exercise is a manifestation of his or her interpersonal difficulties, and that these should be further explored in therapy. If so, the therapist can gently discuss with the patient the factors that seem to make engaging in role playing difficult, taking care not to blame the patient nor frame the difficulty as a therapeutic failure. The therapist can then question how such factors affect the patient's relationships outside of therapy.

The therapist may find that the patient is:

- Anxious about meeting the therapist's expectations.
- Fearful of negative evaluation by the therapist.
- Anxious about his or her ability to 'perform.'

In all of these cases, the therapist can explore the way that these and similar issues affect the patient's relationships outside of therapy.

As with all interventions, the therapist can anticipate problems in advance by considering the patient's attachment style. Those patients who tend to be insecurely attached may find the more confrontative forms of role play, such as the therapist playing the patient, either distressing or anxiety provoking. In these cases the therapist may opt to postpone the role play or consider a less confrontational form of role play. In some situations the therapist might opt to use a one-sided form of role play, such as asking the patient to imagine that his or her spouse was present and could be directly addressed. Such a modification, however, will nearly always lose some of the affective impact of a true role-playing intervention, as the patient will often be looking to the therapist for the 'right' way of saying things rather than being more spontaneous and engaged in his or her part.

The therapist cannot accurately depict the significant other

The therapist can only base his or her 'rendition' of the significant other upon the account that the patient offers. If the therapist depicts the patient's attachment figure in a way that the patient deems inaccurate, the therapist can use the opportunity to explore the basis of the inaccuracy. This can often lead naturally into asking the patient about how the significant other behaves and communicates, followed by an invitation to the patient to play the role of the other to demonstrate the point. It may also be an opportunity to ask the patient, once he or she describes the significant other in more accurate terms, to describe how he or she responds to the difficulties presented by the other person.

For instance, if the patient tells the therapist that he or she is not accurately portraying the anger that the patient's spouse usually displays, the therapist can ask the patient for more details about how that anger is expressed. This can be followed with queries about how the patient deals with the anger – what does he or she do when confronted by the spouse? How does the anger affect the relationship? How does the patient feel in response, and how is that communicated?

In summary, though the therapist should certainly attempt to 'get it right' the first time, there is a great deal of material that can be gleaned from this particular type of poor acting.

The therapist depicts the patient in a manner that is upsetting for the patient

When role playing, an ounce of prevention is worth a pound of cure. This situation should be avoided at all costs, and can best be averted by keeping to *the absolute rule that the therapist's task in playing the patient's role is to reinforce the patient's strengths and to model new communication techniques.* In IPT, the therapist should never portray the patient in a negative fashion, nor use the patient role to point out the patient's faults. There is simply no justification for doing so, as it will invariably come across to the patient as demeaning. Further, this type of indirect and critical communication is a very poor example for the therapist to set. In cases in which feedback to the patient about his or her communication style would be helpful, the therapist can provide this directly and constructively while the patient is playing him or herself, rather than when the therapist is playing the patient.

Case example: Sarah

Sarah was a 34-year-old woman who had been referred for IPT for marital problems. She complained that after the birth of her daughter Jenny, her husband James had failed to contribute to the care of the baby as he had agreed to do. While Sarah initially reported that this had been the first major dispute during their relationship, there were, after a careful history was taken, several other conflicts which became apparent. It appeared that in each, Sarah's typical style was to attempt to avoid the conflict by ignoring it, and that she rarely was able to confront James about her anger. It appeared that the couple had been able to 'bypass' the specific postpartum problem in this fashion with Sarah avoiding the issue. In contrast to previous situations, however, her anger, though not expressed to James, had gotten to the point that she was considering leaving the relationship. She had yet to express this to James, however, who had apparently only noticed that she was much more sullen and withdrawn than usual.

In her accounts of her interactions with James, Sarah had found it difficult to describe in detail the character of James' interactions with her. More importantly, she had trouble identifying the specific aspects that distressed and angered her. In order to further clarify this, the therapist proposed a role-playing exercise in which Sarah depicted her husband. The following exchange took place during the role play:

Therapist (as Sarah): James, I want to talk about Jenny.
Sarah (as James): [Sarah has picked up a newspaper and is holding it to obscure her face] Hmmm?
Therapist: Can we talk about Jenny?
Sarah: Um Hm.
Therapist: Does that mean yes?
Sarah: What?
Therapist: Does that mean yes we can talk?
Sarah: [still buried in the newspaper] About what?
Therapist: Jenny.
Sarah: [still behind newspaper] Our daughter Jenny.
Therapist: YES!!!!
Sarah: Mmm Hmm.
Therapist: [secretly wishing that a projectile was close at hand] Could you stop reading the paper for a minute and participate in the discussion? When I feel that you aren't paying attention to me when I'm trying to talk to you, it makes me feel very angry.
Sarah: No, I'm listening.

The therapist then suggested they stop the role play, asking Sarah:

Therapist: Is that how it really is?
Sarah: (with satisfaction) Oh yes.
Therapist: If he truly communicates like that, I can understand why you must feel so frustrated.
Sarah: Anyone who had to live with that guy would be frustrated, believe me!

Therapist: When he behaves like that, how does it make you feel?

Sarah: Incredibly angry!!! I feel ignored and unimportant, as if I don't matter at all.

Therapist: So what do you do?

Sarah: I usually just walk away – there's no point in talking to him.

Therapist: How well do you think that he understands how angry you are?

Sarah: Probably not at all – he doesn't seem to notice when I leave, or at least it doesn't seem to bother him.

Therapist: I wonder if there might be another way of communicating how you're feeling – let's try the role play again. By the way, you made it pretty tough on me when you were playing your husband – if you could help me out just a bit I think we could get a little farther.

Therapist (as Sarah): OK – let's get back to the discussion.

Sarah (as James): I thought I was discussing things.

Therapist: I think we need to get some things out on the table. I want you to know that I feel ignored and very angry when I try to talk to you and you don't look at me. I would appreciate it if you would put your paper down when we talk.

Sarah: But I like to unwind when I get home! All I need is 15 minutes by myself with the paper. You hit me with stuff right when I get in the door.

Therapist: Fair enough. If I agree to give you that 15 minutes uninterrupted, will you agree to spend some time talking with me about how we are splitting up the childcare duties?

Sarah: I guess so.

Therapist (out of role play again): What did you think of that?

Sarah: Well first, I don't think he'd be so reasonable. But it is true that I usually try to corner him right when he gets home – I'm so exhausted by that time that I just want to hand Jenny off and take a break myself.

Sarah was able to gain some insight into her husband's position, and to reflect on the ways in which she might be communicating poorly with him. In addition, the role play afforded the therapist the opportunity to model some new communication for Sarah. In subsequent role plays, the therapist was able to help Sarah develop communication and behavioral strategies to engage James more effectively, which allowed her to communicate her feelings and needs more clearly to him.

CONCLUSION

Role playing is one of the most demanding techniques in IPT, as well as being one of the most rewarding. It is invaluable as a tool for gathering information, particularly about the patient's communication and style of interpersonal interaction. As a tool for effecting change, it provides a supportive *in vitro* environment for the patient to develop and practice communication and interpersonal skills; this is particularly useful where there are issues of interpersonal sensitivity. As role playing is a demanding and confrontational intervention, its use as a 'tool' to help the patient resolve his or her interpersonal problems requires a significant degree of clinical judgment.

13

Problem Solving

INTRODUCTION

Problem solving is a fundamental intervention in IPT, and is a primary method for helping patients to bring about change in their interpersonal relationships. Problem solving is of help with all of the problem areas, but is particularly useful in dealing with Interpersonal Disputes and Role Transitions. An overview of the process of problem solving is depicted in Figure 13.1.

Problem solving, absent the technical jargon, is a directive technique in which the therapist attempts to help the patient develop solutions to a specific interpersonal problem and to implement the best of those solutions. It involves developing an accurate understanding of the problem, brainstorming with the patient to develop possible solutions, and implementing the solution that seems to be best suited to the situation. Between sessions the patient then attempts to carry out the solution, and reports back to the therapist at the next session with the results of that trial. The results are discussed in therapy, and if needed, modifications are made or new ideas are discussed.

Though the primary goal of the problem-solving intervention is to relieve the patient from the immediate stressor, a desirable side effect is to literally teach the patient to apply the problem-solving technique to other interpersonal situations that he or she might face. There is an old adage that states that giving a man a fish feeds him for a day, while teaching him to fish feeds him for a lifetime. This is a wonderful analogy for problem solving in IPT – the idea is both to help solve the immediate problem and to teach the patient the process of problem solving so that he or she is better equipped to deal with future interpersonal problems.

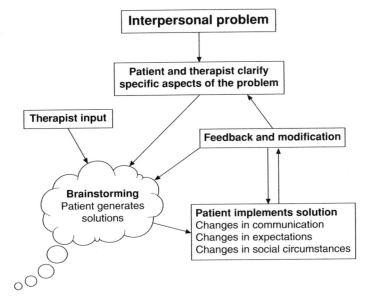

Figure 13.1 *An Overview of Problem Solving in IPT. The patient and therapist clarify a particular interpersonal problem. The patient is then encouraged by the therapist to generate solutions to the problem, implement them and monitor progress, modifying where necessary. The feedback process may lead to new problems which can be clarified, another round of brainstorming solutions, or to modifications of the solution that was implemented. This process enables the patient to develop a greater sense of mastery over the interpersonal problem.*

AN OVERVIEW OF PROBLEM SOLVING

Problem solving has four basic components:

1 Conducting a detailed examination of the problem.
2 Generating ('brainstorming') potential solutions.
3 Selecting a course of action.
4 Monitoring and refining the solution.

Conducting a detailed examination of the problem

This should include all relevant aspects of the history of the problem, as well as the patient's attempts to resolve it to date. Approaches that the patient has taken to similar problems in the past, successful or otherwise, should also be explored. Throughout the process, the problem should be linked to the patient's symptoms. The therapist should also help the patient to define the problem as specifically as possible. Attempting to address a general complaint that 'my marital relationship is going badly' is extremely difficult, as opposed to addressing a specific problem such as 'my spouse and I are having trouble talking about our finances.' The more specific the problem, the easier it is to address. It is the therapist's task while problem solving to help the patient break the problems down into manageable pieces.

Consider the case of a married woman with a depressive illness who is working to resolve an interpersonal dispute with her husband. She and the therapist would, as a matter of course in dealing with disputes, have examined the need to practice more effective communication. The specific problem is the inability of the couple to find time to communicate. In this case, the therapist is active in narrowing the focus of the problem:

> **Patient:** My husband never seems to want to spend time with me – he's not interested at all in my day or what's happening with me.
> **Therapist:** Sounds like the two of you don't talk much.
> **Patient:** My whole life and schedule is totally messed up – he doesn't understand at all.
> **Therapist:** I can imagine how difficult it must be to juggle all the responsibilities you have. Turning again to the dispute with your husband, can you tell me how you have tried to approach your communication problem with your husband thus far?
> **Patient:** Well, I have told him his work has to come second to his marriage!
> **Therapist:** I see. Did that get anywhere?
> **Patient:** No, he just became defensive.
> **Therapist:** Maybe if we concentrate on the specific communication problem the two of you are having, rather than attempting a total overhaul of both your schedules, the problem might be easier to address, and may also go a long way towards resolving the dispute with your husband.

Generating ('brainstorming') potential solutions

These should be the patient's own ideas as far as possible, and the 'ownership' of the process should remain with the patient. The therapist should aim, wherever possible, to have the patient generate the ideas to be discussed, as the aim of the intervention is not merely to resolve the acute crisis, but also to help the patient develop problem-solving skills.

'Brainstorming' solutions to interpersonal problems is basically a technique within the general rubric of problem solving. The patient should be encouraged to develop any and all ideas – even ones that at first may seem impractical. The goal at this stage is to develop a list of alternative solutions from which the patient can choose the one most likely to be effective.

During this process, the therapist can also introduce new solutions to the patient without directly telling the patient what to do. For instance, the therapist may share with the patient the solutions developed by other patients with whom the therapist has worked. The therapist could, if therapeutic judgment suggests it will be helpful, also offer suggestions which are framed as questions. Questions such as 'Have you considered. . .?' or 'I wonder if this approach might be helpful?' are relatively less directive than statements which tell the patient what course to follow. Introducing suggestions at this point also allows the patient to consider them as one of many options, and allows the patient to retain a sense of autonomy when choosing the option he or she wishes to follow.

Selecting a course of action

The bottom line in IPT is that the patient take action to resolve his or her interpersonal problems. This may take many forms – often a change in communication or an

```
┌─────────────────────────────────────────────────┐
│                                                 │
│        Problem − Boss won't give me pay rise    │
│                                                 │
│     Solution          Pros      Cons     Net +  │
│                                                 │
│     Ask directly       IIII      II       III   │
│                                                 │
│     Resign and          I        IIII      −    │
│     find another job                            │
│                                                 │
│     Go to union        IIII      IIII      −    │
│                                                 │
│     Rewrite job         III       II       I    │
│     description                                 │
│     ──────────────────────────────────────      │
│                                                 │
│        Winner              Ask Directly         │
│                                                 │
└─────────────────────────────────────────────────┘
```

Figure 13.2 *Written Summary of Evaluating Options.* *The process involves listing all options and then evaluating their relative pros and cons to derive a suitable option. In this case, the patient has a dispute with his boss about a payrise. After generating as many solutions as come to mind, the process of systematically evaluating the 'pros and cons' of the situation leads to the selection of the option of 'ask directly.' The patient and therapist will then attempt to improve the patient's communication and monitor how he attempts this with his boss. The next phase involves implementing the solution and monitoring its progress.*

extension of social support – but action must occur. The process at this point may involve evaluating the relative 'pros and cons' of the potential solutions, and then deciding upon a course of action. Unless there is a direct threat to the patient's well-being, the therapist is nearly always best served by encouraging the patient to make an autonomous decision about which course to follow.

If it suits the individual patient, the discussion can be summarized in written form (Figure 13.2). Doing so may, with some patients, provide further impetus to complete the task. In some cases the therapist could even give the paper to the patient as a homework reminder.

Monitoring and refining the solution

At the beginning of the session after a solution is chosen and a course of action is agreed upon, the therapist should always query the patient about the implementation of the solution. This reinforces the therapist's expectation that the patient will be working on the problem between sessions, and that implementation of the specific solution is expected as well. This also implies to the patient that he or she has the capacity to make changes and to resolve his or her problems.

The patient should report back to the therapist with information about how he or she implemented the proposed solution. The patient may have enjoyed some degree of success in the application, or he or she may have encountered some difficulties or unforeseen contingencies. The therapist should direct the patient to 'walk the therapist through' the application of the proposed solution, including the details of conversations and interpersonal interactions. Throughout the entire process the therapist should positively reinforce the patient's attempts at implementing solutions, emphasizing his or her relative strengths and minimizing or 'shoring up' the patient's relative weaknesses. For example, the therapist might say:

Therapist: Last week we developed a plan that you would talk to your wife about your desire to change jobs. How did it go?

Patient: Not too bad, but not so well either, I guess.

Therapist: I'd like to hear about all of it – can you walk me through the process from start to finish.

Patient: What, the whole thing?

Therapist: Sure, the whole thing, step by step, from beginning to end. It would even be good to start with how you brought the subject up with her.

THE TECHNIQUE OF PROBLEM SOLVING

The spectrum of interventions

There is a continuum of specific interventions that fall within the scope of problem solving. The spectrum extends from more directive interventions, such as the therapist offering direct advice to the patient, to interventions which encourage the patient to be autonomous and both develop and choose the solutions to be implemented. Determining which level of intervention to use depends on a number of factors, including the timing within the therapy, the patient's attachment style, the patient's ability to realistically develop solutions, and the degree to which the patient can tolerate directives from the therapist.

As with all therapeutic interventions, the therapist should be guided by the patient's attachment style when engaging in problem solving. When working with patients with more secure and flexible attachment styles, the therapist is likely to be able to operate along the entire range of the spectrum. A more securely attached patient is likely to be better able to use suggestions and directives from the therapist than a less securely attached individual, but is also able to function more independently and is also likely to be able to more effectively generate his or her own solutions. As is the case with other techniques, security of attachment is a clear prognostic indicator.

On the other hand, patients with more avoidant or ambivalent attachment styles may have more difficulty with therapist-directed interventions, which may be seen as non-empathic or authoritarian. A patient who is insecurely attached may also develop an excessive dependency on a therapist who is self-disclosing or directive. The therapist should be mindful of the possibility of generating problematic transferential reactions if he or she uses self-disclosure or explicitly directive interventions untempered by clinical judgment. When working with less securely attached individuals, the therapist is usually best served by moving the patient towards the more autonomous end of the spectrum of intervention, doing so by providing lots of positive reinforcement and encouragement, but without offering direct advice.

The use of more directive problem-solving techniques also raises the risk that the therapist's own personal feelings or judgments will unduly influence the patient's choices. This is a threat particularly when the patient's problem resonates with the therapist's own life experience and the therapist offers directives to the patient that are based on this, rather than attending to the patient's unique situation. As in any kind of therapy, the therapist is well-advised to be well aware of his or her personal reactions to the patient.

DEVELOPING NEW SOLUTIONS

Solutions to problems can be developed using many specific interventions. Various interventions which range from directive to autonomous are described below.

Therapist directives

The therapist may choose to be explicitly instructive with some patients. Being more directive usually works best with more securely attached patients who are able to tolerate and use direct advice, but it is sometimes necessary with patients who are simply unable to generate any solutions to their problems. The therapist should always be aware, however, that the patient who claims to be unable to generate any ideas may be setting a trap for the therapist similar to those that he or she has laid for unsuspecting significant others in social relationships. Pushing the therapist to generate the 'answer' to the problem may allow the patient to be passive and may foster more dependency.

Some patients, however, because of state-dependent factors such as severely depressed mood, are simply temporarily unable to generate enough momentum to brainstorm with the therapist. If this is the case, particularly early in therapy, the therapist may want to offer more behaviorally oriented suggestions or directives to the patient. When doing this, the therapist should model the process of problem solving using explicitly the process of listing options and evaluating the relative pros and cons of each. The therapist should frame this as a process to which the patient can contribute. Some useful statements may include:

- 'I'd like to offer you some suggestions as to how you might approach this problem – you can contribute your own as you feel you are able.'
- 'Which of the ideas that I mentioned seem plausible to you?'
- 'What ideas can you think of that I may have missed?'

Therapist-directed brainstorm

Most patients have an intrinsic capacity to generate solutions to their problems. Their responses to queries about previous attempts to solve their problems is often a good indicator of how willing they are to exercise that capacity.

With those patients who are actively engaged in problem solving, the therapist should explicitly invite the patient into the process. Positive feedback and encouragement will further foster the patient's attempts to develop a solution and implement it. This should enhance the patient's sense of competence. Useful phrases include:

- 'Why don't you run some ideas by me, and then we can try to find some solutions to this problem by looking at the pros and cons of each of them.'
- 'That approach sounds like it would work really well for you. What might be some of the advantages/disadvantages of that particular idea?'

For each idea generated by the patient, the therapist should lead the patient through the process of evaluating the pros and cons for the option, and then decide upon the most suitable approach.

Homework

The '*in vitro*' process of therapist directed problem solving will often benefit from an '*in vivo*' component in which the patient applies the solution to the problem outside of therapy and monitors the process. This can literally be assigned as homework, or the directive to the patient to attempt the solution between sessions can be implied. In either case, the patient should report back to the therapist about the attempted solution at the next session.

As therapy progresses, the patient may also demonstrate increased competence in the process of brainstorming as a means of developing solutions to problems and establishing their comparative merit. At that point, the therapist may give the patient a homework assignment to apply the method to other problems outside of the therapeutic relationship. This might be framed in the following way:

> 'You certainly have been able to approach problems and evaluate potential solutions here in our sessions. I would like to suggest a homework exercise that might help you consolidate this skill even further. You mentioned that there were problems related to your mother-in-law, though we haven't had a chance to discuss them yet in therapy. Why don't you, between now and our next session, try to apply the problem-solving techniques we have been discussing with respect to your wife to the problem with your mother-in-law?'

The therapist might also review with the patient the appropriate steps to take in the process:

- Step 1: Ask 'What exactly is the problem, and how can I break it down into smaller problems?'
- Step 2: List all the possible solutions, no matter how implausible.
- Step 3: Identify the pros and cons and decide on a solution that you can implement.
- Step 4: Apply the solution and review what happens so that it can be fine-tuned if needed.

Therapist self-disclosure

For patients who are at a lesser risk of developing problematic transference, and for situations that are not too personal, the therapist may elect to disclose some of his or her own experiences with similar problems, or may discuss other approaches that other patients in similar situations have applied. With proper timing and judicious use, self-disclosure can enhance the therapeutic alliance and increase empathy; the risk, of course, is that poor timing and judgment about when to use disclosure can lead to disastrous consequences. Therapeutic judgment should rule the day, with non-disclosure being a viable default in nearly all cases.

Comparatively neutral topics that may be suitable pretexts for self-disclosure – if the therapist chooses to use it – may include minor household or workplace problems, common difficulties in child rearing (based on real experience where possible!) and scheduling appropriate time for family or recreation.

Patient-initiated brainstorm

In many cases the patient will readily engage in the problem-solving process, and will report progress to the therapist. In this situation, the therapist should support and encourage the patient, reinforcing the gains made and the fact that the patient has been diligent in tackling the problem directly. The therapist can also review the process by which the patient came to a particular solution, further reinforcing the process:

> 'That does seem like a good idea. I am curious – can you "walk me through" the process you used to come to that decision?'

Drawing on the patient's past experiences

One of the most useful and helpful ways to facilitate problem solving is to simply ask the patient the questions:

- 'What have you done to resolve similar situations in the past?'

and

- 'How could you apply this to your current problem?'

These questions reinforce the idea that the patient is capable of solving his or her problems, reinforce the patient's strengths, and help the patient to develop solutions that are autonomous.

In circumstances where the patient insists that the problem is unique in their life, the therapist may generate some response from the question:

- 'What usually works for you when you find yourself in other difficult situations?'

POTENTIAL DIFFICULTIES USING PROBLEM SOLVING

There are several potential difficulties that the patient might encounter when the problem-solving approach is used.

Difficulty engaging in the problem-solving process

As with any of the IPT techniques, excess passivity by the patient should be discouraged. The observed behavior may be due to the effects of illness, or may reflect fears about change. The latter should certainly be explored further, with extension to the ways in which the patient's conservative nature affects his or her relationships outside of therapy.

When met with resistance initially, it is reasonable for the therapist to be a bit more directive and active in the process as a temporary measure, in order to facilitate getting the process underway. The therapist should ensure that further instances of problem solving occur in the treatment in order to encourage the patient's autonomy and enhance his or her sense of competence. Alternatively, the therapist may choose to select a more neutral problem that is less difficult or challenging, and encourage the patient to achieve mastery with a relatively easy problem first, thus lending encouragement and momentum to further problem solving.

Lack of a solution to the problem

There are some circumstances in which the problem does not have a clear solution, or in which the patient is simply unable to generate a solution to the problem. In the first instance, the patient and therapist should return to clarification of the problem and re-evaluate the patient's expectations for change. It may be that a minor alteration in the severity of the interpersonal problem, or a less substantial change in the way the patient deals with it, may be sufficient to bring about relief from symptoms. At other times, appropriately implemented solutions may fail to bring about improvements in the patient's interpersonal problems, and the focus of intervention may need to shift to altering the patient's expectations about the situation.

Implementation of the solution worsens the situation

Change may have an adverse effect rather than a beneficial one. Interventions in interpersonal problem areas may intensify problems, lead to dissolution of a relationship, or lead to worsening of the patient's symptoms. The 'pros and cons' of any potential solution require careful consideration, as well as the need for caution. If the intervention has a risk of 'backfiring,' then the patient and therapist should generate contingency plans for this possibility. If the adverse outcome was unexpected, the therapist should inquire about the details of the implementation of the solution, and also what transpired afterwards. In all circumstances, the therapist should reinforce that the patient should persist with the problem-solving approach, and that the setback can be used as new information which can be used to understand the problem more fully and to develop modified and improved solutions.

Case example: Anne

Anne was a 46-year-old self-employed woman who had been referred for management of a depressive illness in the context of a significant interpersonal dispute with her husband. Anne described her husband as having an 'awful temper,' and as having a tendency to 'put her down' and 'speak badly to her.' The therapist and Anne identified that the problem was that her husband would become angry and verbally hostile when he was frustrated, and this led to outbursts which caused Anne great distress. Anne described that her typical response to his rages was to feel intensely angry herself, but rather than express that anger to her husband, she would withdraw and try to pretend that nothing had happened.

The therapist and Anne discussed the difficulty:

Therapist: It seems the problem is what you should do about his angry outbursts.
Anne: How to stop them?
Therapist: Well yes, but perhaps more how to deal with them.
Anne: Uh huh. . . .
Therapist: What have you tried to do in the past when he gets angry?

Anne: I usually run for cover and end up with a migraine.

Therapist: What has been the result?

Anne: Well, he quiets down, but we usually don't speak for days. I end up feeling worse because I know that it's just going to happen again – it's only a matter of time.

The therapist suggested that they attempt to solve the communication problem together, and that the next step was to brainstorm about potential solutions. She first asked Anne how she had dealt successfully with similar problems in the past. Anne described how she often dealt with difficult and irate customers, which seemed to her to roughly parallel the problem with her husband. Anne generated her possible responses to an angry and hostile customer. She came up with the following options:

- Asking the customer to leave.
- Ignoring the hostility and continuing as if there were no conflict.
- Asking the customer to refrain from aggressiveness in her place of business.
- Inquiring what the customer was angry about and offering a compromise.

The therapist then asked Anne to apply the same problem-solving approach to her husband's hostility. Anne stated that she felt the best option with her husband was simply to ignore the hostility and continue as if nothing had happened. The therapist felt that this was a poor choice, as it seemed largely to be the same strategy that Anne had unsuccessfully used to that point. Nonetheless, she encouraged Anne to try this the next time her husband became angry. The therapist was primarily concerned at this point with engaging Anne in the problem-solving process, and in fostering her sense of ownership of the solution.

At the next session, Anne reported that ignoring the problem had not been helpful, and that her husband's outbursts seemed to have worsened. The therapist inquired about what specifically had not worked, and Anne reported that she had not been able to 'ignore his temper long enough.' Despite further discussion about the available options, Anne insisted on persisting with the option of ignoring his anger. The therapist then chose to encourage Anne to refine the way in which she implemented the approach of ignoring her husband, again likening it to the way in which Anne had customarily dealt with these types of problems at work.

At the next session, Anne reported that she had come to an important realization: there was a key difference between her customers and her husband. She didn't have to live with her customers, and if they got too unruly, she could ask them to leave. In contrast, she was literally 'stuck' with her husband, and the relationship problems were too important to ignore. It had become apparent to Anne that her approach was not bringing satisfactory results.

Anne: The problem is still there, and I am not happy.

Therapist: OK, I understand. Why don't we go back and reassess the options you have.

Anne: OK.

Therapist: You recall the options we discussed? [Opens file and produces original paper leaf with options]

Anne: Oh yes.

Therapist: What are your thoughts about what you would like to try?

Anne: I suppose that the best option would probably be to ask him what he is angry about, but when he's in one of his rages, he simply isn't reasonable. I just don't think that will work.

Therapist: I agree – trying to talk to someone when they are in that state won't get you anywhere. This brings to mind, however, a woman I was working with several months ago. Her circumstances were quite different from yours, but she did have problems communicating with her husband when he got angry. She landed on the idea of approaching him about the anger after he had cooled down, since he just wasn't reasonable when he was mad. I wonder if that might be of some help to you?

Anne: I am skeptical, but I simply can't ignore it any longer.

Therapist: When might be a good time to approach your husband so that you can talk with him about what's happening?

Anne reported at the next session that she had spoken with her husband about her response to his anger. He had been somewhat responsive, but had another 'episode' during the week, which left Anne feeling discouraged. However, she did note that though her husband was still 'rude,' his anger was less intense. Though still unhappy with the situation, Anne did report feeling a bit more hopeful that things might change. Several sessions later, her expectations about the relationship were discussed:

Therapist: It sounds like you have done a nice job of talking with your husband about your frustrations and your response to his anger outbursts.

Anne: I think so. He has listened, and it has gotten better. But I'm still not satisfied – he still gets angry, and every time he does, I keep getting frustrated.

Therapist: Realistically speaking, how much more do you think that his behavior will shift?

Anne: Probably not much more – it's hard to know – I suppose only time will tell.

Therapist: Well, perhaps we should shift the focus of our discussion a bit. What are your expectations about how he will behave?

Anne: I think originally I was expecting that he would stop altogether, and that there wouldn't be any more of the outbursts. He seems to be working on it, but I just don't know if he can completely contain them. He has always had a pretty quick temper. Maybe it's unrealistic to think that he can control them completely.

Anne and the therapist focused on her explicit expectations of her husband and their relationship, and how these might be modified given that her husband was unlikely to change completely. As therapy continued, Anne was able to come to a more balanced view of her husband – as his outbursts diminished, she began to realize that there were many good things about their relationship. She ultimately elected to remain in the relationship, and though at the end of therapy she continued to express some dissatisfaction with his temper problems, she felt on balance that the relationship had improved and that she had the ability to address his temper directly when it flared.

CONCLUSION

Problem solving is a very effective way of generating productive change in the patient's social relationships. The therapist should ensure that the patient is active and contributes to the process as much as possible. A successful problem-solving intervention usually serves to give the patient a sense of mastery over his or her problems, as it allows the patient to experience the benefits of his or her self-initiated efforts. It is also likely to lead to a significant degree of symptom relief. The ultimate goal when problem solving in IPT is to assist the patient to creatively solve his or her problem as well as to develop the skills to address other interpersonally based problems in the future.

14

Homework

INTRODUCTION

The term 'homework' has many connotations, conjuring up for some unpleasant reminders of tests and papers, often put off until the last minute. Psychotherapeutically, homework has a long but mixed history, and its use has ranged from the 'requirement' that it be applied in behaviorally oriented therapies to a complete exclusion in psychoanalytic treatments.

The use of homework in IPT follows directly from the theory undergirding the treatment and from the interpersonal orientation of the therapy. In essence, homework should be utilized when, in the therapist's judgment, it increases the likelihood that the patient will make productive changes in his or her interpersonal functioning and communication. The time-limited nature of the treatment makes the logic of homework obvious – if it can facilitate more rapid improvement, then it should be used.

It should also be remembered that brief psychotherapy is inevitably directive,[1] particularly a therapy like IPT which is explicitly directed towards improvement in current functioning. The therapist's job is to persuade or influence the patient to make changes to bring this about. This includes working to enlist the patient as a cooperative participant in the process, and in many cases involves helping the patient become the primary agent of change. Nevertheless, this cooperative endeavor always includes directive intervention on the part of the therapist – it is simply a matter of degree whether this takes the form of more subtle techniques within the therapy session or takes the form of overt homework assignments.[2] Homework is a natural extension of the therapeutic process used in IPT.

HOMEWORK IN IPT: WHAT IS IT?

Homework is nothing more complicated than a task that the patient is to do in the interval between sessions. In general, the goal of homework assignment is to *increase the likelihood that the patient will engage in constructive communication change, that his or her symptoms will be decreased, and that his or her interpersonal functioning will be improved.*

This broad definition leaves open a multitude of possibilities, all of which may be used as long as they adhere to the basic tenets of IPT. Homework assignments are congruent with IPT as long as they:

- Are interpersonal in nature.
- Are consistent with the time-limited nature of IPT.
- Do not involve an intervention based upon the patient–therapist relationship.

A variety of techniques which are consistent with these principles might be used in IPT. For instance, an intervention in which the patient is asked to schedule pleasurable activities would be outside of the scope of IPT, but an assignment in which the patient is to schedule pleasurable activities *with a significant other* is well within the scope of IPT. Requesting that the patient engage in a relaxation procedure as a stand-alone intervention would be outside of the scope of IPT, but asking the patient to *explain to a significant other* why time alone and meditation are important to the patient is completely consistent with IPT.

The general rule is that tasks which involve communication and interaction with others are within the scope of IPT. These homework assignments can be categorized as:

1 Direct communication assignments.
2 Appraisal assignments.
3 Activity and behavioral assignments.

Direct communication assignments

These are perhaps the most obvious of all of the homework assignments, and simply involve having the patient engage in direct communication with others. A patient with marital disputes about finances, for example, might be given the assignment to have a conversation with his wife about his concerns at 7:00 p.m. on Wednesday evening. A patient with social phobia might be given the assignment to go to a social engagement and to attempt to speak to at least one other person while there. The essence is that the assignment is directed towards a specific direct communication.

Appraisal assignments

Rather than assigning a direct communication, the patient may be asked instead to monitor and record his or her communications. The purpose of this is two-fold. First, it provides important information about the patient's interactions and communication patterns to both the patient and therapist. Second, it has the effect of raising the patient's awareness of his or her communication. Asking the patient to record his or her conversations draws attention to the communication, and makes the patient more aware of what he or she is saying, the degree to which he or she feels understood, and also draws attention to the responses of others. In essence, it enlists the patient's observing ego. This is a very effective way of helping the patient develop some insight into his or her communication patterns, and the self-monitoring which occurs may also be a very effective mechanism for change.

Activity and behavioral assignments

Having the patient engage in specific activities, such as exercise, is by itself outside of the scope of IPT. There is no doubt, however, that such activities may be very helpful to selected patients. Assignments like these can be brought into line with IPT by focusing the primary point of the intervention on improving communication and building social support.

Practically speaking, this means that giving a narrow assignment to practice relaxation techniques is not consistent with IPT, while requesting that the patient ask someone else to participate with him or her in relaxation does address the goal of increasing social contact and support. Similarly, asking the patient to exercise would be too limited for IPT, while assigning a patient the task of finding someone to exercise with, or of joining a health club to exercise with the goal of meeting other people as well as exercising, would be within the realm of IPT.

'Paradoxical' assignments

These types of assignments, though they have been widely used in strategic therapies to great effect, are not within the realm of IPT. Though they may be directed at relationship change and communication specifically, they should not be utilized in IPT because they do not allow the therapist to model direct communication. In IPT, the therapist should constantly model effective communication for the patient – a paradoxical directive does not model this, and therefore undermines one of the basic principles of IPT.

HOMEWORK IN IPT: TO WHOM SHOULD IT BE ASSIGNED?

The obvious answer to this question is, 'to anyone whom the therapist believes will benefit from a specific assignment.' There are several guidelines which are useful in IPT which are examined below.

The primary consideration in IPT is to assign homework to patients who are likely to complete it. While this seems patently obvious for all therapies, it is extremely crucial in IPT. This is because if a homework assignment is not completed, the non-compliance is then likely to become the dominant issue in the therapy. Not only does this shift the focus to the patient–therapist relationship, as the resistance to the homework assignment must be discussed within the therapeutic relationship, it also detracts from the focus on immediate symptom resolution and improvement in interpersonal functioning.

As a form of a directive, the assignment of homework subtly shifts the therapeutic relationship. In essence, assigning homework shifts the therapist to a more powerful role in which he or she is directing the patient about which course to take, with the expectation that the patient will complete the task assigned. While this shift is quite tolerable to some patients, with others it will shift the therapeutic relationship in ways that make the alliance more difficult to manage. With more passive-aggressive patients, for example, the assignment of homework is likely to elicit passive-aggressive behavior towards the therapist. Not only is the homework not likely to be completed, but the assignment itself – putting the therapist in a more dominant position – is likely to cause problems in the therapeutic relationship.

In a similar fashion, assigning homework to some dependent patients may also cause problems in the therapeutic relationship. If the therapist takes on a more dominant role, he or she may elicit even more dependent behavior on the part of the patient. As opposed to the passive-aggressive patient, who often will not even attempt the assignment or complain that 'the dog ate it,' dependent patients will often complain that the assignment is too difficult, and use the failure as a means of reinforcing their dependency on the therapist.

There are many patients, however, who benefit a great deal from homework. In general they tend to be quite motivated, relatively securely attached, and may even ask the therapist for additional work between sessions. In the best of circumstances, the patient will even go beyond the assignment, or modify it in creative ways that bring about even more positive change.

By way of analogy, imagine that the therapist is a battlefield general who is able to influence his or her troops, but unlike a real general, is unable to enforce direct orders by court-martialing or involuntarily committing non-compliant patients. Thus, the therapist/general can rely only on personal persuasion, charisma, charm, and good looks (as well as therapeutic techniques) to get the patient/soldier to climb out of the trench, face his or her anxiety, and confront the imagined foe. For more courageous patients (i.e., those more securely attached), giving a direct command to face the enemy is sufficient, and is the best and most direct way to bring about change. For other soldier/patients, a direct order will increase anxiety and fear, and result in the patient digging in even deeper to seek protection. Dependency will be exacerbated. For some soldier/patients, the therapist-general's command to climb out of the relative security of the foxhole will be met with disdain, with the patient saying in a passive-aggressive way, 'I'll show the arrogant dag who's boss.'

While the analogy may be a bit too militaristic for some, it nonetheless illustrates the principle that the therapist should very carefully select those patients to whom he or she assigns homework. To do otherwise is to risk causing iatrogenically more transferential difficulties in a therapeutic context in which examination of the transference is not only outside of the scope of the treatment, but detracts from the aims of the therapy. As a general rule of thumb, patients who are more securely attached are more likely to benefit from directives, while those who are less securely attached should be approached with caution. In all cases, the goal of homework is to increase the chance that the patient will improve his or her functioning.

HOMEWORK IN IPT: HOW SHOULD IT BE DELIVERED?

There are a number of methods by which homework can be assigned, but they all ultimately depend upon the therapist persuading the patient to undertake the task. The difference is simply a matter of degree, with the spectrum running from therapist-generated to patient-generated tasks. The point at which the therapist intervenes along that spectrum, however, has a great deal of impact on the likelihood that the homework will be completed; great care should be taken to ensure that the level of intervention matches the individual patient.

The most desirable assignment is one which is initiated by the patient. An astute and motivated patient might, for example, remark to the therapist that it would be helpful if he or she initiated a conversation with his or her partner to resolve a conflict. The therapist need only concur and encourage the patient in such a situation. Patients like this are, unfortunately, few and far between, though they are much sought after by therapists. Nonetheless, the more the homework is generated by the patient, the more likely it is to be accomplished.

The therapist can encourage this kind of patient-initiated problem solving by using non-specific directives with the patient. For example, the therapist might ask questions such as:

- 'What do you think would be helpful to accomplish between sessions?'
- 'How do you think you can best solidify the communication changes we've been working on?'
- 'How do you think this problem might best be addressed between now and next week?'

This type of non-specific directive accomplishes two things. First, it clearly implies to the patient that he or she is expected to work between sessions. While doing so, however, it also gives the patient a great deal of autonomy in developing solutions. Gentle guidance on the part of the therapist, or collaborative work to refine the homework following the patient's suggestion, can also occur. Special care should be taken to ensure that the patient's 'assignment' is not overly ambitious – homework should always be such that it is within reach of the patient and can be successfully completed. The goal of homework in IPT is not to frustrate the patient but to maximize productive change.

Further along the spectrum towards specific therapist-generated directives are those which take the form of psycho-education. For instance, in the case of a depressed patient, the therapist might note to the patient that it is well known that increasing activity and decreasing isolation is helpful to most depressed patients. Acknowledging the fact that it is difficult, the therapist might then ask the patient for ideas about how these general goals could be accomplished between sessions. The therapist is in essence influencing the patient to begin to generate specific solutions which can be collaboratively refined. Giving the patient ownership and working collaboratively will increase the likelihood of completion.

More specific directives can be given by the therapist using examples gleaned from other patients. Confidentiality should of course be maintained, but the therapist might find it useful to mention strategies that other patients have used to deal with similar problems. A postpartum woman who is dealing with a conflict with her spouse, for instance, might be influenced to address the conflict with her partner more directly if the therapist describes a similar case in which such a problem was successfully addressed by another patient. The use of details which are similar to that of the patient will enhance the power of the intervention, as the patient recognizes similarities with his or her own situation.

As with all interventions, care must be taken with such approaches. The more specifically directive the approach of the therapist, the greater the risk of rupturing the therapeutic alliance. Though the specific intervention noted above may be quite beneficial and help some patients feel better understood, others may feel alienated, feeling that the therapist is not understanding them as individuals.

The most specifically directive intervention is simply for the therapist to tell the patient exactly what to do between sessions. While some patients will benefit a great deal from this, and a few will even honestly ask for homework to do, the therapist must take great care to ensure that taking a more dominant role does not precipitate transference problems.

In summary, the therapist is generally best served by using the least directive approach that is feasible. Allowing a patient to take the lead encourages the patient to take responsibility for the task, and increases his or her sense of ownership. Moreover, it keeps the therapist from assuming that he or she ultimately knows what is best for the patient instead of listening to the patient for advice on how to solve the problem.

Case example: Tom

Tom was a 40-year-old business executive who had come to therapy for help with marital problems. His wife of 15 years was threatening to leave him, stating that he was too invested in his work and didn't prioritize her or the family. Tom had a very high-powered job with a legal firm, and though he claimed he 'intellectually recognized' that his wife had a good point, he also felt that she didn't understand how stressful his job was.

In the first several sessions the therapist learned that Tom had a number of social relationships, mostly at work, and mostly with men; however, like Tom, most of them were also devoted to their work, and expected others to be equally obsessed. The culture was that one was not supposed to show weaknesses, and further, any discussion of emotion was taboo. Tom also described himself as having difficulty with emotional expression outside of this setting – though very articulate, he described never having had close relationships in which he could discuss his feelings. Though he desperately wanted to do so, particularly with his wife, he found it extremely difficult to do so, much less to initiate such a conversation about his feelings.

The therapist noted that Tom was very goal-oriented, and that he tended to be fairly dominant. This was apparent in both subtle and direct ways within the therapy itself. Near the end of the first session, for instance, Tom rather adamantly told the therapist that they 'needed to meet again the next week,' before the therapist had even had the chance to bring up the topic of future appointments. Tom always had a particular agenda to discuss, and always brought in a written list of materials to cover, somewhat like a business meeting. Typically, the sessions would begin with Tom setting out his agenda and informing the therapist that this was how they would spend the session.

At the end of the third meeting, the topic of homework arose at Tom's instigation:

Tom: We've met for 3 weeks now, and you still haven't given me any assignments to do. That would never happen in my company – if you were working for me, I'd be giving you a lot of stuff to take home!

Therapist: (fighting off the temptation to say, 'I'm glad I don't work for you!') Many people I work with do find that having something specific to accomplish between sessions is very helpful in achieving their goals. Before thinking about a specific task, let's think those through. What are your goals for the next week?

The therapist was well aware of several things at this point in therapy. First, Tom's attachment style was somewhat avoidant and, given his personality style, Tom was likely to disengage from therapy if he felt that the therapist wasn't being responsive to his requests. At the same time, the therapist also recognized that giving a direct and specific assignment to Tom was fraught with danger, as Tom was used to being in charge and was not likely to respond well to the therapist taking a more dominant position within the therapy.

The therapeutic challenge, then, was to assist Tom to develop an assignment for himself that both maintained a productive therapeutic alliance and helped him to become more able to discuss his feelings and to communicate better with his wife. As Tom experienced some success with this, the therapist was hoping that he would begin to develop some insight into his communication style as well, ultimately leading to a more permanent change in communication and a deepening of his relationships. The therapist came into the homework discussion hypothesizing that Tom would benefit from talking directly to his wife about his feelings of conflict and stress about work and their relationship, but knowing that simply giving Tom a directive to do so would likely be disruptive to the therapeutic alliance as well as unlikely to succeed.

The therapist chose, therefore, to use Tom's own vocabulary at this point in the therapy, choosing to more subtly direct Tom rather than confront him directly about the need for him to express his feelings more openly. Using words like 'people I *work with*,' '*goals*,' and '*tasks to accomplish*,' the therapist framed the issue in terms that were comfortable to Tom, all the while moving him slowly but inevitably towards improving his communication.

Tom: Well, my main goal is to save my marriage. And my wife has made it pretty clear that she isn't happy.
Therapist: The goal to save your marriage sounds like a very good general goal – kind of like a business plan, I guess. How do you usually approach a general goal like that?
Tom: In my business, we start by breaking it down into smaller steps. Then you can set some specific deadlines to get each one done.
Therapist: Sounds good – what specific steps do you see that need to be accomplished in this case?
Tom: First, I need to set up some time to talk with her – I still don't quite know what she sees as the specific problem. She just keeps saying that she doesn't feel 'close' anymore. Then I guess I'd better communicate what I'm thinking more clearly to her.
Therapist: Sounds good so far – what is it that you'd like to tell her, exactly?
Tom: The main thing is that I don't feel like she understands all the stress that I'm under. Work is difficult enough, but now to have to deal with this kind of dissatisfaction at home too . . . and I want her to know that even though she may not think so, I do still love her very much.
Therapist: It seems to be helpful to you to have a kind of written agenda to get things done – I noticed that you have used that for our sessions. Would it be helpful to write down what you want to tell your wife?
Tom: Great idea doc! (*takes out a sheet of paper from his briefcase and proceeds to write several notes*)
Therapist: Now that you've got a good idea of where you're heading, what is the next step?
Tom: Setting some specific deadlines. Why don't we say that I should have a good conversation with her by this time next week?

Therapist: Sounds ambitious, but you seem like the kind of guy who gets things done when he sets his mind to it. Do you think figuring out a specific time would be of help?

Tom: Now I know why they pay you the big bucks, doc. Yeah, Thursday night is usually fairly free – no meetings or any activities with the kids. I'll talk to her after we get the kids to bed.

Therapist: Sounds like a plan. I'll look forward to hearing how it turns out.

Tom approached his wife the next Thursday. He reported in the next session that the attempt wasn't very successful – his wife had been put off by his 'demand' that they talk, and more so by the fact that he had a written agenda for the conversation. According to Tom, she had said that having an agenda made her feel like he wasn't listening to her. Though the attempt was not as successful as it might ideally have been, the therapist pointed out that Tom had made a strong effort. Further, Tom was now more open to other suggestions about how he might approach his wife differently.

CONCLUSION

The intent of homework is to increase the likelihood that the patient will engage in communication or social activity that will lead to improved functioning and symptom resolution. Though homework is not required in IPT, it is extremely helpful for many patients. The therapist should tailor both the assignment and the way in which it is delivered in order to maximize the likelihood that the assignment is carried out, as refusal or resistance to homework is likely to shift the focus of IPT away from improvement in external relationships to a focus on transferential issues. When used, homework in IPT should be interpersonal in nature, and ideally should be directed by the patient as much as possible.

REFERENCES

1. Haley, J. 1990. *Strategies of Psychotherapy*. New York: Triangle Press.
2. Haley, J. 1987. *Problem Solving Therapy*. San Francisco: Jossey-Bass.

15

Use of the Therapeutic Relationship

INTRODUCTION

The therapeutic relationship is of extreme importance in IPT. In fact, one might well argue that it is the most important part of the therapy, a view clearly supported by research in the area.[1-3] If the alliance is not maintained, the patient will abandon therapy, leaving the therapist with a treatment manual full of techniques, but no patient.

The nature of IPT, however, does limit to some degree the ways in which the therapeutic relationship can be used as a point of intervention. IPT is characterized by the fact that the therapeutic relationship is usually not directly discussed. To do so is likely to lead the patient away from immediate symptom resolution and improvement in functioning in here-and-now relationships. While working with the transference directly may be very helpful for well-selected patients, it is outside of the scope of IPT, and is not clinically necessary for many patients.

Nonetheless, the therapeutic relationship can be used in several extremely important ways in IPT. The first is as a means to gather information. Second, the therapist may need to 'manage' the relationship – i.e., to attend to the patient's attachment style and personality and shift his or her communication accordingly so that there is more congruence in the therapeutic relationship.

THE THERAPEUTIC RELATIONSHIP AS A SOURCE OF INFORMATION

One of the primary tenets of IPT is that individuals enact attachment and communication patterns consistently across all relationships. This includes, of course, the therapeutic relationship. Patients tend to impose their 'working models' upon the therapist, and act towards the therapist in ways which directly reflect their attachment styles. Hence the therapeutic relationship is an important source of information about the ways in which patients behave and attach to others in relationships outside of therapy.

Those patients with more secure attachments will generally have more flexibility in their therapeutic relationships. They are able to enter into therapy seeking help in an effective and appropriate way. In addition to being able to ask for help, they are able to use feedback from the therapist effectively. Their working model, which essentially reflects the belief that others can generally be trusted, is imposed upon the therapeutic relationship, and enables them to develop trust rapidly.

In contrast, patients with less securely attached styles have more difficulty in establishing a therapeutic bond. This is usually displayed as a problem with seeking help or asking for it directly. Insecurely attached patients have more difficulty developing trust in the therapist because their previous relationships have taught them to be wary of others. This may be manifest as more of an anxious ambivalent dependency, or as avoidant behavior. In either case, the information is crucial to the therapist as it reflects the troubles these patients are having in relationships outside of therapy.

Using the therapeutic relationship as one source of information, the therapist can then begin to develop more accurate hypotheses about what kinds of difficulties the patient is having outside of therapy. Questions to investigate these hypotheses can then be asked about outside relationships.

Managing the relationship in such a way as to maximize the veracity of this information, and the speed with which it is obtained, is an art. The therapist must balance the need to obtain information with the need to develop a working relationship with the patient, which may require more direction on the part of the therapist. Information about the patient's attachment style, based on the therapeutic relationship, can best be obtained in an unfiltered way if the therapist is non-directive, passive, and non-disclosing. This is in essence the principle that is used in psychoanalysis – the patient is more likely to develop an unfettered transference reaction to the therapist if the therapist is as opaque as possible.

While this may be beneficial for some patients with a high degree of frustration tolerance, it is difficult for many patients, and also unnecessary for many. A deliberate attempt by the therapist to foster a transference reaction will move the therapy away from a focus on current functioning. As many patients want primarily to resolve their immediate crises, and do not need a thorough reworking of their internal psychic functioning, the best course is for the IPT therapist to avoid such deliberate provocation.

The therapist must therefore carefully balance the techniques used to gain more information from the patient by leading him or her to react to a neutral therapist with the need to focus on current functioning, and the time limit imposed by IPT. It is also important to consider that the information gleaned from the therapeutic relationship is only one source of information – the patient's own report of interpersonal patterns and information from others is equally important.

THE IDEAL THERAPEUTIC RELATIONSHIP

Psychotherapists have long struggled to find a metaphor that captures the ideal therapeutic relationship. Elements include teacher, collaborator, confidant, advisor, confessor, expert, and many others. In IPT specifically, authors have spoken about the need to maintain a 'positive transference,' though this is rarely defined in concrete terms. What exactly does this mean?

The most concise way to describe the ideal relationship in IPT is to couch it in the terms Kiesler and Watkins use to describe interpersonal relationships.[4] The therapeutic relationship should be characterized by the following:

- *There is a high degree of affiliation.* In other words, the patient and therapist like each other, are genuinely interested in what the other has to say, and care about each other's welfare. This parallels very closely elements that Rogers described as important in therapy: warmth, empathy, and genuineness.[5] Ideally, however, this should be reflected by both the therapist and the patient.
- *There is a high degree of inclusion.* Kiesler and Watkins used this term to describe the degree to which the relationship matters.[4] In other words, the relationship has to be important to both patient and therapist. Both must be invested in the relationship, and both must put value in what the other has to say. If the therapeutic relationship is of no importance to the therapist, he or she will not invest energy in it. If it is not important to the patient, he or she will withdraw from it. In either case, therapy will ultimately fail without inclusion.
- *The therapist is accorded a degree of expertise.* This directly implies that the patient put him or herself in a less dominant position, because he or she is coming to the therapist for advice or help in solving a problem which he or she is unable to solve alone. Ideally, the patient will view the therapist as having something of value to offer, and will be receptive to the therapist's feedback and put it to use. This does not imply that the patient is passive; rather, the patient is more like a junior partner or apprentice who is seeking help from an expert, with the ultimate goal of achieving autonomy.

It is this last point that is often the sticking point in therapy. More aggressive or detached patients may be unwilling to give up their desire for control, even temporarily, and will approach the therapist confrontationally or passive-aggressively. Conversely, more ambivalent or dependent patients will attempt to create a relationship with the therapist which does not ultimately lead to independent functioning and autonomy. Though able to engage in therapy readily, as they are quite willing to accord the therapist the 'expert' role, they attempt to lock the therapist into that role so that they can continue to be dependent and passive. Patients must ultimately move from that position as therapy is completed in order to function autonomously.

A corollary of this is that the ideal therapeutic relationship is not static over the course of therapy. While affiliation is ideally fairly stable, neither inclusion nor dominance should be. As therapy nears conclusion, the patient and therapist will ideally move towards a relationship in which the patient is on a par with the therapist – the patient should be able to problem solve on his or her own, should be able to recognize patterns and initiate change independently, and in essence should be preparing to leave the relationship. Correspondingly, investment in the relationship also diminishes over time. Ideally, the patient will look back on the therapeutic experience as one that was greatly beneficial, but not 'need' it in the same way, nor be invested in it in the same way, as during the therapy.

Sports analogies seem to be useful for many therapists and patients, though there are a multitude of others that can be used as well. Such analogies can be reflected directly to patients as a model for understanding what is to occur in therapy, and as a way of understanding both their role and the role of their therapists.

The patient is like an athlete, a swimmer for instance, who comes to an experienced coach with a specific problem. The overall goal is to swim more efficiently and faster. The patient may be aware of specific problems – perhaps he or she was a good swimmer but suffered an acute injury, and now needs help in order to regain functioning. The analogy here is obvious: an acute crisis has temporarily impaired an otherwise functional individual.

Perhaps the patient was able to swim well, but has noticed that as the competition is getting tougher, a long-standing technical difficulty, such as a hitch in stroke, is inhibiting peak performance. Perhaps early life experiences were such that the patient never quite learned the technically correct way to swim. Perhaps the patient's stroke was modified to adapt to earlier stressors, but the techniques which were once adaptive are no longer. While the modified stroke allowed the patient to continue functioning earlier, it is now an impediment, and the patient needs help in recognizing the problem, making adjustments, and practicing to reinforce the changes.

Patients such as these have often developed attachment styles as a result of difficult early life experiences. These styles allowed them to function to some degree at that time, but are now no longer functional, and are in fact getting in the way of developing meaningful interpersonal relationships. A coach/therapist in this case would help the patient to recognize the problem by listening to the patient's report, watching the patient swim a few laps, having the patient make a few adjustments, and having the patient jump back into the pool for further observation. As improvement began, the coach would also have the patient practice to reinforce the change.

Inherent in this analogy is the notion that the coach doesn't do all of the work. The patient is expected to do the majority of the work in IPT – the therapist can give pointers, share experience, and help motivate, but the patient has to get in the pool and swim the laps. Therapy, as with athletics, is only as successful as the training that is done.

Thus, the ideal relationship in IPT is one in which the patient is able to allow the therapist to work from this expert position, while at the same time the patient is invested in ultimately establishing independence and autonomy.

MANAGEMENT OF THE THERAPEUTIC RELATIONSHIP

The time-limited nature of IPT makes management of the therapeutic relationship both easier and more difficult. It is easier because in many ways it puts less direct pressure on the therapist. In long-term therapeutic relationships, transference issues almost inevitably arise, and discussion of the therapeutic relationship and transference elements of therapy is often difficult for both therapist and patient.

On the other hand, management of the therapeutic relationship is more difficult because, as opposed to simply waiting for the transference to emerge, the therapist must work actively and with intent in order to create and maintain a positive therapeutic alliance, and to prevent the development of problematic transference. This requires both recognizing potential problems that might occur, as well as taking steps to keep them from happening. The therapist ideally walks a very fine line between maintaining a benevolent expert role and being a taskmaster, and between allowing an appropriate degree of dependency and fostering self-sufficiency, all the while keenly attending to the idiosyncratic attachment style of the patient.

Another sports analogy serves well to describe this situation. Conducting therapy in this way is similar to playing billiards. A novice therapist can become proficient at making a single shot. With more experience, a therapist may not only be able to make a shot, but also be able to place the cue ball in a position to make the next shot. More experience and the therapist can make the first shot, place the cue ball for the next shot, and also place the cue ball so that if the shot is missed, the opponent is faced with a difficult shot. Understanding the strengths and weaknesses of one's opponent is crucial to achieving this level of play. A seasoned therapist develops a vision of the whole table, and can literally visualize how the whole game will be played – how every shot will be made – before the first shot is taken. An experienced therapist knows which shot to take first, how to place the cue ball, and how to set up the whole game while accounting for the strengths and weaknesses of the patient.

While obviously not a competition, the analogy holds true to a large degree for psychotherapy. A seasoned therapist literally develops a feel for how the entire therapy will progress, adjusting his or her approach to the particular patient in order to make subsequent interventions more likely to succeed. Adjusting one's own play to facilitate the success of the patient is the art of IPT.

Defining the therapeutic relationship in IPT

The first thing that the therapist can do to attempt to approach the ideal therapeutic relationship described above is to lay down ground rules for the conduct of IPT. This takes place largely in the assessment phase of treatment, and is analogous to discussing the rules prior to beginning to play billiards. During the assessment, the therapist can educate the patient about how IPT is to proceed, describing the concept that patients are expected to work between sessions, are responsible for bringing material to be discussed, and are to collaborate with the therapist to solve their acute problems. The time-limit should also be raised as an element of therapy, as it is one of the most important 'rules' of the game. If, when asked for feedback, the patient indicates that he or she cannot abide by these rules, or if the therapist is suspicious that the patient will not be able to follow them (because of personality, attachment, or other factors), then another kind of treatment should be offered. In essence, the therapist should not start the game until the patient agrees to the rules.

The therapist can also set the stage for the therapeutic relationship with the patient by presenting the therapy with confidence. Rather than being neutral about the patient's chances to improve with treatment, the therapist should be confident and reassuring, and should present the treatment to the patient in that way. Assuming the air of an expert – a kind and benevolent one, but an expert nonetheless – is a very effective way of setting up the kind of positive relationship that is desirable in IPT.

This can also be done by framing questions to the patient in a way which reflects the therapist's interest in the patient and his or her ability to understand the patient. Clarification and reflection, when carried out with genuine interest, go a long way towards establishing a high degree of affiliation and expertise. The more active approach taken by the therapist will also facilitate the positioning of the therapist in the expert role. Early in therapy it is useful to establish that the therapist will be asking direct questions about the patient's experiences; this also establishes the therapist's position.

CONCLUSION

The goal in IPT is to approximate as closely as possible the ideal therapeutic relationship described – in other words, to develop and maintain a positive transference. In order to do so, the therapist must be active, and must also take the patient's attachment style into consideration. The process rests on technique to some degree, but the most important elements in establishing a productive therapeutic alliance are experience and clinical judgment. There is no substitute for either.

REFERENCES

1. Martin, D.J., Garske, J.P., Davis, M.K. 2000. Relation of the therapeutic alliance with outcome and other variables: a meta-analytic review. *Journal of Consulting and Clinical Psychology* **68**, 438–50.
2. Zuroff, D.C., Blatt, S.J., Sotsky, S.M., *et al*. 2000. Relation of therapeutic alliance and perfectionism to outcome in brief outpatient treatment of depression. *Journal of Consulting and Clinical Psychology* **68**, 114–24.
3. Barber, J.P., Connolly, M.B., Crits-Christoph, P., Gladis, L., Siqueland, L. 2000. Alliance predicts patients' outcome beyond in-treatment change in symptoms. *Journal of Consulting and Clinical Psychology* **68**, 1027–32.
4. Kiesler, D.J., Watkins, L.M. 1989. Interpersonal complimentarity and the therapeutic alliance: a study of the relationship in psychotherapy. *Psychotherapy* **26**, 183–94.
5. Rogers, C.R. 1957. The necessary and sufficient conditions of therapeutic personality change. *Journal of Consulting Psychology* **21**, 95–103.

Section 4

Problem Areas

16

Interpersonal Disputes

INTRODUCTION

Disputes, arguments, disagreements, and differences of opinion are a part of all human relationships – the 'seasoning,' so to speak, of human life. From time to time, more piquant life-seasonings may lead to problems.

Interpersonal disputes may be selected as a problem area in IPT when such disputes are relevant as either a cause or consequence of the patient's distress. Attachment theory[1] hypothesizes that disruptions in attachment, such as those caused by interpersonal disputes, makes vulnerable individuals more likely to suffer interpersonal problems. Interpersonal disputes are relevant when they cannot be resolved, when the relationship is significant to the patient, or when there is little social support available to the patient to assist in resolving the dispute. The general approach to interpersonal disputes is displayed diagrammatically in Figure 16.1.

Interpersonal disputes are either resolved or remain chronic. In the latter case, they may be grudgingly tolerated in the relationship, or lead to its dissolution. IPT is designed to assist the patient to revisit the process of resolution of the dispute. It is important to note that the IPT therapist should not enter into therapy with a prejudice about the outcome of the relationship. There are a number of possible outcomes for any given relationship:

- The patient may elect to end the relationship and move to other social supports.
- The patient may decide to maintain the relationship with a change in expectations and an increase in social support external to the relationship.
- The patient may elect to maintain the relationship after making changes in the relationship.

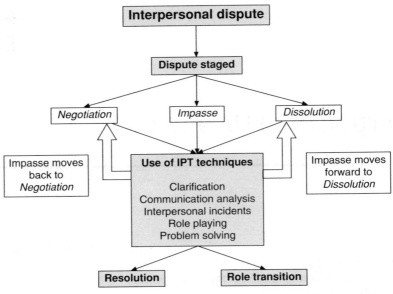

Figure 16.1 *Interpersonal Disputes. During the negotiation phase of the dispute, the patient and therapist attempt to clarify the dispute and the affect associated with it. Communication styles are analyzed to identify problematic communication. Modification of communication or expectations about the dispute can be achieved using role playing or problem solving. If the dispute is at the impasse phase, the therapist should help the patient clarify the history of the dispute and the patient's current view of the problem. The associated affect generated can then be used as a motivation for change. If this is successful, the therapist can continue working on the problem as with negotiation. If the dispute is at the dissolution phase, the therapist must clarify that this is actually the case. This will usually lead to some degree of associated affect. Once this has begun, the therapist and patient can deal with the problem area as a role transition.*

In each case, the objective in IPT is for the patient to make an objective, well-reasoned decision about how to manage the relationship, as opposed to an uninformed, impulsive decision.

Interpersonal disputes can be overt and temporally related to the onset of illness, or may be subtle and not immediately apparent in the compilation of the interpersonal inventory.

Table 16.1 *Types of Interpersonal Disputes*

- Overtly hostile conflict: *domestic violence, verbal abuse.*
- Betrayals: *infidelity, impropriety, conflicting loyalties within a family.*
- 'Disappointments': *unmet expectations at work or school.*
- Inhibited conflicts: *anger at partner's illness or disability.*
- Subtle mistreatment: *verbal abuse, denial of intimacy.*
- Developmentally determined conflict: *separation-individuation issues.*

Overtly hostile conflicts such as abusive or violent relationships are usually obvious in the early stages of history gathering, but may not be disclosed by the patient. In some cases, the dispute is in the form of a 'betrayal' of trust such as an impropriety or, in the case of intimate relationships, an affair. 'Disappointments' may occur at any stage of a relationship and are often more subtle, particularly when expectations are not clearly communicated in a relationship. In some cases factors peculiar to the patient, such as personality or cultural context, or peculiar to the dispute, such as physical or psychiatric illness in a partner, may preclude it becoming overt. Some disputes are subtle and may only become apparent in the treatment accidentally; for instance, a patient may inadvertently disclose a conversation that reveals the dispute.

Interpersonal disputes may also be developmentally determined to some degree. In many of these cases, the disputes arise as part of the life cycle and the therapist should aim to help the patient place the dispute within this context. Role transitions may also be used as a problem area in such cases.

ASSESSING INTERPERSONAL DISPUTES

Interpersonal disputes may become evident while the initial history is being taken, and in many cases may well be the presenting problem. Some disputes may only clearly emerge or become apparent during the construction of the Interpersonal Inventory. While historical information spontaneously offered by the patient may be the most valuable source of information, it is often necessary for the therapist specifically to elicit information about the relationship with questions such as:

- 'How do you express anger to others?'
- 'How have things been with your spouse/partner?'
- 'How have you been getting along with your family?'
- 'How are things going with colleagues at work?'
- 'Are you having difficulty communicating with people around you? Anyone in particular?'
- 'Have you found yourself unhappy or disappointed with anybody around you?'
- 'Are you finding yourself in more arguments with people than usual?'
- 'Are you happy with the way people treat you? Anyone in particular?'
- 'How well do you think that others understand you?'

Occasionally, patients will describe an apparent interpersonal conflict, yet conceptualize it as a 'role transition.' Conversely, the therapist may view the patient's problem as one of 'role transition,' while the patient thinks of the issue as an 'interpersonal dispute.' While it is of value to come to an agreement about the nature of the problem, the therapist should not rigidly impose a problem area upon the patient at the expense of the therapeutic alliance, particularly given the overlap of the problem areas. The purpose of the problem areas is not to be dogmatic and to make a correct 'diagnosis' but rather to maintain the therapeutic focus on interpersonal problems. The specific problem area is less important that maintaining a general interpersonal focus.

When working on an interpersonal dispute the therapist should answer the following questions:

1   *When did the patient first become aware of the dispute?* Has the patient recognized that there is a dispute? Has he or she been able to link the dispute and the onset of psychological distress?

2   *What were the patient's expectations of the other person or situation and how did these change over time?* The therapist should establish whether the patient's expectations are unrealistic in the context of the relationship. He or she should clarify the ways in which the changes in expectations have resulted in improvement or worsening of psychological symptoms.

3   *What attempts has the patient made to try to resolve the dispute, and what has kept a resolution from occurring?* The therapist should discuss the ways in which the patient has attempted to resolve the dispute prior to therapy, including the ultimate effects of these attempts. On occasion, the patient's attempts will have exacerbated the problem. Exploring these attempts is a good way to further establish the patient's style of communication and degree of motivation for change.

4   *How does the patient communicate his or her needs in the relationship in general, and how has this changed over the course of the dispute?* The therapist should try to establish how the patient's communication style has contributed to the development of the dispute. Observations of the way in which the patient communicates with the therapist, as well as information gathered using communication analysis will help to establish how dysfunctional communication has contributed to the development and persistence of the dispute. This should also provide guidance regarding which specific interventions, aimed at improving the patient's communication style, may help bring about a resolution of the dispute.

5   *What is the patient's attachment style, and how has it contributed to the development of psychological symptoms in the context of the dispute?* The patient's attachment style should inform the therapist about the way in which the patient's distress has developed. Hypotheses about the patient's attachment style may be drawn from the history the patient gives of his or her interaction with caregivers and peers, descriptions of adult relationships, and in the way in which the patient interacts in therapy. The patient's attachment style should influence the interventions chosen by the therapist; it also has implications regarding the development of the therapeutic relationship.

6   *What does the dispute suggest about how the patient will function within the therapeutic relationship?* In general, the development of the therapeutic relationship will be influenced by the same factors that operate on the patient's other relationships. The therapist should take care to note the style of communication the patient uses in therapy, the patient's expectations of relationships in general, and how these expectations are communicated, in order to anticipate and deal with parallel problems which may develop in the therapeutic relationship.

STAGING THE INTERPERSONAL DISPUTE

Interpersonal disputes can roughly be described as being either acutely distressing, smoldering and persistent, or as leading to the ultimate dissolution of a relationship. Determining which of these stages a dispute is in is of great help to the therapist in understanding the patient's perception of the problem, and in understanding the patient's goals for the relationship. In IPT this is achieved by 'staging' the dispute.[2] Interpersonal disputes are conceptualized in IPT as one of three stages:[2]

- *Negotiation*: disputes in the negotiation stage are characterized by ongoing attempts by both parties to bring about changes. The negotiation phase typically involves the expression of more affect, and is more readily recognized by the patient as a source of emotional distress. Assessment of the patient's interpersonal communication and specific interpersonal incidents is often helpful in addressing the patient's communication style and its role in the cause and maintenance of the dispute.
- *Impasse*: this refers to a stage at which the patient's attempts at resolving the dispute have stalled. Efforts to resolve the dispute are less likely to be ongoing. While neither party is making active attempts to end the relationship, communication has usually become more entrenched. Patients may not spontaneously report disputes at the impasse stage; the therapist should therefore obtain information about potential disputes during the initial history using more direct inquiry.
- *Dissolution*: this refers to a stage at which the conflict is at such an advanced stage that the relationship is beyond repair. This may not be the opinion of both parties, however, as there are occasions when one person will be ending the relationship as another desperately clings to it. In the dissolution stage, the goal of the IPT therapist is to help the patient 'move on' from the relationship. In these circumstances, the interpersonal problem may be reframed as a role transition, representative of the movement of the patient out of the relationship. In such a case, the therapist can be of most assistance in helping the patient grieve the loss of the old relationship and in the generation of new social supports.

During the negotiation phase of a dispute, the patient and therapist should clarify all aspects of the dispute as well as the affect which is generated by the dispute. This should include both the content affect which the patient reports when describing various conflicts, as well as the process affect observed, as the patient discusses the dispute in therapy. The therapist should also address the patient's communication style to help identify the ways in which the patient's communications are contributing to the dispute. Modification of communication or expectations about the dispute can be achieved using role play or problem solving.

During the negotiation phase of a dispute, the patient will typically have a higher degree of motivation for change, and may be more willing to actively contribute to the problem-solving process in therapy. In the impasse and dissolution stages of disputes, patients may often have variable degrees of motivation and insight, and may be less willing to engage in the process of change.

If the dispute is at the impasse phase, the therapist should help the patient clarify the history of the dispute and the patient's current view of the problem. The process and content affect generated can then be used to motivate the patient to change. If this is successful, the therapist can continue working with the patient on the problem as if it is in the negotiation phase.

The *strategy* of working with interpersonal disputes in IPT is to help patients move from the impasse stage, where by definition the conflict is smoldering but unresolved. This can be done by either helping the patient become more invested in the relationship and moving the conflict back to the negotiation stage of dispute, or by helping the patient recognize that he or she is less invested in the relationship and moving the conflict forward to the dissolution stage.

If the dispute is in the dissolution phase, clarification that this is actually the case will lead to some degree of associated affect, often in the form of grief or remorse about the relationship. This should be explored in detail, as it may lead the patient to new insights about the relationship. If the relationship continues to be at the dissolution stage, the therapist and patient can deal with the problem as a role transition or a grief and loss issue as well.

Utilizing techniques which help the patient generate solutions to his or her relationship disputes enables the patient to improve his or her ability to deal not only with 'acute' aspects of the specific relationship dispute, but also to develop skills to deal with future problems which might develop within the current relationship. This will ultimately not only help to prevent the relationship from deteriorating after treatment has ended, but should also help with new relationships.

Thus, even in those cases in which the patient is in a relationship which he or she ultimately chooses to end, the goal in IPT is to help the patient to better understand how he or she has contributed to the conflict. If this is accomplished, the patient will be better positioned to enter into new relationships without making the same mistakes. This is particularly crucial given that patients tend to manifest the same attachment style, and develop relationships in the same way, across time. If insight is not forthcoming, the patient is likely to step from the frying pan of one bad relationship into the fire of another just like it.

INTERPERSONAL DISPUTES: TECHNIQUES

After having established that a dispute exists and subsequently identifying its stages, the therapist and patient should work to resolve the dispute to bring about the satisfactory dissolution of the relationship. Disputes in the impasse phase should be moved one of these two directions. When discussing disputes, the patient will often experience emotions such as sadness or anger. It is vital for the therapist to help the patient recognize these emotional reactions, particularly with disputes in the impasse stage, in which the patient may have little motivation for change (Figure 16.2).

Clarification

The use of open-ended questions and empathic listening will help build a therapeutic alliance with a patient who is experiencing interpersonal disputes. This is obviously the foundation of all interventions in IPT, but is particularly important when dealing with disputes. This is in large part because the patient often comes into therapy feeling frustrated that the other person involved in the dispute doesn't understand the patient's perspective, and this feeling is likely to be imposed upon the therapist, barring a good alliance. Further, clarification will help identify specific aspects of the patient's dispute, which is crucial given that the patient's report to the therapist is likely to be biased. With less insightful patients, the report will often reflect an implicit message that the other person is to blame, and at least part of the communication to the therapist about the dispute is an invitation to the therapist to side with the patient against the 'oppressive other.' The therapist should therefore take care to expand on these areas further, as

Interpersonal Disputes

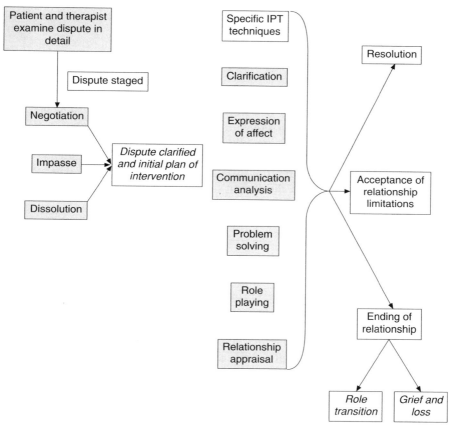

Figure 16.2 _Therapeutic Interventions in Interpersonal Disputes._ _The history of the dispute is examined in detail. After staging the dispute, the therapist helps to bring about a resolution by altering the patient's communication patterns, using problem solving, or helping the patient modify his or her expectations about the relationship. The dispute either begins to resolve, or the patient decides to leave the relationship, leading to a role transition. Regardless of the outcome of the dispute, a primary goal of the therapy is to help the patient emerge from the dispute with increased social support._

'what is not said' is often extremely important in determining the true nature of the dispute. This is frequently the case during the impasse phase.

Expression of affect

When relating the history of the dispute, the patient may begin to experience emotions such as sadness or anger. It is vital for the therapist to help the patient recognize these –

this can often be accomplished by exploring both process and content affect as the history unfolds. The affect can best be elicited simply by having the patient discuss the relationship; in particular, focusing on specific interpersonal incidents in which conflict has occurred will often help the patient to recognize and express emotional reactions. Once identified, these emotions can be used to motivate change in the conflicted relationship.

Communication analysis

Disputes may arise out of poor or maladaptive communication, or the dispute may lead to ineffective communication in a situation in which the communication was once much better. The therapist should direct the patient to report verbatim conversations and interpersonal incidents that he or she has had with others. This will provide material so that the patient's communication style can be analyzed, and hypotheses can be drawn about the ways in which the patient's communication is contributing to the perpetuation of the problem.

Problem solving

Once the history of the patient's relationship problem is well understood, and once the therapist has a good understanding of the patient's communication style, then the therapist and patient can collaborate on generating potential solutions to the specific interpersonal dispute. Both old strategies for dealing with similar problems as well as new approaches should be discussed. It is important for the patient to be as active as possible in this process in order to help gain a sense of mastery over the problem. This should also help the patient to develop the skills to address other problems in the future.

Role playing

Role playing can be a valuable intervention when dealing with interpersonal disputes. The therapist may choose to play the role of the significant other to gain further insight into the patient's communication style, and then give feedback to the patient so that his or her communication can be discussed. The patient may also play the role of the significant other, which is often a good way to help the patient gain insight into the other's experience. Role playing may also be used to help the patient develop assertiveness or communication skills, providing an 'in vitro' environment in which to practice these skills.

Relationship appraisal

Disputes are often based on expectations about the relationship that are non-reciprocal. Unrequited love, expectations of performance, or conflicts about the role that each person is to assume lead to conflict because of differences in expectations. In addition, conflicts can be exacerbated because the patient's expectation of the other exceeds what he or she is capable of doing, or exceeds what is possible to do in the given situation.

For instance, a woman having postpartum difficulties may expect her husband to take over the childcare responsibilities when she returns to work. If he is working as well, this may simply prove to be unrealistic, as it is literally not possible for him to fulfill her expectations. A patient with a spouse who is relatively detached and who may have avoidant traits may expect her spouse to be able to communicate deep emotional feelings – this too may be an unrealistic expectation given the limitations inherent in the spouse. Conversely, the husband's expectations that his wife will only need the amount of communication that he is comfortable with may also be unrealistic.

In these situations, the therapist may need to examine the expectations of the patient in detail, and determine whether they are realistic. If they are not, then the patient is bound to be disappointed no matter how much his or her communication improves. The therapist can give direct feedback to the patient about the expectations in some circumstances, or in others may want to let the patient take the lead. In either case, the goal is to help the patient realistically appraise his or her situation.

This particular technique bears many similarities to approaches taken in cognitive therapy. Technically speaking, it is similar, as the therapist is challenging the patient's expectations as might be done in CBT. Theoretically speaking, however, the two are very different. In IPT, the therapist makes no assumption that he or she is challenging the patient's underlying cognitions or maladaptive schemas; rather, in IPT the therapist is helping the patient to examine nothing more than his or her expectation about a specific relationship. In IPT, the therapist is always concerned with expectations about relationships.

INTERPERSONAL DISPUTES: TROUBLE SHOOTER

The patient reports an absence of disputes

During the initial phase of history gathering, a patient may fail to acknowledge the presence of significant interpersonal disputes, despite the fact that elements of the history strongly suggest a serious conflict is present. Possible reasons for this may include the patient's personality, psychological defenses, cultural factors, or reluctance to self-disclose during the early stages of the therapeutic relationship.

In these circumstances, the therapist should retain a high index of suspicion for the presence of a dispute without 'pathologizing' the situation and potentially damaging the therapeutic alliance. In other words, disputes should be reframed as common and reasonable parts of relationships; moreover, their presence should not imply that the relationship is doomed or dysfunctional. The therapist should look for inconsistencies reported by the patient, as well as examining the patient's communication and problem-solving styles. If an interpersonal conflict become apparent, the therapist can impress upon the patient that working on the dispute can improve the relationship and help relieve symptoms.

The patient who appears unmotivated for change

Needless to say, a patient who is unmotivated can be very difficult to work with in IPT. Such patients are, of course, difficult to work with in any format. Amotivation can be a significant phenomenological feature of a mood disorder, or it may be a reflection of the characterological qualities of some individuals, such as those with avoidant or dependant personalities. If the therapist and patient recognize amotivation as a feature of the patient's illness, the initial stages of therapy should focus on achieving more limited goals or achieving mastery over smaller, more manageable aspects of the patient's interpersonal problem. As the patient experiences success, his or her motivation may well improve in tandem with mood. The therapist should continually emphasize the patient's gains, and use this to reinforce motivation over time.

If the amotivation is characterological, the therapist should give serious consideration to the appropriateness of a focal, structured therapy such as IPT, and should examine the potential benefits of a longer-term dynamic treatment – a 'treatment failure' may be catastrophic for the patient and reinforce his or her sense of hopelessness.

An important distinction in this regard is the patient's motivation to *engage* in therapy and his or her motivation to *work* in therapy. Dependent patients, for example, are often quite willing to seek help (i.e., to engage in treatment) but may not be motivated to change once their dependency needs are met by entering a therapeutic relationship. Fortunately, with therapeutic effort such patients can usually be influenced to change once they are engaged in the therapy process. In addition to the obvious method of using the time limit to encourage change, the techniques described in previous chapters can be extremely helpful in increasing motivation in these situations. On the other hand, patients who have difficulty in engaging in therapy are often neither good candidates for IPT nor any other type of therapeutic intervention.

Put simply, patients who are able to walk through the door for the first appointment and return for subsequent sessions are at least motivated to engage in therapy, and therefore have the opportunity to benefit from treatment. Those who are do not seek treatment, who are not able to tolerate therapy, or who are sporadic in their attendance and commitment to therapy usually won't do well. There is simply no therapeutic technique that is effective if the patient is not present.

The patient with overwhelming social adversity

The presence of overwhelming social adversity, such as financial deprivation, chronic and seemingly intractable interpersonal disputes, or multiple traumatic losses, may precipitate a sense of hopelessness for both the patient and therapist. If, however, despite apparently overwhelming social problems, such a patient appears motivated for change, sees the relevance of an interpersonal focus, and has the capacity to work towards realistic goals, IPT is a worthwhile endeavor. In fact, remarkable success can be achieved in circumscribed interpersonal areas with such patients. Our experience with indigent patients and others with difficult social circumstances suggests that there is no reason to assume that these reasons alone will adversely affect outcome.[3]

In cases such as these, the therapist should avoid suggesting that all of the patient's problems will be addressed, and can instead work collaboratively to set modest and achievable goals. Working towards outcomes such as developing attachments and social supports outside of the problematic relationship, or improving assertiveness and problem solving skills, is appropriate. The therapist should also provide the patient with a warm and collaborative relationship which supports the patient in his or her efforts to deal with these difficult situations. The combination of empathy and an interpersonal problem focus may well contribute to improving psychiatric symptoms in illnesses previously regarded as 'chronic' or 'treatment-resistant.'

The patient who undermines the therapeutic process

Passive-aggressive behavior, acting out, or splitting, are major problems for a focal, time-limited treatment such as IPT. It is reasonable to assume that these behaviors reflect both the patient's problematic attachment style and his or her dysfunctional way of communicating attachment needs. The silver lining to these behaviors is that they can, when they occur in therapy, be a veritable gold mine of information, as the patient's interactions with the therapist will reflect his or her interactions with others. If the therapist can identify these behaviors in a constructive and non-critical way in the patient's interactions outside of therapy, then he or she can then help the patient to alter problematic interactions in communication or interpersonal behavior in these relationships.

If the therapist recognizes these behaviors as an intrinsic part of the patient's personality, and therefore likely to occur frequently during treatment, using IPT may lead to only limited improvement. There are circumstances, however, in which such behavior is related to a particular situation (i.e., is 'state-dependent') and is potentially amenable to IPT, if considered in the context of a problematic relationship. The therapist must be explicit in formulating the treatment contract and must continually reiterate the need to maintain an interpersonal focus and a time limit in this situation.

If the patient's disruptive behavior persists and threatens to undermine the course of treatment, it should be confronted directly and framed as breaking the therapy contract or as preventing the patient from dealing with important problems in the time available in treatment. Difficult behavior within the therapeutic relationship should be promptly extrapolated to real relationships in the patient's life to avoid shifting to a transference based treatment which would depart from the IPT model. If the patient's behavior in relationships outside of therapy remains the focus of treatment, significant progress can be made in helping the patient understand his or her contribution to the interpersonal problem.

Case example: Donna

Donna was a 41-year-old woman who sought counseling for a marital conflict. During the Interpersonal Inventory, Donna reported that she felt a profound lack of intimacy in her relationship with her husband, Blake. Donna reported that their communication was quite limited, that they didn't seem to have much in common any more, and that their sexual relationship was very poor. Donna reported that she had attempted to talk to Blake about this, but reported that the conversation, 'just didn't get anywhere.' The problem area of 'interpersonal disputes' was chosen, and the dispute was described as at an 'impasse.'

During the initial phase of IPT the therapist had difficulty getting Donna to engage in the therapeutic process. The therapist found herself frustrated and at times irritated with Donna, as she typically answered queries with only brief or incomplete responses. The therapist began to work on the hypothesis that this same style of communication was impairing Donna's relationship with her husband.

Therapist: Donna, tell me about the last time you felt that you and Blake really talked.

Donna: (long pause, then softly) A few weeks ago.

Therapist: What happened?

Donna: (long pause, then softly) Um, … we … um … talked about our relationship a bit.

Therapist: Was it like this?

Donna: Hmm?

Therapist: Was it like you and I are talking now?

Donna: (softly) I don't understand.

Therapist: It seems that when we talk together, there is a lot of non-verbal communication, but not much is spoken.

Donna: … Um, yes.

Therapist: Donna, how do you think your feelings about your relationship with Blake have affected your ability to speak your mind, like you used to?

Donna: (pause, then softly) Quite a bit, I suppose.

Therapist: I wonder if Blake understands how your feelings about him have affected your ability to communicate. How well do you think he understands what you are experiencing?

Donna was able to link her feelings of isolation from Blake with her communication problems, particularly identifying with the thought that Blake had no idea about what she was feeling. As the focus of the treatment shifted to her communication, Donna also reported feeling angry and frustrated with herself and with Blake, but felt at a loss as to how to proceed. The therapist and Donna agreed that it was important for Blake to know that she was feeling isolated and alone, and that this had affected her desire to communicate, which in turn had a deleterious effect on the relationship.

A conversation was enacted using a role play in which the therapist played Blake. During the process the therapist became even more aware of how inhibited and misleading Donna's communication had become. She commented on this experience while role playing, and asked Donna if Blake had been critical of this. The therapist and Donna continued to rehearse her communication over the next few sessions, using the role play technique to improve her ability to communicate how she was feeling.

Towards the end of the therapy, Donna reported a number of conversations to the therapist, in which significant improvements in her communication style were evident. Donna reported an improvement in her dispute with Blake and also a significant improvement in her sense of isolation. The therapist encouraged Donna to begin to utilize other social supports during this time, including several friends who were receptive to providing her with support.

The patient with an impaired significant other

There are often instances in which the IPT therapist will encounter a patient with a significant other who may have psychological difficulties – social adversity often affects families as well as individuals. The burden of caring for or interacting with an impaired partner or family member can often lead to interpersonal problems for the caregiver. Family therapists often talk of the 'identified patient,' in which a particular family member presents for treatment for a problem that has complex origins in the social milieu in which the family lives, implying that there may be systemic sources of psychopathology within the family. These kinds of systemic problems are often encountered in IPT.

The clinician has a number of options in cases such as this, including inviting the impaired partner to a session, conducting couples therapy, seeing the partner separately, or providing a referral for the partner if warranted. When the significant other is reluctant to address his or her psychological problems, the therapist may have to help the patient reframe the behavior or responses of the significant other as maladaptive communications, and encourage the patient to find out what they are intended to convey. In cases in which the significant other refuses treatment, changes made by the individual seeking treatment will hopefully affect both parties in the relationship, and may also have benefits for the significant other. Even in the most egregious cases in which the significant other is impaired and not willing to seek treatment, the therapist should never withhold treatment from the individual who is seeking it simply because the significant other will not attend.

Case example: Peter

Peter was a 44-year-old man who presented to a psychologist with a history of feeling excessively sad and hopeless over the previous few months. He told the psychologist that this had developed as a result of an argument he had with his 19-year-old daughter, Cassandra. He described his symptoms as fluctuating with the vicissitudes of the problems with Cassandra. Though Peter's symptoms were not intense enough to constitute a depressive episode, his distress was marked, and as a result he was highly motivated for treatment. Peter's previous physical and mental health had been good.

The problem between Peter and Cassandra appeared to be related to the breakdown of Peter's marriage to Cassandra's mother 3 years earlier. Since that time Cassandra had spent most of her time with her mother, who had apparently depicted Peter's contribution to the failure of the marriage in a one-sided manner. Cassandra herself had experienced difficulties with her health (complaining of chronic fatigue) and had also exhibited a number of problematic behaviors including several self-harm incidents, substance abuse, and suicidal ideations. Despite the seriousness of her distress, Cassandra had not sought help. Peter had encouraged Cassandra to get some treatment, but had received an indifferent and at times a hostile response from her.

Peter also complained that he felt stressed because of demands being placed upon him by his partner, Jane. Peter and Jane had been together for twelve months and Jane had been offered a job in another city. As a consequence, Jane had been pressuring Peter to marry her in order to 'cement their relationship' and to 'let us get on with our lives.'

After compiling the Interpersonal Inventory, Peter and the psychologist agreed that the difficulties he was currently experiencing with Cassandra and Jane were best conceptualized as interpersonal disputes. Peter was most concerned with his difficulties with Cassandra, and opted to focus on these first.

Peter and the therapist were able to clarify the nature of the dispute with Cassandra in detail. Peter felt that his expectations of Cassandra were that she should, 'try and hear my side of the story' and also, 'look after herself more effectively.' He also felt she should realize that his suggestion that she seek treatment was well intended, and was a reflection of his concern for her. He felt that he had great difficulty communicating this to Cassandra.

As Peter described the situation in detail, the therapist noted that he became quite tearful and agitated. The therapist called attention to Peter's process affect, noting the discrepancy in his rather factually presented story in the presence of obvious sad affect. Recognizing and admitting to his sadness helped motivate Peter to further address the dispute. The therapist and Peter discussed an Interpersonal Incident with Cassandra that had taken place prior to the session.

Therapist: Can you tell me about the last time you and Cassandra spoke?

Peter: Yes – it was a disaster.

Therapist: That's an interesting word to describe it. Perhaps we could consider that interaction in detail, so that we can better understand the problems with communication and how you might resolve them.

Peter: OK. I'll try to remember what happened.

Therapist: Fine. Can you describe the context of the conversation?

Peter: Yes. I rang Cassandra.

Therapist: What did you say exactly when you spoke to her?

Peter: What I said? 'Cassandra, it's Dad.'

Therapist: And what did Cassandra say then?

Peter: She said, 'What do you want?'

Therapist: How did you respond to that?

Peter: I think I said, 'What do you mean what do I want?'

Therapist: Was that how you sounded?

Peter: (confused) What do you mean?

Therapist: As you're relating it to me, it sounds very neutral and without emotion. What was the emotion that was communicated?

Peter: Well, now that you mention it, I was pretty hot. I think I was shouting.

Therapist: OK. Can you tell me how Cassandra responded to you after that?

The discussion revealed that Peter had reacted to Cassandra's hostile responses in kind, and that his responses had inflamed the situation further. The therapist and Peter agreed that his communication with Cassandra needed further work, and the next few sessions focused on consciously communicating his feelings directly to Cassandra.

When exploring his relationship with Jane, Peter felt that he expected Jane to, 'give me some space' and to, 'let me deal with the problems with my daughter first.' Peter felt slightly more confident in his ability to communicate these expectations to Jane, but felt that she still didn't understand his point of view. Peter and the therapist opted to work on clarifying his expectations of Jane and on rehearsing his communication to her. The therapist and Peter agreed that the particular problem was how to reconcile Jane's wish to move interstate without the need to force the issue of her wish to marry Peter, who stated, 'I am still getting over my last marriage.' The therapist and Peter discussed a number of potential solutions including: (i) a trial period of living apart with arrangements to meet every weekend; (ii) Jane looking for similar employment close to home; and (iii) Peter relocating to another city with and without getting married.

Peter rejected the last option, given that it would further distance him from Cassandra and make the resolution of that dispute more difficult. Peter then communicated this to Jane and a decision was reached to live apart temporarily. He then applied similar problem-solving strategies to his conflict with Cassandra, in particular brainstorming about how to approach her most effectively, and how to communicate his desire that she seek help for her problems. Peter was able to communicate with Cassandra in a way that acknowledged her anger but also conveyed his message clearly. Cassandra then agreed to see a psychologist. With the resolution of both disputes, Peter felt a significant improvement in his functioning.

The case highlights the fact that in working with interpersonal disputes it is important for the patient and therapist to clarify as explicitly as possible the core expectations of the other person in the dispute. This should be coupled with an exploration regarding the way in which the patient communicates his or her expectations and attachment needs to the other person in the dispute. Once this is done, problem-solving work can commence with the goal of improving communication.

CONCLUSION

Interpersonal disputes are frequently encountered in IPT, and are the bread and butter of therapy, as nearly all interpersonal relationships engender conflict at some point. The goals in IPT are to identify the dispute, stage it appropriately, and then help the patient move either towards resolution of the conflict or dissolution of the relationship. The therapist should pay particular attention to the patient's style of communication and his or her expectations about the relationship, as both are frequent contributors to the problem as well as factors that maintain the dispute.

REFERENCES

1. Bowlby, J. 1969. *Attachment*. New York: Basic Books.
2. Klerman, G.L., Weissman, M.M., Rounsaville, B.J., Chevron, E.S. 1984. *Interpersonal Psychotherapy of Depression*. New York: Basic Books.
3. O'Hara, M.W., Stuart, S., Gorman, L., Wenzel, A. 2000. Efficacy of interpersonal psychotherapy for postpartum depression. *Archives of General Psychiatry* **57**, 1039–45.

17

Role Transitions

INTRODUCTION

Change is a frequent occurrence in everyone's life. In many ways, adaptation to change both determines and is determined by one's physical and mental health. In most circumstances change is dealt with successfully, and individuals adapt to new conditions without developing psychological problems. In others, individuals with poor interpersonal resources or who are faced with overwhelming change have difficulties.

All interpersonal relationships occur in complex psychosocial contexts. When the context changes, as in a role transition, the nature of the relationship changes. An example of this process is the role transition faced by a young adult who graduates from high school and leaves home to go to college. While there may be no major intrapsychic changes in the person or in those around him or her, the context of relationships with parents, siblings and others changes. This process brings about dynamic changes in those relationships. The young adult moves to become less dependent upon his or her family of origin, moves toward more adult responsibilities, and begins to relate differently to parents in his or her new role. In other circumstances life-cycle transitions or deterioration in health status may be significant contextual changes. In IPT, the process of change within relationships which occurs as a consequence of contextual changes within the patient's life is conceptualized as a role transition.

Though some transitions, such as loss of health, may be seen as wholly negative by the patient, most change involves some good and bad elements. When working with a patient who is experiencing a role transition, the therapist focuses directly on the ambivalent feelings that the patient is experiencing while undergoing the transition, bringing the patient's attention to both positive and negative reactions to the change.

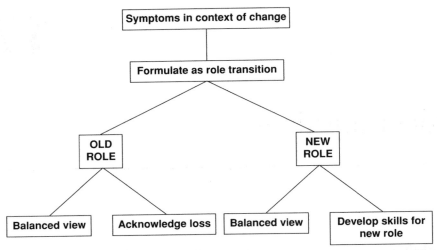

Figure 17.1 *Role Transitions*. *The therapist helps the patient identify significant role transition during the Interpersonal Inventory and then proceeds to help the patient accept the loss of the old role and acknowledge the affect associated with the transition. The patient and therapist then appraise the new role, identifying the challenges it presents and implementing solutions to the problems the change has created in order to help the patient better adapt to the new role. The therapist also works to help the patient develop a more balanced view of both the old and new role.*

The therapist's task is to help the patient to recognize these ambivalent reactions and to deal with them effectively (Figure 17.1).

THE NATURE OF ROLE TRANSITIONS

Role transitions can be developmental life events, such as adolescence, pregnancy, or aging, or situational changes such as unemployment or divorce. As in all life events, role transitions need to be seen in the context of the person's interpersonal and sociocultural environment, and in light of psychological factors such as personality and attachment style. Seemingly minor role transitions can be experienced as major losses by a patient who has poor social support or attachment difficulties. In other situations the loss of a comfortable old role and the advent of a seemingly formidable new role literally forces the patient to move from conditions in which he or she felt comfortable and able to function into a new environment which is perceived as overwhelming, difficult or anxiety-provoking.

Table 17.1 *Types of Role Transitions*.

- Life stage role transitions: *adolescence, parenthood, aging, retirement.*
- Situational role transitions: *job loss, promotion, graduation, migration.*
- Acquisitive role transitions: *career advancement, new house, financial windfall.*
- Relationship role transitions: *marriage, divorce, step-parenthood.*
- Illness-related role transition: *diagnosis of chronic illness, adaptation to pain or physical limitations.*

ASSESSING ROLE TRANSITIONS

Role transitions may be apparent during the gathering of the initial history, or may only emerge after careful exploration of an event or aspect of the patient's life and its significance to the patient.

Table 17.2 *Questions to Elicit Role Transitions.*

- 'Have you recently changed your working or living circumstances?'
- 'What changes have occurred recently in your working life?'
- 'Have there been recent changes in your home or social life?'
- 'Have you recently passed any milestones in your life?'
- 'Have you recently started (or talked about starting) a family?'
- 'Are you expecting any major changes in your life over the next few months?'
- 'Have there been any changes in your physical health?'

In some cases, historical or demographic factors may be associated with role transitions.

Table 17.3 *Potential Indicators of Role Transitions.*

- Age: *life stage role transition; illness-related role transition.*
- Gender: *life stage role transition; family role transition.*
- Marital status: *relationship role transition; acquisitive role transition.*
- Employment: *situational role transition; acquisitive role transition.*
- Ethnicity: *situational role transition.*
- Medical history: *illness-related role transition.*

Occasionally, role transitions may not become apparent until well into the course of therapy. As the patient and therapist clarify and develop a better understanding of the patient's interpersonal problems, or as interpersonal work proceeds and changes to relationships occur, the use of the role transition problem area may become more appropriate. Examples of this may be the reformulation of a relationship dispute in the dissolution stage as a role transition, or the acceptance of a diagnosis of depression as a chronic recurrent illness requiring a role transition in the patient's thinking about his or her health.

A novel and useful conceptualization which involves a change or transition in the patient's self concept is that of an 'iatrogenic role transition,' which was first described by Markowitz in his work with patients suffering from dysthymic disorder.[1] Markowitz conceptualizes the patient's current dysthymic role as 'illness,' and the new euthymic role to which he or she is transitioning as 'wellness.' After presenting the dysthymic 'illness state' as an old role, the patient and therapist clarify all of the interpersonal effects that the illness has had upon the patient's life. The patient and therapist then construct an interpersonal model which would characterize the patient's life if the effects of the mood state were no longer present. The therapist focuses upon helping the patient develop skills which will help the patient act, think and feel less depressed in this 'wellness state,' a new role which is literally assigned to the patient. This ingenious process of 'putting the cart before the horse' is clearly a desirable alternative to labeling a patient as having interpersonal deficits. When using this approach, however, the therapist must make sure that the patient can actually make the transition to wellness – to suggest to a patient that he or she can transition from a dysthymic state works well only if the patient can overcome the mood disorder.

ROLE TRANSITIONS: THERAPEUTIC STRATEGIES

The essential therapeutic tasks when working with role transitions are to:

- Develop a productive therapeutic alliance.
- Work with the patient to clarify the transition, including both the old and new roles.
- Help the patient grieve the loss of the old role and its associated social supports.
- Help the patient to conceptualize the old role and new role in a balanced and realistic way.
- Help the patient to develop new social supports and new social skills, if needed.

Defining the 'old role'

The process of more fully understanding the patient's roles relies heavily upon the technique of clarification. The therapist should generally maintain the focus of discussion upon the transition, and explore details about the specific aspects of each role. The therapist should also ask questions which clarify how the patient has come to see things as they have historically.

When discussing the 'old role,' the therapist's tasks are four-fold:

1 *To understand the patient, and to help the patient better understand his or her circumstances.* To an independent observer, a role transition might not appear to be a loss experience at all, and in some cases it may be seen as an overall positive change. In contrast, the therapist must work to understand the nature of the role transition from the patient's perspective, and to understand its meaning in the patient's life. As the therapist does so, not only will the patient's perspective become clearer to the therapist, but the patient should also come to understand his or her circumstances more fully.

2 *To recognize the loss and subsequent ambivalence or anxiety about the role transition.* As an understanding of the patient's perspective develops, the therapist is more able to empathize with the 'loss' experience that the patient has experienced in the change of roles. As empathy develops, it can be communicated to the patient and can validate the patient's sense of loss, and his or her anxiety or ambivalence about undertaking the new role. The communication of empathy will foster the therapeutic alliance, and the recognition of anxiety about the future is also greatly therapeutic.

3 *To engage the patient's affect so that change is facilitated.* The patient's emotional reactions – sadness at the loss of the old role and anxiety about the new role – should be acknowledged by the therapist and used as a motivating factor to help the patient resolve the role transition.

4   *To help the patient to conceptualize the old role and new role in a more balanced and realistic way.* The therapist should attempt to clarify the patient's perception of the positive and negative aspects of the old role in order to help the patient develop a more balanced view of it. In this way the patient may come to see that the 'loss' of the old role may have its advantages as well as its disadvantages. The same is true for the new role – the patient should be encouraged to explore and articulate the positive and negative aspects of the new role. Helping the patient to recognize his or her ambivalence and to develop a balanced view of both roles is the goal.

A classic role transition is that which occurs after childbirth. A new mother may see that her life before children had the advantages of freedom, career progression and ample leisure time. Intrinsic to the old role is a comfortable and familiar social support system which may be dramatically affected by change in child status. She may also feel that parenthood leaves her tired, with little freedom, and with less time to spend with her partner. After conceptualizing the passage into parenthood as a role transition, the patient and her therapist review and clarify the positive and negative aspects of both the old and new roles. While doing so, the woman may recognize that, from a different perspective, she greatly enjoys being a mother, and in her old role had lost touch with friends who had entered parenthood. Despite the loss of some social support, she may recognize that having a child leads to new social connections as she spends more time with friends who have children (Figure 17.2).

Like all role transitions, this is an area in which the therapist can really be effective in helping the patient to describe his or her experience. Becoming a parent is a profound transition, and one which is often difficult to describe. A therapist who is genuinely interested in the patient's unique experience can bring about tremendous change simply by encouraging the patient to talk about what having a new child is like – empathy, warmth, interest, and caring go a long way. Asking questions such as 'What is it like to be a new parent?,' 'What is it like to hold your child?,' 'What about parenthood is different than you expected?,' 'What does it feel like to care for your baby?,' and especially 'What is it like to love someone like you do your child?' are literally life-changing ways to get the patient to think and talk about the experience.

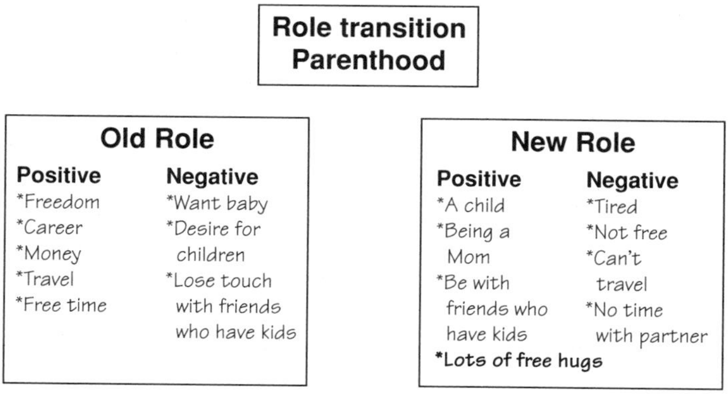

Figure 17.2 *Role Transition of Motherhood.* *The patient and therapist review the positive and negative aspects of the old and new roles to develop a more balanced view of both.*

5   *To help the patient develop new social supports.* The transition to parenthood is also an excellent example of the need to address social support in the new role. In addition to coming to a more balanced view of the transition, the patient should also be encouraged to develop new social supports. New relationships provide both emotional support and help to meet the patient's attachment needs in the new setting.

Dealing with the 'new role'

In general, the patients who present for treatment tend to view their new roles as negative and laden with challenges that they may feel incapable of meeting. Patients with less secure attachment styles may overestimate the scope of their challenges and underestimate their capacity to meet them. New roles become stressors for these patients as they attempt to cope with challenges they feel that they are not able to overcome. The therapist must help such patients to reappraise the challenges of the new roles and their ability to deal with the transitions, and should also help such patients to begin to develop new social supports.

Consider the case example of a man who has developed depression in the context of being diagnosed with adult-onset diabetes mellitus. His appraisal of the new role he has been forced to assume – 'a diabetic' – may be that it is a process of increasing ill health and disability, full of difficulties such as the need to adhere to demanding lifestyle modifications, to take medications, and to make multiple visits to doctors, podiatrists, and dieticians. Many people would see this new role as an overwhelming challenge that they felt poorly equipped to meet. In this particular case, the therapist should first help the patient to grieve the loss of the old role, and discuss how the change has affected his sense of self and his relationships with others. The therapist should also help the patient to develop a more balanced view of the new role. While this may be difficult in a situation in which the patient's appraisal that the new situation is mostly negative is accurate, the therapist can often discuss the life change as a point at which the patient can reassess his or her priorities and make a conscious decision about how to structure relationships and life in general. Many patients are able, after grieving the loss of health, to use the change as a point of transformation – a 'wake up call' – and to use it to reassess their life goals and priorities.

The therapist should also help the patient to consider some of the other potential positive aspects of the new role, such as the opportunity to adopt a healthier lifestyle, and the recognition of a potentially lethal medical condition which had previously been unrecognized and can now be safely treated. The therapist should also help the patient reassess the challenges of the new role, such as adherence to lifestyle adjustments such as dietary requirements, and should help the patient develop the interpersonal support needed to put these into practice. For instance, the patient may want to enlist his wife for both interpersonal support and practical support with his new dietary habits. Other friends may be enlisted for help with exercise and other lifestyle changes.

In addition, the therapist can help the patient to begin to communicate his experience with illness. In addition to enlisting social support in a way that is helpful for the patient, he can also begin to more fully meet his attachment needs by communicating his experience in a way in which others can understand and to which they can respond. As a therapist, asking questions such as 'How well do you think others understand your experience?' and 'What can you do to help others to understand your experience more fully?' are of great benefit.

ROLE TRANSITION: TROUBLE SHOOTER

Patient does not recognize the role transition

As with all interpersonal problem areas, the patient's perceptions and expectations of particular events in his or her life may be vastly different from the inference drawn by others. It is the task of the therapist to help the patient recognize that his or her distress is temporally related to a particular event or change in circumstances, and to help conceptualize this connection as a role transition. As with other problem areas, it is not necessary to 'diagnose' a role transition – the interpersonal areas should be used flexibly with the primary goal of maintaining an interpersonal focus.

For example, a woman who has become depressed in the context of her daughter leaving home for college may not choose to conceptualize this as a role transition, but see it instead as a grief and loss issue, or perhaps a dispute with her daughter who is attempting to establish herself as an adult in a context outside of the family. The therapist should acknowledge the patient's view of the problem, and work with the patient collaboratively rather than attempting to diagnose or 'sell' the idea of role transition at the risk of damaging the therapeutic relationship.

This is particularly true as there is a great deal of overlap between all of the problem areas in IPT. For instance, a divorce could be considered a grief and loss issue, a role transition issue, or an interpersonal conflict, and may even be intertwined with interpersonal sensitivity issues. The death of a significant other similarly may involve grief and loss issues, or involve transition issues as new responsibilities are assumed and new social supports are needed. The primary purpose of the problem areas in IPT is to focus both the patient and clinician on specific interpersonal problems and to maintain the interpersonal focus of treatment. For the clinician to insist on diagnostic specificity is simply to assume that the clinician is more familiar with the patient's problems than is the patient, an assumption which impedes the clinician from truly listening to the patient. The therapeutic alliance should never be sacrificed in order to force a patient into a particular conceptualization of his or her problem.

An astute therapist can use the discussion about how to conceptualize the patient's interpersonal problem as a means of enhancing the alliance by further clarifying the issue with the patient. For example, rather than definitively interpreting for the patient that his or her problem is a role transition, the therapist can 'offer' a tentative view which the patient can then accept or reject. This has the benefit of conveying to the patient a desire to understand his or her problem more fully, and will go a long way towards enhancing the alliance. Further, this also allows the patient to be more invested in the therapy, and encourages the patient to offer the therapist important clarifications or additional information about how he or she perceives the problem.

The therapist might say to the preceding patient, for example:

'We have approached the problem with your daughter as a "dispute," and your communication and problem-solving skills have really improved. I can still sense that you are distressed by the problem and you have said on a few occasions that, "maybe she needs to get on with her own life." Perhaps it would be helpful to think about how the change in your relationship with your daughter has affected you and how you might be feeling about being the mother of a college student. What are your thoughts about reconsidering some parts of this problem as a role transition in addition to your original view of it as a dispute?'

Patient does not recognize or accept positive or negative aspects of a role

Patients frequently over- or under-emphasize the positive or negative aspects of a role. The effects of the patient's mood upon his or her thinking patterns may be particularly significant in influencing this assessment. In these circumstances the therapist can:

- Review and further clarify the aspects of the old or new role.
- Highlight the likely effect of depression or anxiety on the patient's view of the role.
- Highlight to the patient that despite his or her feelings about the lost or gained role, the transition has occurred, and the best chance of improving his or her symptoms is to work to overcome the difficulties in adapting to the new role.

The last point is particularly salient in IPT. The bottom line in the therapy is action – the therapy is designed to help the patient cope and function maximally given the change.

There is little affect with which to work

Some patients have intrapsychic conflicts that make it difficult for them to experience emotion within the therapy sessions. This may be addressed by examining an Interpersonal Incident in which the patient may have experienced distress or other relevant affect. The patient will likely exhibit some degree of affective shift using this technique. If the patient continues to have problems despite this technique, the therapist can focus upon more the practical aspects of helping the patient to adapt to the new role, in the expectation that this, even absent the affective involvement, will aid in the reduction of symptom severity.

As a general rule in all therapy and in IPT in particular, the more affect that is experienced by the patient, the more likely change is to occur. Thus, asking questions – with genuine interest – about how the patient feels or reacts emotionally to situations should be a focal and frequent intervention.

Case example: Terry

Terry was a 49-year-old married business executive who had been admitted to a general hospital with severe chest pains. Investigations showed that Terry had suffered a significant anterior myocardial infarction. Terry was also found to have elevated blood glucose and to be moderately hypertensive. After 3 days in the hospital's coronary care unit, Terry was seen by an endocrinologist, who diagnosed type II diabetes mellitus and instituted management with diet and oral hypoglycemic medication. After being examined by his cardiologist, Terry was also started on antihypertensive medication.

After being visited by his cardiologist, Terry complained to the nursing staff that he was unhappy with the consultation and wanted a second opinion. This was arranged, and another cardiologist confirmed the diagnosis of hypertension and also concurred with the recommended treatment. Terry became angry with the second cardiologist, and attempted to discharge himself against medical advice. A psychiatrist was called to see Terry in the coronary care unit. She gave Terry an opportunity to ventilate his frustrations and discuss his feelings about the situation. He reluctantly agreed to remain in the hospital, and she left Terry her details should he wish to contact her again.

Several days later, Terry was discharged from the hospital and referred to a cardiac rehabilitation facility. After about three weeks, the psychiatrist received a phone call from the cardiac rehabilitation nurse who had observed a deterioration in Terry's mood. The therapist arranged for an outpatient appointment with Terry. At the second consultation, the therapist noted that Terry now endorsed numerous symptoms consistent with a depressive disorder. Terry told the therapist that he had not had any previous difficulties with his mental health, and that he had been physically well prior to his heart attack. Terry felt that he was unable to deal with the 'triple whammy' of ischemic heart disease, hypertension and diabetes, as well as the fact that he was now taking so many medications that he 'rattled.'

After further discussion with the therapist it became apparent that Terry was quite driven in his work – he had been a highly successful businessman running his own chain of electronic stores for twenty years prior to his illness. Terry spent a great deal of time during the initial sessions discussing with the therapist how he had built up his business from 'small beginnings' and how it had become a successful chain of stores. Terry described himself as a 'hard-nosed professional' who had no time to be ill. To illustrate this, Terry stated to the therapist 'in small business the weak are killed and eaten by their competitors.'

When the therapist inquired about Terry's feelings about being diagnosed with heart disease and with diabetes, she noted a marked shift in Terry's affect. Terry became tearful and dysphoric when discussing the impact of the event on his life. The therapist reflected the following to him:

> 'Terry, it seems that you have developed a number of symptoms that I think indicate you have developed a clinical depression. You have obviously been a strong and capable man throughout you life, and this catastrophic development in your physical health seems to have really overwhelmed you. I can certainly understand that this is your first experience with ill health, and it is a massive one at that. There are many reasons why people become depressed, but it seems that for you that this particular event has been the main cause.
>
> I think that you would benefit from some counseling that focuses on how you can best adjust to your new health circumstances, and the impact that your health problems are having on your life. I think that there is also good reason to consider trying an antidepressant medication, and I think this would be of benefit to you. However, I also understand that you are reluctant to take yet another pill. I think that if we were to meet for twelve sessions of Interpersonal Psychotherapy we would be able to address this issue in a more structure way which would be of great benefit to you.
>
> What are your thoughts about this view of your problem?'

The therapist's presentation captured many of the elements of a good conceptualization, and highlights the importance of the delivery. First, she allowed Terry to respond to her tentative hypothesis regarding his role transition. This was particularly important given the fact that Terry described himself as fiercely independent. The therapist realized that she needed to give Terry even more of a sense of control than other patients might need. Second, there was a clear sense of developing a collaborative relationship in the therapy. The therapist was able, however, to maintain her role as a 'benevolent expert,' setting up a positive transference relationship which could be maintained through the brief course of therapy.

Terry agreed to the therapeutic contract, and he and the therapist constructed an Interpersonal Inventory. In the inventory Terry acknowledged his transition into a chronic physical illness as a significant problem. Terry stated that he felt a strong sense of grief and loss at the change from his previous 'perfect physical health.' The therapist agreed that there were certainly significant grief issues present, and she agreed that would be a reasonable way of conceptualizing the problem. The therapist also suggested the possibility that viewing the loss of health as a role transition would also be helpful, as it offered a way in which Terry could grieve the loss of his 'healthy self' while also helping him to acknowledge the need to adjust to his new circumstances.

Terry initially described his old role as being one of 'strength, capacity and invulnerability.' Terry recalled in particular being able to work 16-hour days, 7 days a week. 'I could get by on no sleep and only little amounts of food. I could eat stress for dinner and spit it out without any problem.'

The therapist then asked if Terry had any reservations about how his life was before the heart attack, and what he might have changed. In particular, she asked about how his previous lifestyle was affecting his role as a husband and father. Terry responded that, 'It wasn't all beer and skittles, but at least I was able to get things done my way.' The therapist further clarified with Terry how his previous role may have had some negative aspects, including some detrimental effects on his marriage and his relationship with his children. Terry was able to acknowledge that these may have been drawbacks of his old role, and as a result, he was able to feel less aggrieved by its loss. He was also able to see the transition as a way of reprioritizing these relationships.

With recognition of some of the negative aspects of the old role, some patients often also have a sense of grief or loss. This is of the 'I wish I had done things differently' type. Thoughts such as 'I wish I had been a better father' or 'I wish I hadn't got divorced' often lead to a sense of guilt or remorse.

The art in IPT is to help the patient to express these feelings in a supportive therapeutic relationship while at the same time recognizing that the time limit and relationship focus of IPT require that the therapist maintain the pace of the therapy. While grieving and dealing with remorse is an essential part of the therapy, the ultimate aim of IPT is to help the patient address the question: 'given my change in circumstances, how can I function most effectively right now.'

The ideal outcome would be for the patient to come to an epiphany and see the crisis as an opportunity for re-evaluation and change. The therapist, taking care to be empathic, can often reflect this directly to the patient. For instance, the therapist might say:

'Despite the loss of your health you have experienced, the "silver lining" is that it has now forced you to think about how you want to structure your life. It has taken you off the "fast track," and you can now spend some time thinking about how you want to structure your relationships. That is what we should focus on in the remainder of therapy, so that I can help you to follow through with the changes you would like to make.'

The therapist and Terry shifted to focus on the new role. Terry acknowledged that his cardiac rehabilitation specialist had strongly urged him to limit the number of hours he worked, improve his sleep, allow time for exercise, and modify his diet. This would require that he work more routine hours and be home for prepared meals rather than eating restaurant and take-out food. These lifestyle modifications were seen by Terry as important to his health. Terry also felt 'washed out' by his medication. The therapist and Terry engaged in a role play regarding how he might approach his cardiologist (with whom he had the initial disagreement) about changing his anti-hypertensive medication or looking at alternative interventions without getting angry or appearing demanding.

The focus of discussion then shifted to Terry's business and the need for him to modify his hours. The therapist suggested that Terry might benefit from a problem-solving approach:

Therapist: Perhaps we could brainstorm a few solutions to the problem.
Terry: Guess so, wouldn't hurt.
Therapist: OK. You've said that the problem is basically the business needs to be manned at least 12 hours a day to maintain the edge over your competitors.
Terry: That's right.
Therapist: And that you really need to be only working 6–8 hours per day as well as taking time out to eat a healthy lunch and make sure that you're home in time to do some exercise.
Terry: That's right.
Therapist: OK. Well, what do you see as potential solutions to this.
Terry: Well, I guess one might be to hire some help.
Therapist: What would that involve?

The therapist and Terry then developed four or five potential solutions to the problem. In each instance they evaluated the pros and cons of the particular option, and Terry chose the one he thought most reasonable. Terry went about implementing this and reported back to the therapist.

As Terry was able to make the appropriate lifestyle modifications needed for his health without compromising his business, he described his mood as improving. Terry stated that he still felt a great sense of loss when he reflected on his previous physical health status, but he was able to state that 'at least I know I'm human.'

IPT offered Terry a way of concretely understanding the change in his life occasioned by his physical health problems. Terry had been provided with an opportunity to reflect on his old role and mourn its loss. He had also been provided with a collaborative working relationship which helped him formulate strategies to deal with his new role, with which he felt poorly equipped to deal. In the final analysis, the therapist was able to help Terry regain sense of control over his situation, which was a core loss for him.

CONCLUSION

Role transitions are frequent presenting problems in IPT. Patients are usually able to make connections with the life events which have led to their distress, though they may not conceptualize the problem in quite the same way as the therapist. The strategy in dealing with role transitions is to assist the patient to mourn the loss of the old role, and to develop a more balanced view of both the old and new roles. Encouraging the patient to develop new social supports in his or her new environment is also crucial.

REFERENCE

1. Markowitz, J. 1998. *Interpersonal Psychotherapy for Dysthymic Disorder*. Washington, DC: American Psychiatric Press.

18

Grief and Loss

INTRODUCTION

The psychotherapist Irvin Yalom wrote 'Grief is the interest owed on the debt of attachment.'[1] Loss is a fundamental part of human experience and is encountered in all phases of the life cycle. The intrapsychic processes that mediate an individual's progress through grief and loss have been mapped by many authors, all sharing a view that the human being who suffers loss endures intense, and sometimes extreme anxiety, despair, and detachment. Individuals who are able to adapt to the loss in a productive way ultimately move on to initiate new relationships which provide meaningful social support, though they never truly 'replace' the lost person.

In IPT, the model proposed by Bowlby[2] serves as the most suitable with which to work psychotherapeutically with grief (Figure 18.1). Bowlby described that humans moved through three stages of loss, which he labeled as, protest, despair, and detachment. In IPT, the goal is to help patients work through these phases and continue on through a resolution of their grief. The resolution involves helping patients to develop insight into their loss and their experience of it, and also involves sharing that experience with others. The latter is absolutely crucial in IPT. This process of sharing with others will begin to engage social support, diminish patients' sense of isolation, and begin to help patients develop new attachments. While the working through of the loss intrapsychically is extremely helpful and is a necessary part of IPT, it is the communication of the experience to others and the development of social support surrounding the loss which characterizes IPT.

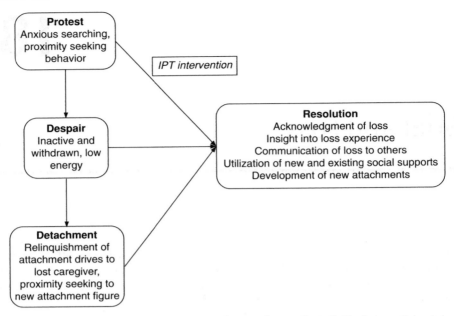

Figure 18.1 *Model of Loss using IPT and Attachment Theory.* *The individual moves through a pathway of response to loss as described by attachment theory. The IPT therapist intervenes in this process by creating a therapeutic relationship in which the patient can discuss the loss. The patient then extends this by communicating his or her experience to those in his or her social network. The patient also works to improve the utilization of existing social supports and to initiate new supports.*

The intrapsychic 'working through' of the loss experience in therapy is an example of the process of utilizing new social support, though the sharing of experience is initially confined to the therapeutic relationship. Therapist warmth and empathy are crucial to this process. Once this begins within the therapy, the IPT therapist then works to help the patient extend the expression of his or her loss experience to social supports outside of therapy.

THE NATURE OF GRIEF AND LOSS

It is often useful for the therapist to formulate many types of non-bereavement losses as grief issues. In addition to the death of a significant other, loss of physical health, divorce and loss of employment are examples of interpersonal stressors which might be seen by the patient as grief issues. In general, it is usually best for the therapist to place the patient's problems within the area which is the most meaningful for the patient. Moreover, in IPT grief need not be considered as 'normal' or 'abnormal' – it is the task of the therapist to attempt to understand the patient's experience, not to pathologize or label it.

Once a grief issue is established as a focus of treatment, the therapist's tasks are to:

1   Facilitate the patient's mourning process.

2   Assist the patient to develop new interpersonal relationships, or to modify his or her existing relationships so as to obtain increased social support.

Though new or existing relationships cannot 'replace' the lost relationship, the patient can reallocate his or her energies and interpersonal resources over time.

Several strategies are useful in dealing with grief issues. Primary among these is the elicitation of affect from the patient, which may be facilitated by discussing the loss and the circumstances surrounding the loss, both of which serve to assist the patient to realistically reconstruct the relationship. A discussion of process and content affect may be quite useful during this process.

Grief issues commonly involve layers of conflicted feelings surrounding the lost person. Assisting the patient to develop a 'three-dimensional' picture of the lost person, including a realistic assessment of the person's good and bad characteristics, is a necessary process in the resolution of the grief. Often, the patient will initially describe the lost person as 'all good' or 'all bad,' and be unaware that this idealization (or devaluation) covers other contradictory feelings which may be difficult to accept. The development of a balanced view of the lost individual greatly facilitates the mourning process. In essence, part of the grief work involves moving the patient to a securely attached way of experiencing, thinking about, and describing the lost individual as a 'whole person' with both positive and negative qualities.

This same process can also be used for other losses – for example, the loss of a job, a divorce, or loss of physical functioning. In such instances, the patient will also need to grieve the loss, and to move towards establishing new social relationships which will provide more support. Encouraging the patient to develop a more realistic view of the loss may also be of help.

THE FEATURES OF GRIEF AND LOSS

The experience of grief and loss shares much phenomenologically with depression, and their clinical differentiation is often challenging. While clinicians need not pathologize the experience of grief, constant vigilance should be maintained for the development of depression and other psychiatric difficulties in the context of grief. This is particularly the case in such circumstances as 'traumatic bereavement,' 'conjugal bereavement,' or the death of a child. In other words, the closer the attachment, and the more traumatic the circumstances surrounding the loss, the more vigilant the therapist should be. While diagnosing depression in a bereaved individual is a complicated process, a few phenomenological features are useful clues to the presence of depression. These include:

- *Marked self-reproach*: in contrast to individuals suffering from depression, those who are grieving are able to retain an intact sense of self and maintain their sense of self-esteem, and generally do not develop excessive guilt.
- *Suicidality*: while bereaved individuals may experience a sense of 'indifference to life' for a time after the loss, this seldom evolves into suicidal ideation or intent.
- *Psychomotor retardation or agitation*: psychomotor agitation and retardation have been noted to be indicators of severe endogenous or 'melancholic' depression, and do not typically appear as physiological features of grief.

- *Marked psychotic symptoms*: individuals with auditory or visual hallucinations should be evaluated for underlying psychotic processes.
- *Marked lack of reactivity*: many bereaved individuals will describe a marked loss of interest in their usual activities, but the complete absence of reactivity should be regarded as clinically significant.

Additional features which are characteristic of both grief and depression include:

- Depressed mood or sadness.
- Irritability.
- Poor sleep.
- Loss of appetite.
- Loss of interest in usual activities.
- Indecisiveness.
- Anxiety symptoms such as panic attacks or obsessional thoughts.

COMPLICATED GRIEF

In IPT, there need not be a distinction between 'normal' and 'abnormal' grief. The primary goal of the therapist is to understand the patient's experience with grief, not to pathologize it or to describe it to the patient as, 'nothing more than a normal reaction.' Patients request treatment for a variety of grief and loss issues; it should be assumed that patients who present for treatment with such issues will benefit from IPT, particularly if the grief or loss is identified as a significant issue from the outset of treatment. As it is not necessary for a patient to have a psychiatric diagnosis to profit from treatment with IPT, self-identification of a grief issue by the patient serves as sufficient grounds for evaluation for treatment.

Grief and loss problems are conceptualized in IPT as resulting from two factors, both of which may be operative for the patient who seeks treatment surrounding a loss. The first factor is that the patient's social support system is not sufficient to sustain him or her through the loss experience. The second is that the patient may not be communicating his or her needs for support in such a way that others can respond effectively. Both of these factors are obviously strongly influenced by the patient's attachment style, as it influences the extent of the social support which the patient will have available, as well as his or her capacity to utilize it.

In IPT, the therapist takes the temporary role of a support figure for the patient, and forms a relationship in which the patient can work through conflicted feelings about the loss. While this process might take place in social relationships, it often needs to occur first in the therapeutic relationship, particularly if the patient has difficulty utilizing his or her social support system. Similarly, those patients who have a limited social support network may also need to use the therapeutic relationship in this situation.

Nonetheless, as grief and loss are often associated with more severe difficulties, it is useful clinically to fully evaluate all of the patient's reactions to the loss. The term 'complicated grief' can be used to describe circumstances in which the grief reaction has been delayed, is prolonged, or is associated with more severe mental illness. The commonly acknowledged forms of complicated grief are:

- *Delayed grief*: a grief reaction which has its onset at a time distant from the actual loss.
- *Absent grief*: the individual does not appear to have experienced, or does not acknowledge experiencing, a grief reaction at the time of the loss or thereafter.
- *Hypertrophic grief*: grief which leads to more severe psychiatric problems such as depression or anxiety disorders.
- *Prolonged grief*: an individual's difficulties with the grief experience have not diminished over time.
- *Grief associated with latent trauma*: a loss, particularly a traumatic loss, which is associated with unmasking latent post-traumatic stress disorder (PTSD) or dissociative symptoms that relate to previous trauma. Often the lost attachment figure may have been involved with the trauma, e.g., the perpetrator of abuse.

IDENTIFYING GRIEF AND LOSS

There are several useful clues to the presence of a grief issue in a patient presenting for treatment:

- The relationship with the lost person.
- The nature of the loss – trauma, suicide, disappearance.
- The context of the loss – financial implications, lack of social support, cultural context.
- The age of the lost person – child, parent of young child, child sibling.
- The age of the bereaved – young spouse, child.
- The absence of affect – suggesting complicated grief.

WORKING WITH GRIEF AND LOSS IN IPT

The basic tasks of working with grief in IPT are (Figure 18.2):

- Identifying a grief or loss issue.
- Clarifying the circumstances surrounding the loss.
- Linking the loss to the onset of psychiatric symptoms or social dysfunction.
- Helping the patient accept the painful affects associated with the loss.
- Helping the patient initiate new attachments and develop more effective social supports.

Clarifying the circumstances of the loss

In the initial sessions of IPT, and particularly during the process of completing the Interpersonal Inventory, the therapist must often rely heavily on the technique of clarification in order to help the patient to better understand the circumstances of the loss. As clarification can be both an active and a passive process, the therapist must exercise judgment as to which is the most suitable; this will usually be determined by the

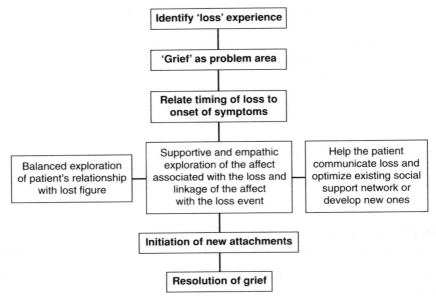

Figure 18.2 *Working with Grief and Loss in IPT.*

patient's affective state. In circumstances in which the patient is in a markedly dysphoric state in therapy, the therapist should usually be less directive while encouraging the expression of affect with empathic remarks. In contrast, if the process affect is minimal, more directive questions about the circumstances surrounding the loss, and the emotional reaction of the patient to those events is quite helpful. Specific questions about grief which may be helpful include:

- 'How were things with (the lost individual) around the time they died?'
- 'What are your feelings about (the lost individual)?'
- 'What are the most difficult things about (the lost individual) not being present anymore?'
- 'What kind of support do you have?'
- 'What have you shared with others about your experiences of the loss? (*This question is particularly important as it focuses the patient on developing social support and extending their experience.*)'

As the patient participates in the process of clarification, he or she has the opportunity to begin to share the experience with the therapist, who serves as a temporary empathic and understanding attachment figure. The extension of this process should also be a part of IPT, as the therapist should encourage the patient to begin to share the experience with others as well. The communication which occurs in therapy sets the stage for the communication which occurs later in the patent's social relationships. *In essence, the therapist is literally helping the patient to reconstruct the experience in such a way that it can be communicated meaningfully to other people.*

Specific questions about the actual loss experience and the events surrounding the loss may be of great help in this process:

- 'How did you find out (the lost individual) had died?'
- 'What was your reaction to this news?'
- 'What was the funeral like?'
- 'What was your mourning process like at the time?'
- 'What kind of support did you get at that time?'
- 'What would you have liked from others at that time?'

This is because the process of thinking about and describing concrete events and the circumstances surrounding them leads easily into the process of describing emotions and psychological reactions to the loss. Beginning with the facts usually leads the patient fairly rapidly into the emotions that accompany them.

Linking the loss to the onset of psychiatric symptoms or social dysfunction

In many circumstances, the onset of psychiatric symptoms or social dysfunction occurs proximate to bereavement. For the therapist to be able to help the patient link the timing of the loss to the onset of problems, the patient must develop a better understanding of the significance of the loss and how it may figure in the origin or course of symptoms. The therapist and patient may need to devote a number of the middle sessions of IPT to discussing the patient's changing conceptualization of the bereavement, as well as the affective component of the loss. Techniques such as examining process affect and eliciting Interpersonal Incidents will foster this process. As the patient understands the aspects of the loss more fully, recognition of the link to symptoms usually becomes more clear.

In other cases, the loss may have occurred in the past, and its significance may not be clear to the patient in the early stages of treatment. Often the patient's reactions to losses are reactivated by current circumstances, and the connection may be unclear initially to the patient. For instance, a woman may have lost her mother years before, and may have dealt with the loss and functioned quite well since the loss. However, when she has a child of her own, the loss of her mother becomes reactivated as the new circumstances – the new baby – bring the loss back to mind. Many women have the expectation that their mothers will be there to help with a new baby, both physically and with emotional support. Thus, the loss becomes more acutely intense in these circumstances at a point distant from the actual loss. In such cases, the therapist should help the patient connect the current events with the feelings of grief and loss, and continue to work as with grief in other circumstances.

Helping the patient accept the painful affects associated with the loss

The presence of painful and strongly felt affect is for many patients the most distressing aspect of grief. Invariably, a patient's psychological coping mechanisms will moderate how this manifests clinically. While the IPT therapist should not aim to overwhelm the patient's usual defenses, there is often a need for the therapist to 'push' the patient to describe his or her experience despite the temporary anxiety or dysphoria it may produce, so that the painful affects and memories can be fully experienced by the patient. In order for the patient to experience the affect associated with grief within the session, he or she will need to feel secure within the therapeutic relationship.

Because of this, the importance of developing a productive therapeutic alliance cannot be overstated. While recognition of grief and therapeutic techniques are all helpful to the patient, the therapist must establish a caring and empathic relationship with the patient. There is great value in simply discussing one's experiences of grief in an empathic and understanding relationship – this is the therapist's primary task when working with grief. Once the patient begins to communicate his or her experience with loss in therapy, the therapist can help direct the patient to begin to share his or her experience with others outside of therapy as well.

In order for the experience of affect within IPT sessions to be therapeutic, two conditions must be met:

1 *The patient must be able to recognize his or her affect.* This may be difficult for patients who have a tendency to utilize 'neurotic' defense mechanisms such as isolation of affect, dissociation, or somatization.[3] In such cases, the patient's emotional reaction to the loss may simply be too great to bear, and as a consequence is literally ignored or sequestered outside of the patient's awareness. The therapist can respond to this by pointing out to the patient occasions of discrepancy between process and content affect, as a means of bringing emotion to the patient's awareness in therapy.

2 *The therapeutic relationship must offer a 'secure base' to enable the patient to explore his or her affective experience.* Bowlby has described a 'secure base effect' in attachment relationships, in which the sense of emotional security in the relationship allows an individual to explore and take emotional risks that might otherwise be difficult.[4] This is absolutely crucial in IPT (and also in all other kinds of therapy), and forms the basis for the therapeutic alliance. All of the interventions used in IPT rest upon this foundation.

Helping the patient initiate new attachments

As the patient moves through the process of understanding and integrating his or her grief experience, the desire to develop new attachments should naturally evolve. As noted previously, Bowlby described that during grief experiences, 'protest' gives way to 'despair,' and then the individual moves to a phase of 'detachment.' It is in this last phase that the individual relinquishes ties to the lost attachment figure and begins to seek new attachments. The therapist can help the patient to initiate and develop new attachments that help to replace the support provided by the lost attachment figure, fulfilling some of the emotional, physical and social needs that were met by the lost person. As progress continues, the patient and therapist will develop an understanding of what care needs were met by the lost attachment figure and perhaps more importantly, what care needs now exist.

This is by no means to suggest that someone can replace the lost person. The therapist must take care never to state or even imply to the patient that the lost person can be replaced – to do so will destroy any sense of empathic resonance that has been established. Instead, while the lost person can never be replaced, it should be acknowledged that human relationships and social connections are intrinsically important to everyone, and that the patient still has the need and the capability to maintain old relationships as well as to develop new ones. Relationships give meaning and purpose to life, and the isolation that often occurs following a loss can leave the patient bereft of meaning as well as grieving the lost individual.

Grief work in IPT therefore involves helping the patient to begin to reconnect with others, and also to form new relationships. This can be done in large part by encouraging the patient to begin to share his or her experience of the loss with others. This accomplishes two things: it helps develop needed social support, and as the patient describes the experience to others, he or she will continue to understand it more fully and integrate it more fully into his or her experience.

GRIEF AND LOSS: TROUBLE SHOOTER

Gradual or incomplete loss (anticipatory grief)

In some circumstances patients present for help with grief in the context of an incomplete or gradual loss. Patients whose spouses or parents are disabled with progressive dementing illnesses, or are dying of chronic or malignant illnesses are examples of this kind of grief. Despite the incomplete nature of the loss, the grief and loss problem area is still very appropriate to use as a means of focusing treatment in IPT – the specific grief issue can be termed 'anticipatory grief.' Helping patients to cope with anticipatory grief issues is a very productive way to use IPT, as patients can process their grief and feelings about the impending loss in real time. There may also be opportunities to discuss the upcoming loss with the person who is dying, giving patients the opportunity to attempt to resolve interpersonal issues with the involved person, rather than regretting not having done so.

When the anticipated death is caused by a process that allows the patient's dying significant other to interact and communicate with the patient in a meaningful way, the patient and therapist may be able to achieve much in the realm of prevention of a complicated grief process. The patient can address the issues in the relationship that are conflicted both in therapy and with the significant other, working to put emotional affairs in order. Many patients will value the opportunity to explore this aspect of the loss, and this clinical situation is often one of the most fertile grounds for achieving change in IPT.

All of the techniques used for grief reactions can be used when dealing with anticipatory loss. For example, asking the patient to describe his or her reaction to the news of cancer, to the gradual deterioration that is occurring, or to the progressing dementia, can be very helpful. Asking what the patient expects to happen over the next few months or years, and even expectations about the funeral, are also useful. The utility of discussing these issues should be clear – dealing with them in an anticipatory fashion allows the patient to construct support before the fact, and to talk about what kind of support is needed and how it might be obtained ahead of time. This allows the patient and therapist to literally preempt potential problems that must be dealt with retrospectively in cases in which the death has already occurred.

Working with dying patients

The value of IPT for chronically ill and dying patients has been demonstrated by Markowitz and colleagues, who have worked extensively with patients with HIV-AIDS.[5] Their experience has been that some patients choose 'grief' as a problem area in the Interpersonal Inventory, largely acknowledging the issue of anticipatory grief regarding their own deaths. Though the work of Markowitz *et al.* has been limited to those patients with HIV who are depressed, clinical experience leaves no doubt that IPT is of great benefit to patients with other types of terminal illnesses, and is of benefit to patients who seek help in coping with such illnesses whether or not they meet diagnostic criteria for depression.

The IPT therapist can use the anticipatory grief approach when working with patients who are anticipating their own deaths. The goals of the treatment are to help the patients enlist social support during the end stages of their illness, and to communicate their experience to others. Further, creating a therapeutic relationship in which they can literally grieve their own anticipated loss is also extremely important. Several writers have described the pathway to accepting death,[6] perhaps the most well-known being Kubler-Ross,[7] who described a process of 'anger' giving way to 'denial' which proceeded to 'bargaining' and ultimately 'acceptance.' The therapist can serve as a sounding board for the patient, as well as encouraging the patient to extend communication outward to his or her social support network.

The relevance of this approach to IPT is that these phases of grief regarding the loss of self may also result in other interpersonal difficulties. The therapist can help the dying patient to address parts of his or her anticipatory grief experience by identifying unresolved or latent disputes with others. The role transitions that others will undergo after the patient's death can also be addressed.

The patient who has difficulty experiencing affect

Some patients' affective experience may be so tightly defended psychologically that there appears to be little or no meaningful affect with which to work. If the therapist believes that the patient's psychological defenses are leading the patient to display physical symptoms rather than affect, the therapist may choose to connect these symptoms to the loss experience. For instance, a patient with a more avoidant attachment style who tended to be alexithymic might present with somatic features such as pain or headache following the death of a parent. Such an individual will likely tolerate the therapist's attempts to link these physical symptoms with his or her loss experience if they are framed as part of the stress response that people experience after losses. A discussion about the patient's experience of stress would then lead naturally into the more affective components of the experience.

It is of paramount importance to pace the therapy appropriately with patients experiencing grief and loss. Rather than insist that the patient 'must' resolve his or her grief issues, the primary goal of the therapist should be to create an environment in which the patient can begin to share his or her experiences. This involves active listening, warmth, acceptance, and the conveyance of positive regard to the patient. The therapist is essentially creating a temporary attachment relationship with the patient to facilitate this process.

The therapist must not push the patient too quickly or beyond what he or she is able to tolerate. The goal of IPT is not to iatrogenically create anxiety about an issue to force the patient to resolve it, and is certainly not to precipitate more symptoms. The pacing should be determined by the patient's ability to tolerate the discussion, rather than the therapist's agenda.

There are several options for doing this with patients who have difficulty in recognizing conflicted feelings about a loss. The first is to change the contract such that the sessions are spaced further apart, giving the patient time to process his or her experience. The second is to arrange a temporary reprieve from therapy, with an appointment for the patient to return at some point in the future. In either case, the therapist should not 'dismiss' the patient, but should make specific provisions for contacts in the future.

A medical analogy is helpful in clarifying this further. With the exception of surgery, in which the patient to be operated upon is literally anesthetized and unconscious, there are no medical procedures in which a physician can impose his or her agenda on the patient. Even patients who are undergoing various procedures, such a lumbar punctures or endoscopy, will often tell their doctor to 'slow down,' or remark 'that hurts.' Physicians are obligated to slow down or even desist in such cases, rather than press on unaware of the patient's distress. A therapeutic alliance demands that the patient give informed consent for the treatment.

In the same way, when patients have difficulty in expressing or recognizing emotion, the therapist should not artlessly impose his or her agenda or interpretations upon the patient. The patient is in essence saying 'slow down' and 'that hurts.' No psychotherapeutic treatment should inflict the therapist's agenda upon the patient. Pacing should be determined by the patient in conjunction with clinical judgment.

The patient replaces the lost attachment figure with the therapist

When offering the patient a supportive relationship that is in essence a 'secure attachment base,' the therapist is to some degree temporarily replacing the patient's lost attachment figure. However, it is important to be clear that this attachment is a completely appropriate response on the part of the patient to a severe interpersonal stressor. Not only is such use of therapy medically and psychologically sanctioned, it is exactly the kind of use for which IPT is designed. Therapy always involves some degree of dependence on the therapist. Patients who do not have social support networks on which they can depend during crises, or who are unable to effectively enlist the support that they do have, are behaving productively when they use therapy to help resolve their crises.

The issue is not, therefore, the replacement of the lost person with the therapist, but rather the replacement of the lost person exclusively with the therapist. To allow or encourage an exclusive therapeutic relationship does run counter to the goal of IPT, in which the patient is encouraged to establish social and interpersonal supports outside of the therapy relationship. This highlights the importance of the therapeutic contract and time limit of IPT. If the level of the patient's attachment to the therapist is intense and prolonged, the likelihood of relapse at the time of termination of therapy is increased. The therapist therefore needs to be vigilant for this kind of overly dependent attachment throughout treatment.

Direct inquires about the patient's attempts at social connections, as well as assistance in finding appropriate venues for support, such as support groups or religious groups, are helpful in facilitating extra-therapy support and building attachments outside of the therapeutic relationship. The therapist can also give homework assignments to the patient to attend or become involved in such activities.

Case example: Rob

Rob was a 38-year-old man referred to a psychiatrist by his local doctor for a depressive illness with which he had struggled for the last 6 months. Rob's local doctor had prescribed an antidepressant for him, although this had done little to alleviate the severity of his symptoms of depression. Rob described having a few male friends, but otherwise had little social support, and had not been engaged in any meaningful intimate relationships. Though living in his own apartment, he had a great deal of contact with his mother, who lived in the same city.

Rob described that he and his mother were constantly at odds, particularly since his father had died of colon cancer about a year earlier. Rob told the therapist that he had not been particularly close to his father, but felt 'sad that he had died.' He felt that there may have been some connection between his father's death and his depression, but had trouble describing in any detail how it was affecting him. The therapist was able to identify with Rob that the onset of his mood symptoms did seem to correspond to his father's death, and that Rob's psychological distress was clearly impairing his ability to function.

Rather than diagnosing his grief as 'normal' or 'abnormal,' the therapist simply noted that Rob had identified issues related to the loss of his father, was having difficulty functioning since that time, and was seeking help. IPT was presented as a treatment likely to be beneficial in dealing with Rob's loss. The therapist and Rob agreed to twelve sessions of IPT focusing primarily on grief and loss issues; Rob also wished to devote some time to resolve the dispute with his mother.

During the Interpersonal Inventory, Rob told the therapist that he had not been close to his father as a teenager, and had difficulty recounting any specific interactions with his father during his childhood or teen years. He reported that he had contact with his father throughout his adult life, but spoke to him mostly about 'guy stuff' such as sports or home improvement. Rob stated he didn't feel losing his father was a particularly devastating blow, but he noted that he had at times tried to 'convince himself' that it should have been. The therapist continued to explore Rob's relationship with his father with the goal of helping him to develop a more balanced view of the relationship.

Therapist: Rob, we have talked a lot about how things were with your father, including some of your regrets about the relationship. Perhaps we could talk more about the positives?
Rob: If there were any.
Therapist: I can't help but imagine that there were at least a few. You said as a boy you and he spent time together.
Rob: Yeah. We did a lot together.
Therapist: How did things change as you got older?
Rob: Well, we just didn't really 'connect' like we did when I was a kid.
Therapist: How did you connect back then?
Rob: Well, we didn't really. We just sort of talked about nothing.

Therapist: Tell me about a time you remember when that happened.

Rob: Well, there was one time when I invited my dad to a basketball game. I was about twenty or so, and was at college. My dad came up to visit, and we went to see the Hawkeyes. I was really hoping that we'd be able to have a good conversation . . . we hadn't really connected for a long time. Mostly what I remember is how we just spent time together, not really talking about anything important, but just being together to watch the game and talk about sports. I really regret that I didn't do more of that later – my dad was never one to initiate things, so I would have had to do it. I never really did though, and now I wish I had. . . .

Rob spontaneously recognized that he was feeling very different when relating this story, and began to discuss his feelings of loss, guilt, and regret with the therapist. Rob was also able to discuss his feelings about his dad not being the 'perfect' dad for whom he had wished.

By the middle sessions of treatment the therapist noted that Rob had, with only one or two exceptions, continued to display little or no emotion when discussing his father's loss. Rob told the therapist he felt uncomfortable discussing more emotional subjects, and had 'not really cried' about the loss of his father. The therapist then asked Rob about the funeral.

Therapist: What do you remember of the funeral?

Rob: Pretty horrible really. I have never liked funerals.

Therapist: You're right – funerals are almost always sad occasions, though many people do find them comforting as well. What was the most difficult moment for you?

Rob: When they closed the curtain and the coffin disappeared.

Therapist: What were you thinking?

Rob: (starting to cry) that . . . I would never see him again.

The therapist sat quietly with Rob while he wept and then began to compose himself. Rob told the therapist that he hadn't been able to cry about his father or the sadness he felt until that moment in therapy. The therapist then highlighted to Rob that it had only been recently that he had begun to describe his relationship with his father in a more balanced way, and that the emotion had soon followed.

In later sessions, Rob and the therapist discussed the newly recognized impact of his father's loss. Rob recognized that he derived comfort from connecting with male friends, with some of whom he had begun to share his experiences with the loss of his father. One friend in particular seemed to be able to connect well with Rob – this friend had also lost his father and had a similar experience with a father with whom it was difficult to feel connected. As he became more aware of his own reactions to his father's death, his relationship with his mother also improved. Both had been able to talk about his father to one another on several occasions – this was the first time they had done so since his death. Rob's depressive symptoms improved, and at the end of the IPT treatment he reported feeling 'sad rather than depressed.' This was an important qualitative difference for Rob, as he was able to identify and characterize his emotions, and he reported being able to experience them more fully. The 'sadness' felt appropriate to him, and he no longer had pervasive problems in functioning at work or socially. He told the therapist that the ability to explore his relationship with his father was critical to how he felt and that he was glad to have had the chance to 'put things right in his mind.'

CONCLUSION

In IPT, grief and loss can be broadly conceptualized. The problem area includes reactions to an actual death, anticipatory grief of another, or of one's own death. Loss of physical health, or of relationships as a result of divorce or other causes can also be considered grief issues. As with the other problem areas, the primary point is to use the area to maintain the interpersonal focus of treatment rather than to make the correct 'diagnosis.'

When working with patients who are experiencing grief, the therapist has two essential tasks. The first is to help the patient to begin to describe his or her experience, including emotional reactions in particular. This is done largely through the creation of a therapeutic relationship in which the patient feels secure in dealing with his or her feelings. The second task is to help the patient extend this process outside of therapy. The development of social support is crucial, and can be encouraged by having the patient begin to share his or her experience of loss with others.

REFERENCES

1. Yalom, I. 1989. *Love's Executioner*. New York: Basic Books.
2. Bowlby, J. 1973. *Attachment and Loss: Volume 2. Separation*. New York: Basic Books.
3. Valliant, G. 1977. *Adaptation to Life*. Boston: Little and Brown.
4. Bowlby, J. 1969. *Attachment*. New York: Basic Books.
5. Markowitz, J.C., Kocsis, B., Fishman, B., *et al*. 1999. Treatment of HIV-positive patients with depressive symptoms. *Archives of General Psychiatry* **55**, 452–7.
6. Raphael, B. 1983. *The Anatomy of Bereavement*. New York: Basic Books.
7. Kubler-Ross, E. 1969. *On Death and Dying*. London: Macmillan.

19

Interpersonal Sensitivity

INTRODUCTION

Interpersonal sensitivity relates specifically to a patient's difficulty in establishing and maintaining close interpersonal relationships. It is distinct from the other problem areas in IPT, because it describes a consistent style of attachment and personality rather than referring to an acute social stressor. In many cases, interpersonal sensitivity can be understood as the baseline attachment and personality style upon which an acute stressor is imposed. Interpersonal sensitivity can therefore be conceptualized as a complicating factor in one of the other three problem areas.

For example, a patient may be undergoing a grief and loss experience complicated by his or her interpersonal sensitivity, a mode of interpersonal functioning which is likely to make it more difficult to develop new social connections following the loss. Similarly, a patient may be undergoing a role transition, and the complication of an interpersonally sensitive style may make it more difficult to develop new social skills or develop new social relationships.

There are situations, of course, in which interpersonal sensitivity is the patient's presenting problem. In such cases, the patient's longstanding sensitivity problems have usually rendered him or her with a paucity of social relationships and a lack of interpersonal connectivity, and the resulting distress leads him or her to seek therapy. Intuitively, this kind of longstanding problem would seem to be less amenable to a time-limited treatment, but limited empirical research does suggest that IPT can be helpful for patients with interpersonal sensitivity which is manifest in ways such as social phobia.[1,2] Clinical experience also suggests that such patients will respond well to IPT.

As a result of the differences between interpersonal sensitivity and the other IPT problem areas, patients with interpersonal sensitivities often require a different approach than is utilized with patients who have more adaptive attachment and communication styles. Such patients may have few, if any, interpersonal relationships to discuss in therapy. Relationships with family members, though they may be quite disrupted, may be some of the only relationships in which the patient is engaged. The therapeutic relationship may also take on greater importance, as it too may be one of the few relationships in which the patient is involved. The therapist should be prepared to give feedback to the patient regarding the way he or she communicates in therapy, and should be prepared to utilize role playing as a means of practicing skills that are discussed with the patient. In addition, the therapist often must be active in assisting the patient to get involved in appropriate social groups or activities in the community.

Above all, the therapist and patient must keep in mind the fact that IPT is not designed to 'correct' the patient's social difficulties, but rather to teach the patient skills with which he or she can continue to build new relationships and relieve his or her acute distress.

'INTERPERSONAL SENSITIVITY' VERSUS 'INTERPERSONAL DEFICITS'

It is important in IPT to conceptualize the problem area as a 'sensitivity' as opposed to a 'deficit.' The most significant reason for this is that the term 'deficit' limits the therapist's frame for understanding the patient. In addition, the term 'deficit' has profound negative and counter-therapeutic implications if it is conveyed directly to the patient. Our clinical experience has been that the conceptualization of this area as 'interpersonal sensitivity' provides the patient with a clinical focus that validates his or her suffering in a more empathic and realistic way, as it acknowledges it as a part of his or her life experience rather than depicting it as an interpersonal failing.

Even if the specific term 'deficit' is not used with the patient, its use is problematic for the therapist. Conceptualizing a patient's problem as a deficit pathologizes the problem, and frames the issue as one that the therapist needs to 'fix' as opposed to an experience of the patient which needs to be 'understood' by the therapist. The term deficit is pejorative, and the associated clinical nihilism that is likely to emerge from its use negatively affects the way in which the therapist positions him or herself with the patient.

Finally, interpersonal sensitivity is a more accurate description of the patient's experience than interpersonal deficit. Patients with such problems frequently describe feeling overly sensitive to feedback from others, or fear being scrutinized or evaluated by others. This sensitivity prevents them from establishing the intimate relationships that they would like. Clinical experience with such patients has been that they readily endorse the concept of interpersonal sensitivity, and report that it is an accurate and empathic way of conceptualizing their experiences.

THE FEATURES OF INTERPERSONAL SENSITIVITY

Clinically, interpersonal sensitivity is manifested in a variety of ways. Individuals may report having few friendships or a preference for solitary jobs or recreational pursuits, all of which are reflected in the Interpersonal Inventory. There may be evidence of repeated relationship failures, often with marked similarities. There may also be a general inability to relate to the therapist that impairs the formation of a therapeutic alliance.

Table 19.1 Indicators of Interpersonal Sensitivity

- Few friends.
- Limited contact with family.
- Lack of significant intimate relationships.
- History of repeated relationship failures.
- History of isolative employment, e.g., night shifts.
- Preference for solitary activities.
- Maladaptive behaviors towards the therapist, e.g., submissiveness, hostility.
- Intratherapy problems, e.g., deliberately missed sessions.

THE NATURE OF INTERPERSONAL SENSITIVITY

The manifestation of interpersonal sensitivity is influenced by a number of factors, many of which will not be altered within the scope of a brief and focal treatment such as IPT.

Table 19.2 Common Factors Associated With Interpersonal Sensitivity.

- Attachment style.
- Personality factors.
- Temperament.
- Developmental issues.
- Persisting effects of illness or mood state.
- Relationships which reinforce the sensitivity.
- Cultural factors.
- 'Berkson's bias.'

Attachment style

Attachment style is closely linked to interpersonal sensitivity, particularly the anxious avoidant types of attachment. Insecure attachment may be clinically evident in the manner in which the patient describes his or her current relationships with others, longitudinal patterns of relating to others, and the quality of his or her relationship with the therapist.

The patient's attachment style has profound effects on the therapeutic alliance. The therapeutic relationship with patients with interpersonal sensitivity may be characterized by inhibited communication, difficulty in conveying empathy, hypersensitivity to feedback from the therapist, and problematic behavior such as missed sessions. As a result, the therapist must be extremely attentive to the therapeutic alliance when working with patients with interpersonal sensitivity.

Personality factors

'Personality' is the relatively stable pattern of thinking, behaving and acting that is displayed by an individual over time. Psychiatric classification systems such as *Diagnostic and Statistical Manual of Psychiatric Disorders*, 4th edition (DSM-IV)[3] and *International Classification of Disease* (ICD-10)[4] have highlighted the concept of 'personality disorder' as a substantive clinical entity. This construct emphasizes the presence of persistent maladaptive patterns of interaction that produce clinically significant impairments in social, occupational and interpersonal functioning. While having diagnostic utility, the concept is limited because it does not account for personality features or traits that may only be disabling or clinically significant in certain settings, and may in fact may be adaptive in the person's usual interpersonal environment.

An example of this might be a middle-aged businessman who has some narcissistic personality features which have led to success in his occupational setting. At work, these traits may well be quite functional; however, in other contexts these personality features may be quite disabling. If such an individual has a serious medical problem, such as a myocardial infarction, the traits may well impair his ability to interact with medical staff and comply with treatment. He may become depressed or anxious and is very likely to behave in an interpersonal manner (e.g., being demanding or entitled) which damages his relationship with his medical and social caregivers and may ultimately undermine his treatment. The personality factors that served him well to that point will become a liability.

Alternatively, some personality disorders by their very nature have interpersonal sensitivity as a core feature. This is particularly the case with individuals with avoidant, dependent, or schizoid traits, as well as those with schizotypal personality features. In these circumstances the therapist must consider in the assessment whether the patient's personality traits represent a significant barrier to the delivery of IPT, and whether another modality of psychotherapy would be more appropriate.

Temperament

Temperament refers to the biologically based dispositions that color personality. It was of interest in antiquity and more recently has enjoyed increased attention in both research and clinical contexts. Temperament is evident across the life span and relatively stable over time. Authors such as Cloninger[5] have described temperament-based variables such as 'novelty seeking,' 'harm avoidance,' and 'reward dependence' that may have a neurophysiological basis. These temperamental characteristics undoubtedly have significance in the genesis of interpersonal sensitivity.

Developmental issues

When an individual has suffered from prolonged mental illness, certain developmental tasks may be disrupted. As a consequence, individuals may exhibit behaviors as an adult that are appropriate for earlier developmental stages, but are not adaptive in their current situations. Interpersonal functioning has critical determinants in childhood, adolescence and early adulthood. Individuals who have suffered trauma or become chronically ill during these critical stages may go on to develop interpersonal sensitivity as adults.

The persisting effects of illness or mood state

Acutely depressed or anxious patients may behave in a manner which suggests that interpersonal sensitivity is an issue. Behaviors such as avoidance, irritability or sensitivity to scrutiny may all be present in individuals suffering acute or persistent mood disturbances. These behaviors may not, however, be evident in times of euthymia. In clinical practice it is wise not to assume that problematic interpersonal behaviors are fixed characteristics of patients who are acutely depressed or dysphoric.[6] The need to distinguish features of personality which are 'state-dependent' (behaviors and cognitions arising from disturbed mood) from those that are 'trait-dependent' (behaviors and cognitions that are stable and durable over time) arises commonly in clinical practice.

It is useful in these cases to carefully evaluate the contribution of acute or chronic mood states to the interpersonal sensitivity problem. This is best accomplished in the initial sessions of IPT, in particular during the composition of the Interpersonal Inventory. The therapist should establish the time course of the interpersonal sensitivity, and establish the temporal relationship between the onset of symptoms and the sensitivity. Sensitivity that predates the psychological problems is likely to be characteristic of the patient; sensitivity which is more recent is not.

Relationships which reinforce the sensitivity

There are numerous factors which perpetuate episodes of depression and anxiety, and these may also be operative in the persistence of maladaptive attachment and communication patterns. Over time, an individual's relationships may evolve in a way in which his or her maladaptive behavior is reinforced by significant others, and the individual's style of interaction may be manifest as interpersonal sensitivity. An example would be a patient whose depression leads to a submissive and dependent style of interpersonal behavior. This patient's spouse or partner may develop a complementary 'dominant' behavioral style which becomes ingrained in the relationship. When the illness is persistent, these 'state-dependent' behaviors may become fixed.

Cultural factors

Many communities now boast a broad racial and cultural mix. As a consequence, patients from many different backgrounds may present for treatment. Patients from cultural backgrounds different from the therapist's, or different from the prevailing culture, may appear to behave or react in ways that appear to reflect interpersonal sensitivity, but are in reality entirely appropriate in their own cultural context.

'Berkson's bias'

Individuals with multiple disorders frequently turn to professional caregivers for support and may bias studies examining factors affecting them (Berkson's bias). Social psychiatry researchers such as Henderson,[7] in studying the relationship between social support and depression, have suggested that individuals with 'neurotic illnesses' tend to seek help from professional caregivers and hence fail to establish social support networks within their social milieu.

This is highly relevant to the concept of interpersonal sensitivity as it may help the therapist identify the reasons for the patient's difficulty in developing and sustaining meaningful relationships. It may also help the patient and therapist identify a useful point of intervention – namely, improving the patient's capacity to develop social supports other than professional caregivers. Conversely, the therapist should also be aware that seeking professional support during a crisis is an adaptive and appropriate coping response for many individuals, and should not intrinsically be discouraged or disparaged.

ASSESSING INTERPERSONAL SENSITIVITY

The assessment of interpersonal sensitivity requires that the therapist evaluate the patient's difficulties in establishing and maintaining relationships. In general, there are three avenues by which this can be achieved.

Review of current relationships

The best method of establishing patterns in the patient's current relationships is to gather information about them directly. If the Interpersonal Inventory lacks current intimate relationships, the therapist can focus on non-intimate relationships if they are present. The therapist should also always evaluate the patient's expectations about relationships, and his or her desire to establish relationships. The latter point is extraordinarily important, as it helps distinguish patients with more avoidant qualities – i.e., those who avoid relationships but desire them – from those with more schizoid qualities – i.e., those who neither have nor want relationships. This distinction is crucial in gauging the degree to which the patient will be willing and able to establish and use social support. It also informs the therapist about the potential problems that are likely to emerge in the therapeutic relationship. Those patients with more avoidant tendencies may have problems with therapeutic dependency, while those with more schizoid traits may be difficult for the therapist to engage in treatment.

Review of old relationships

While the focus of the Interpersonal Inventory is usually to highlight current relationships, patients with interpersonal sensitivity may not have many current relationships upon which to focus. In order to more fully establish patterns in the patient's communications and to more fully evaluate his or her attachment style, the therapist may need to focus on more casual relationships or relationships from the past. More emphasis may also need to be placed on family connections, even when these are poor or limited. The goal is to gather information to better understand the patient's difficulties in establishing and maintaining relationships.

Review of the therapeutic relationship

The relationship between patient and therapist is a real relationship, and as such the interpersonal processes which occur in therapy reflect those which occur in the patient's relationships outside of therapy. Processes such as excessive dependency, hostility or other impaired interpersonal behavior inform the therapist about the nature of the patient's interpersonal sensitivity.

While discussion of the therapeutic relationship should be avoided if possible in IPT, the therapist can give feedback to the patient about his or her observations of the patient's particular communication style. This is often done while role playing, such as giving feedback to the patient while practicing a job interview, and the therapist can also give feedback to the patient about his or her interpersonal behavior during therapy. This is particularly helpful with non-verbal communication. For instance, the therapist may remark that the patient's very soft style of speaking makes it difficult for the therapist to fully understand the patient, or that the patient's difficulties with eye contact may make it difficult for others to fully connect with the patient. The therapist can do this as a non-confrontational observation of the patient's communication style, rather than commenting on processes within the therapeutic relationship.

The challenge in giving this type of feedback, of course, is that the therapist is working with a patient who by nature is very sensitive to such comments, and is likely to interpret such remarks as criticism. The therapeutic relationship must be strong enough that the patient can accept and use the feedback rather than experiencing it as a rejection. The art of IPT is developing relationships with patients who have attachment difficulties so that this kind of feedback can be given.

Case example: Bob

Bob was a 31-year-old sales representative who was referred by his local doctor for chronic symptoms of low mood. He was amenable to treatment with IPT as well as antidepressant medication. Among the interpersonal issues identified in the Interpersonal Inventory were problems he had experienced forming intimate relationships with women. He nominated this as an interpersonal problem, and he and the therapist agreed that 'interpersonal sensitivity' described his difficulties well. As Bob had no current intimate romantic relationships, the therapist suggested that they spend time examining Bob's previous relationships.

Bob had been in six relationships during the previous 4 years, all lasting less than 3 months. The first relationship was described as 'distant' despite being highly sexual. Bob had ended the relationship after his partner had suggested that she wanted a more permanent relationship with him. He had no further contact with her. This was followed by a series of similar relationships that had all ended after the women involved had sought more intimate contact with Bob.

During the assessment and initial phases of IPT, the therapist (who was female) made use of the techniques of clarification and empathic listening. She noted, however, that as therapy progressed, Bob disclosed less about his relationship experiences and was less active in the sessions. While the therapist's experience of this transference was not directly addressed in the therapy, she used this information to direct her inquiries about Bob's relationships outside of therapy. The therapist reflected to Bob that there were common themes in his previous relationships – he seemed to be very uncomfortable talking about himself in any depth, and had problems communicating his fears about relationships to his partners. This hypothesis about Bob's interpersonal functioning was largely based on her experience with him in treatment, though the therapeutic relationship was not directly addressed. Bob agreed with this assessment, and began making more of an effort to increase his communication with the therapist.

Towards the end of treatment, Bob was able to begin to develop a more confiding relationship with a woman in his social circle. He reported this to the therapist, and they used the later sessions of IPT to work on his communication style using role playing and communication analysis. Bob's depressive symptoms improved, he continued to apply his newly learned skills to his developing relationship, and the treatment ended as agreed at session 14.

WORKING WITH INTERPERSONAL SENSITIVITY

IPT is designed to help patients resolve *current* interpersonal stressors. In contrast, interpersonal sensitivity is often a pervasive style of thinking and interacting that is characteristic of the patient. Though IPT can be of help with longstanding interpersonal styles, it is generally most effective in helping patients to overcome acute social changes. Consequently, the best focus to use in IPT with patients with interpersonal sensitivity is one which centers on more immediate problems, considering the patient's interpersonal sensitivity as an attachment and communication style which forms the foundation upon which the acute problem is laid. The current problem is, after all, what the patient came to therapy to resolve.

This is not to suggest that IPT should not be provided for patients with longstanding interpersonal problems, for it can be quite effective in such situations. However, the goals of treatment and the expectations of both patient and therapist must be realistic. Attempting to restructure a complex and relatively stable way of thinking and behaving in a time-limited treatment such as IPT will likely only serve to further reinforce the patient's pervasive sense of failure in relationships. In contrast, focusing on the specific manifestations of the interpersonal sensitivity in a current interpersonal loss, conflict, or transition allows the patient and therapist to frame the patient's interpersonal difficulties in an accessible and meaningful way (Figure 19.1).

When dealing with interpersonal sensitivity issues, the therapist should focus on three goals:

1 Optimizing the patient's current interpersonal functioning.
2 Helping the patient to establish new supportive relationships.
3 Helping to resolve the acute stressor which led the patient to seek treatment.

The overall goal of intervention is to help the patient assess his or her interpersonal strengths and weaknesses, to resolve any acute interpersonal crises, and to improve general social functioning. The therapist and patient need to set realistic goals in the realm of social functioning, as progress will likely be limited within the acute treatment time frame. The patient should leave acute treatment with the expectation that progress in this area will continue over time.

In order to assist the patient overcome social isolation, the therapist should encourage the patient to broaden his or her social network by increasing social contact. This may take the form of:

- Approaching others already in the person's environment, e.g., work colleagues, neighbors, church groups.
- Attending self-help groups or support groups for depression, anxiety or other illnesses.

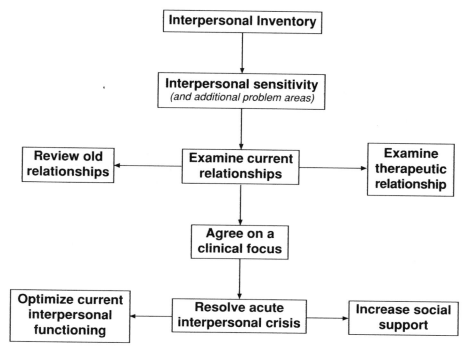

Figure 19.1 *Working with Interpersonal Sensitivity in IPT.*

- Developing new leisure or sporting pursuits.
- Increasing involvement in the local community.
- Volunteer work.

In order to achieve this the therapist may need to:

- Clarify the patient's perceptions and expectations about these activities.
- Generate ideas for increasing social activity using problem solving techniques.
- Help the patient develop skills for the new activity using role playing or communication analysis.
- Model effective interpersonal interaction within the therapeutic relationship.

Using the therapeutic relationship to help the patient improve interpersonal functioning

There are two primary ways in which the therapeutic relationship can be used to resolve problems with interpersonal sensitivity. First, the therapist can model effective interpersonal communication for the patient. In all interactions in therapy, the clinician should model open and trusting communication for the patient. In addition, the therapist can directly demonstrate productive communication for the patient while role playing, particularly when the therapist takes the role of the patient.

Second, the therapist can provide the patient with a supportive, collaborative and empathic relationship which offers the patient an opportunity to improve his or her interpersonal communication *in vivo*. Following the therapist's lead, the patient can practice new communications within the therapeutic relationship. As the patient gains greater mastery of these skills in therapy, the therapist can encourage the patient to utilize these new communications in outside relationships as well.

Case example: Ronald

Ronald was a 39-year-old single bank manager who was referred for treatment of a depressive illness. Ronald described being depressed 'off and on' for many years. He described a longstanding sense of loneliness and an inability to form intimate relationships with women, as well as a consistent feeling of discomfort around his male friends. The therapist and Ronald agreed that interpersonal sensitivity was the most appropriate problem area to focus upon in IPT.

During the initial sessions, the therapist perceived that Ronald communicated in a rather 'salesman-like' and superficial way, which at times made the therapist feel uncomfortable. As therapy progressed, Ronald continued to relate to the therapist in this 'salesman-like' manner in the early parts of each session, but gradually became more genuine and self-disclosing as the session moved on and he felt more comfortable. The therapist judged that enough rapport had developed to comment:

'Ronald, I have noticed that when you come into our sessions you still seem very much in a "work mode" – it's almost as if we were in the bank and I was securing a mortgage from you ... but after the ice breaks, so to speak, you start to relate to me in a much more relaxed manner which I think reflects how you really are underneath that business exterior. Do you find that this happens with other people around you?'

The key in this intervention was the therapist's use of his experience of Ronald within the therapeutic relationship to inform his hypotheses about Ronald's communication outside of therapy, as well as to inform his questions to Ronald about his social relationships. Rather than moving to a discussion of the implications and meaning of Ronald's behavior in therapy, the therapist used this information to help Ronald examine his relationships outside of therapy.

After thinking about the therapist's comment, Ronald agreed that there had been a change in the way he related to the therapist, and that it was common for him to relate to others in this way as well. Ronald admitted that he felt anxious around his friends, and also felt anxious when meeting women in social situations. He also noted that one way he felt he was able to deal with this anxiety was to adopt a 'salesman' persona.

The therapist began working to help Ronald become aware of this tendency in actual social interactions, including those at work. Once Ronald was able to identify when he was acting this way, the therapist moved to helping him identify the new ways in which he wanted to communicate and behave. During this part of the therapy Ronald and the therapist engaged in numerous role-playing exercises. These were designed both to allow the therapist to model new and more genuine communications for Ronald, and to give Ronald the chance to practice them. As Ronald was able to put these into operation, his social interaction increased, his anxiety lessened, and he began to feel less depressed. When Ronald and the therapist concluded IPT after fourteen sessions, Ronald was in the process of joining a sporting organization and was improving his relationships with his friends.

INTERPERSONAL SENSITIVITY: TROUBLE SHOOTER

The therapeutic relationship is poorly developed

A patient tends to form a relationship with his or her therapist which reflects the relationships that he or she forms elsewhere. The therapeutic relationship may therefore be distant, dependent, or even hostile – all can be manifestations of a patient's usual pattern of relating to others. Premature attempts by the therapist to modify this, or to reflect these patterns directly to the patient, may result in the failure of the treatment. The therapeutic relationship must be sufficiently important and meaningful to the patient for such feedback to be tolerable.

The most common occurrence which indicates that the therapeutic relationship is not sufficiently developed is that the therapist's expectations about the patient's behavior within the therapeutic relationship are not met. These include reasonable expectations such as that the patient will speak relatively openly about his or her problems, or that the patient will be responsive to the therapist's questions. In cases in which this does not happen and the patient's willingness to engage in therapy is limited, the therapist should consider the following:

1   *Positive reinforcement of attempts at disclosure by the patient.* This can often take the form of statements such as:

'I feel that I understand you better when you share some of your feelings,'
or
'Your description about how you felt and reacted in that situation helped me to understand you better.'

2   Gently reminding the patient about the agreed clinical foci, and the necessity of open communication in therapy in order to achieve the goals of treatment.

The patient does not follow through with therapeutic directives

It is extremely important in all of the problem areas that the patient attempt new behaviors and new ways of communicating between sessions. This is of particular importance when dealing with interpersonal sensitivity, as the patient will need to at least attempt to implement some of the new communication strategies that are discussed during sessions. The endpoint of IPT is not simply insight – it is behavior and communication change. While insight is certainly desirable, it is an improved ability to effectively enlist social support and to communicate attachment needs more effectively that is the goal in IPT.

The reasons that a patient may have difficulty following through with suggestions such as attempting new interpersonal communications may include:

- The patient's anxiety.
- Ambivalence about the social relationship in which the patient is engaged.
- A sense of inadequacy in initiating social contacts.
- Therapeutic resistance.

In these circumstances the therapist may consider:

1   *Exploring the nature of the patient's anxiety or ambivalence about the behavioral and communication change.* The necessary skills can be practiced in session using role playing, or additional problem solving can be done to find solutions which do not generate the same degree of anxiety.

2   *Linking the difficulties in changing communication to other relationship problems.* Once done, the therapist can highlight that learning to adapt and change is an important means of resolving the patent's interpersonal distress.

3   *Gently reminding the patient that it is crucial to have real interpersonal interactions to discuss during the therapy.* In order to examine the patient's interactions, examples need to be brought to therapy. And in order to have examples, the patient must engage in social relationships between sessions.

The patient drops out of treatment

Despite the clinician's best efforts, some patients, particularly those with sensitivity problems, drop out of treatment. The reasons for this may include:

- Worsening psychological symptoms.
- Logistical difficulties.
- Financial pressures.
- Increased anxiety as a result of therapy.

In this situation, the therapist must first decide whether to contact the patient, and the most appropriate manner to do so if this is indicated. In IPT, there is no rule or precedent that forbids contacting a patient who has dropped out of treatment. In some cases, contacting a patient who has dropped out of treatment may be a pivotal intervention in the therapeutic process. In others, it is clearly not in the patient's nor the therapist's interest to reinitiate contact. Therapeutic judgment should be used in making this determination.

Contacting a patient who has dropped out of treatment is one instance in which the therapeutic relationship should be discussed in IPT. Assuming that the patient is willing to return to treatment, the meaning of the dropout needs to be explored in the next session. What motivated the patient to stop therapy? What were his or her concerns and fears about treatment? What were his or her concerns about the therapist's reaction to the dropout?

The way in which the dropout occurs is also important to discuss. The difference between a patient who calls the therapist directly and states that he or she is concluding treatment and a patient who simply doesn't show for an appointment is highly significant.

The meaning that the patient attributes to the therapist's attempts to get the patient back into treatment should also be discussed. Does the patient see the therapist's action as an intrusion? As a measure of how interested the therapist is in the patient? What effect does the patient believe it will have on subsequent therapy?

Once this information is sufficiently processed, a decision regarding the therapeutic contract should be made. If discussion of the therapeutic relationship has proven fruitful, the patient may be better served if a more psychodynamic form of treatment is offered. If IPT continues to be indicated, then a new treatment contract should be established. The new treatment contract should contain an explicit agreement about what will be done should the patient drop out of therapy at a later date.

The next step in IPT is to extrapolate events and communication to other relationships, particularly those that have been terminated by the patient. Examining the ending of relationships, including the therapeutic relationship, is a powerful way to help the patient recognize patterns in his or her interpersonal interactions.

Case example: Gerry

Gerry was a 35-year-old single man who lived in shared accommodation and worked as a costume designer for a large theater company. He was referred by his local medical officer for worsening depression and anxiety. Gerry stated that he had been quite successful working as a costume designer, and that his work had been much appreciated by those working with him. Gerry told the therapist that as a result of his talent in designing and creating costumes, he was promoted in the theater company to the head of the costume department. This had resulted in changes in Gerry's responsibilities, which now included instructing and supervising several people rather than working alone in his studio.

Gerry described a longstanding pattern of social anxiety to the therapist. He described that literally any form of social contact was anxiety provoking, and stated that at times he would have quite severe panic episodes in response to perceived negative evaluation by others. He found that while he was quite comfortable working on his own in the costume department, the promotion had caused serious problems, as it placed him outside of his 'comfort zone.' His mood had deteriorated, he had developed a great deal of anxiety, and he reported that he had begun drinking in order to try and cope with both.

Gerry had no psychiatric history. His local medical officer had prescribed an antidepressant medication which had been of some benefit in reducing his symptoms of depression, although he still remained depressed and anxious about his work in particular.

Gerry told the therapist that he had been the only child in his family. He spent his formative years growing up in a communist country in Europe. He described his father, a local communist party official, as a 'harsh and distant man.' His recollections of his mother throughout his childhood and early adulthood were of a long suffering, sad woman who was unhappy in her marriage. Gerry had immigrated to his new home as a young adult. He had no intimate relationships apart from a distant association with his flatmate, Helen, with whom he could relate in a limited way. He was also very clear that he had no particular desire for more relationships, and that he was quite happy with his solitary life. He enjoyed his designing work, and found meaning in his hobbies of reading and cinema.

After the initial assessment, the therapist and Gerry discussed options for treatment. The therapist suggested that one option for treatment was cognitive therapy, which was clearly indicated for social phobia. The therapist also highlighted that Gerry's problems could be well conceptualized as an interpersonal sensitivity, and that the recent change in his work circumstances had led to specific difficulties, as he was now in a position in which much more interpersonal interaction was required. The therapist suggested that the immediate crisis – the job promotion – could also be considered a role transition. Gerry agreed to IPT with the goal of resolving the immediate job crisis, and also agreed to continue with antidepressant medication. Gerry also agreed to stop drinking.

The therapist noted in the initial session that Gerry seemed uncomfortable relating to him, and that he felt somewhat bored when interacting with Gerry. He also noted that Gerry seemed unable to accept positive comments from the therapist, such as statements expressing optimism about the benefit of treatment or positive comments about the quality of Gerry's work which was reflected in his promotion. This information, along with data gleaned from Gerry's description of his current and early relationships, made it clear that Gerry was likely to form an avoidant attachment with the therapist and was likely to have difficulties engaging in therapy.

As a result, the therapist consciously altered his style of interaction with Gerry. He used primarily open-ended questions, and made a point of emphasizing that Gerry's responses helped him to understand Gerry much better. The therapist also slowed the pace of therapy, and elected not to give Gerry any homework assignments in the early stages of treatment. He asked Gerry to bring some of his design work to an early session, and spent time having Gerry explain the work he did in detail. The latter intervention was particularly helpful, and as the therapist expressed genuine interest in his work, Gerry began to engage more in the relationship.

Gerry's description of his relationships up until the onset of his symptoms highlighted his avoidance of intimacy. Gerry found initiating and maintaining relationships difficult, and had not found any of his previous relationships particularly gratifying. The therapist asked Gerry about his current relationship with his parents who had remained in Europe; Gerry stated that he had little or no contact with them as he had feared his father's disapproval of his leaving his homeland. There simply did not appear to be much in the way of meaningful relationships, and Gerry did not appear interested in developing any.

As a result, the therapist moved to a discussion about Gerry's experiences in therapy, and his feelings about discussing his problems in that setting.

Therapist: Gerry, I've noticed that over time you have been less anxious and much more open in talking about your experiences here in therapy. What are your thoughts about what has made it easier to do that?
Gerry: You actually seem to be interested in what I have to say.
Therapist: What was therapy like for you initially?
Gerry: I was scared stiff – I wasn't sure it would help, and I didn't really want to talk about anything.
Therapist: Perhaps we could look at how our relationship has developed and see how it has been different from your experiences in other relationships.

The therapist and Gerry then discussed at great length how he had been able to overcome his initial anxiety about talking in therapy. The therapist emphasized the more successful interactions, taking care to give detailed positive feedback to Gerry about specific interactions. The therapist and Gerry spent the next few sessions focusing on ways in which he could build upon his interpersonal strengths, including his general knowledge, his creative talents and his dry but charming sense of humor.

In session 8, the therapist remarked that Gerry seemed ready to begin broadening his social supports by approaching colleagues at work or by initiating new relationships by developing other interests such as art or physical fitness. The therapist and Gerry embarked on some role playing in which Gerry played the role of himself initiating contact with others. A specific assignment to initiate a social contact at work was given to Gerry at the end of the session.

The day before session 9 Gerry called the therapist and left a message that he was canceling all further appointments. The therapist noted that this followed a session in which a role play was used, and in which the therapist's clear expectation was that Gerry would engage in more social contact.

The therapist telephoned Gerry at his home and the following conversation took place:

Therapist: Gerry, I got the message that you wanted to cancel our appointments – is everything alright?

Gerry: (long pause) Well, I went home after our last session and was very upset and started to drink again. I . . . I didn't want to tell you. I just don't know if I can do what you want me to do and socialize with more people. I find this really hard.

Therapist: Gerry, I really appreciate that feedback from you. In retrospect I think I may have been pushing too hard – paying more attention to my agenda for treatment rather than yours. I was very impressed with the way you were able to handle the role play that we did, but I don't think I realized how difficult it is for you to do that with other people.

Gerry: You must be really disappointed with me – I know that you were expecting me to talk to other people, and I just can't do it.

Therapist: I think I can understand now how concerned you must be about my reaction to all of this, but I missed recognizing that at our last session. Again, I appreciate your feedback – had you not said something, it would have left me wondering what had happened. Now I think I understand much better where you're coming from, and also understand that I need to slow down and listen more carefully to what you want to accomplish in therapy. As far as I am concerned we still have four sessions left, and we have work to do. Why don't we plan to meet at our regular time next week and we can continue to work on solving the problem at work.

Gerry returned for session 9, and discussed further with the therapist his concerns that he was being pressured to do what the therapist wanted him to do. Gerry further explained that he thought the therapist was not being attentive to his goals for therapy – Gerry stated that he wanted to resolve his work situation, while the therapist seemed to be aiming to have Gerry 'go to a bunch of tea parties and social events.'

The therapist responded to these comments in two ways. First, he used the occasion to genuinely praise Gerry for giving him the feedback. The therapist recognized that it was difficult for Gerry to do this, but that he had been able to communicate his needs directly to the therapist in a very productive way. The therapist pointed out how this would have been very difficult for Gerry early in treatment, and that he had obviously made a great deal of progress.

Second, the therapist agreed that there was a discrepancy in treatment goals. He further agreed that it was not his role to set the goals, but that his job was to help Gerry make the changes that he felt would be helpful. After some discussion, both agreed that they would focus on dealing with the specific work situation during the remainder of therapy.

They then addressed several specific interactions which Gerry had had recently at work. Gerry reported that though he did not enjoy or want any extra contact with others, he had come to the realization that it was part of his job. It seemed to be helpful to him to consider it as a necessary part of his work and to use this as motivation to fulfill his supervisory responsibilities. Further, Gerry reported that it seemed to be a bit more tolerable to interact with others as a 'boss,' which for him largely meant that he could maintain very strict boundaries. Talk of work, for instance, was tolerable, but within the role of supervisor, Gerry did not feel obligated to talk about anything personal, nor to develop any personal relationships.

At the next session, Gerry reported that he seemed to be able to supervise adequately using this style of interaction. As he had begun to see this as a viable solution to his work problem, he had begun to feel somewhat hopeful that things would 'return to normal' and that he could get back to the solitary pursuits he enjoyed. The therapist went over several of these interactions with Gerry in detail, and highlighted how he had used his interpersonal strengths. Gerry engaged in role plays of several of the more difficult interactions he had faced, including giving negative feedback to one of his workers, and a situation in which an employee had inappropriately asked for extended sick leave.

As the acute phase of treatment approached at its conclusion, the therapist had the following interaction with Gerry:

Therapist: Gerry we are coming to the end of the time we had agreed to meet. It seems to me that you are much less anxious and depressed since you started coming here.
Gerry: Yes I do feel much, much better – work is much more tolerable.
Therapist: I think you have managed to adapt to the change at work quite well. I also appreciate the direct feedback you were able to give to me about feeling pushed to do something you didn't want to – resetting our treatment goals was clearly the right thing to do. I appreciate the effort you made to communicate that to me.
Gerry: It was really unusual for me to be able to talk that way. I'm still not sure how other people might take comments like that, but I appreciate you sticking with me.
Therapist: Before we end, I wanted you to know that I would be glad to meet with you again if you would like. Things seem to be going quite well now, but I can image other circumstances that might be a problem – another promotion for instance?
Gerry: It'll be a cold day in Darwin before I take another promotion if it turns out like this one!

The therapist and Gerry agreed to meet in 6 months to monitor Gerry's progress, and also agreed that Gerry would contact the therapist if he felt he needed help or if he experienced a return of symptoms.

CONCLUSION

The primary therapeutic goals when working with interpersonal sensitivities are to help the patient improve his or her social skills and to develop a social support system which more fully meets the patient's attachment needs. In many cases, patients with sensitivities present for treatment not because of their longstanding relationship problems, but because they are in the midst of an acute interpersonal crisis, such as a transition, a dispute, or a major loss. In such cases, interpersonal sensitivity can be conceptualized as a complicating personality or attachment factor in the context of one of the other IPT problem areas.

REFERENCES

1. Lipsitz, J.D., Markowitz, J.C., Cherry, S., Fyer, A.J. 1999. Open trial of interpersonal psychotherapy for the treatment of social phobia. *American Journal of Psychiatry* **156**, 1814–16.
2. Stuart, S. 1997. Use of interpersonal psychotherapy for other disorders. *Directions in Mental Health Counseling* **7**(10), 4–16.
3. American Psychiatric Association 1994. *Diagnostic and Statistical Manual of Mental Disorders*, 4th edition. Washington, DC: American Psychiatric Association.
4. World Health Organization 1992. *International Statistical Classification of Diseases and Related Health Problems: ICD-10*. 10th edition. Geneva: World Health Organization.
5. Cloninger, C.R. 1987. Systematic method for clinical description and classification of personality variants. *Archives of General Psychiatry* **44**, 573.
6. Stuart, S., Simons, A., Thase, M., Pilkonis, P. 1992. Are personality assessments valid in acute major depression? *Journal of Affective Disorders* **24**, 281–90.
7. Henderson, A.S. 1984. Interpreting the evidence on social support. *Social Psychiatry* **19**, 49–52.

Concluding IPT

20

Completing Acute Treatment and Maintenance

INTRODUCTION

The provision of acute treatment with IPT comes to a conclusion as specified by the therapeutic contract. However, rather than using the traditional psychoanalytic model in which 'termination' is a complete severing of the therapeutic relationship, the completion of acute treatment with IPT simply signifies the conclusion of a specific intensive phase of treatment. In IPT this does not signify the end of the therapeutic relationship – in fact, it is often agreed that the patient and therapist will have therapeutic contacts in the future, and provision is specifically made for these. Clinical experience has consistently demonstrated that a longitudinal therapeutic relationship is beneficial for most patients, and this position is also clearly supported by empirical evidence. Not only are many of the major psychiatric disorders (such as depression and anxiety disorders) relapsing and remitting in nature, but there is also clear evidence that provision of IPT as a maintenance treatment after recovery from depression is helpful in preventing relapse.[1] Because of the therapeutic benefit of maintenance treatment and the evidence supporting its utility, the therapist is obligated to discuss continuing maintenance treatment with all patients treated with IPT.

WHY LIMIT ACUTE TREATMENT?

There are both theoretical and practical reasons for keeping *acute treatment* with IPT time-limited. The time limit is effective in generating change, as it often helps drive the patient to work more rapidly on improving his or her communication skills and on building a more effective social network. In addition, the time limit influences both the patient and the therapist to focus on acute symptoms rather than on personality change or change in attachment patterns.

In addition, to extend treatment beyond the twelve- to twenty-session limit that is typical of IPT may lead to a shift in treatment as transference becomes a more prominent issue. As the relationship between patient and therapist assumes greater importance over time, problematic transference is more likely to develop. In IPT, in contrast to more psychodynamic therapies, the goal is to avoid dealing with transference directly if possible. The development of problematic transference is a function of three factors:

1   *The patient*: the more maladaptive the patient's attachment style, and the more maladaptive his or her communications, the more likely transference will become problematic and need to be addressed.
2   *Treatment intensity*: the more frequently therapy sessions are held (e.g., weekly versus five times per week), the more important transference becomes as a therapeutic issue.
3   *Treatment duration*: the longer treatment continues, the more likely transference is to become a focus of therapy.

Clinical experience and empirical evidence both make clear that IPT should be conceptualized as a two-phase treatment, in which a more intense acute phase of treatment focuses on resolution of immediate symptoms, and a subsequent maintenance phase follows with the intent of preventing relapse and maintaining productive interpersonal functioning.

THE NEED FOR MAINTENANCE IPT

Psychiatrists conducting IPT will also frequently prescribe medication for their patients, and will need to continue to meet with them after acute IPT is concluded in order to monitor medication response. In addition, there may be future life events or stressors during which patients are likely to have difficulties with symptoms or interpersonal functioning, and would benefit from maintenance treatment: a woman experiencing a postpartum depression may have similar difficulties if she is planning subsequent pregnancies; a patient who has had difficulty grieving the loss of a parent may have similar problems at the death of his or her remaining parent; a student having difficulty making the transition to university life may have similar problems when beginning his or her first job. In IPT, therapists should anticipate these potential problems, discuss them with their patients, and plan for treatment in the future should they arise.

In essence, IPT can be seen as following a 'family practice' or 'general practitioner' model of care, in which short-term treatment for an acute problem or stressor is provided until the interpersonal problem is resolved. Once resolved, the therapeutic relationship is *not terminated* – as does a general practitioner, the therapist makes him or herself available to the patient should another crisis occur, at which time another time-limited course of acute treatment can be undertaken. In the interim, the therapist may want, in the same fashion as the general practitioner, to provide 'health maintenance' sessions periodically.

In addition to providing quality clinical care, this model also meets the needs of a managed care practice. In situations in which there is a limit to the number of sessions that can be provided to patients, either because of financial limitations, insurance restrictions, or institutional rules, providing time-limited courses of therapy during crises is a viable way to maximize patient functioning.

This model of intermittent treatment is also extremely helpful in positioning the therapist as a stable attachment figure for the patient. Rather than completely terminating the therapeutic relationship, the therapist can accurately represent him or herself as being available for the patient should other crises occur in the future. Both theoretically and practically there is great benefit within an IPT framework in having the therapist serve as a stable attachment figure for the patient. Many of the patients who come to treatment have attachment styles which incline them to be overly sensitive to threats of abandonment, and forcing a complete 'termination' at the conclusion of acute treatment will iatrogenically move the therapy from symptom resolution to a focus on the termination and the transference involved in this real abandonment by the therapist. *There is no compelling clinical or theoretical reason to come to a complete termination with most patients in IPT while the data clearly support the benefit of maintenance treatment.*

PRACTICAL ISSUES IN CONCLUDING IPT

When to conclude acute treatment

In general, the best approach in IPT is to adhere to the contract that was established in the beginning phases of treatment. The most important reason for this is to maintain therapeutic integrity. One of the most important qualities that the therapist brings to treatment is his or her integrity – the patient must believe that the therapist will follow through with what he or she agrees to do. Without this trust in the therapist, therapy will fail.

On the other hand, the success of therapy is also dependent upon the patient's belief that the therapist is absolutely committed to helping the patient, and that the patient's needs supercede most other considerations. Therapy is designed to benefit the patient, not the therapist. (Exceptions to this rule would include remuneration to the therapist, and educational benefits for clinicians in training.) Moreover, IPT should prioritize helping the patient instead of satisfying the dictates of a manualized protocol. As a corollary, if extending the therapy beyond the number of sessions initially agreed upon is clearly in the patient's best interest, then is should be extended.

The apparent conflict between maintaining the therapeutic contract and extending sessions when needed can be resolved quite simply by renegotiating a new treatment contract with the patient when indicated. Clinical judgment should be used to make such a decision.

Several examples may serve to illustrate the practical issues involved in resolving these issues.

Case example: Joe

Joe was a 38-year-old male who came to treatment for a mild depressive episode which he linked to the death of his father a year previously. Over the course of therapy, it became clear that despite a conflicted relationship with his father, Joe had managed to maintain a mutually supportive marriage of 14 years, had developed a reasonable social support network, and had been productive at work. Joe and his therapist contracted to meet for twelve sessions of IPT.

After making great progress in working through his grief, talking with his wife about his reactions to his father's death, and talking to a male friend who had also recently lost his father, Joe reported that his depression was essentially resolved and that he was doing well.

At session 11, however, Joe requested that therapy be continued indefinitely, as he had 'really enjoyed talking to the therapist, and wanted to meet just in case something else came up.' He began addressing the therapist by his first name, and also began to inquire about the therapist's personal life, such as whether the therapist enjoyed fishing and other outdoor activities like those he himself enjoyed. While much transference 'grist for the mill' was clearly developing, the therapist determined that Joe had benefited from the acute treatment and was functioning well. As Joe and the therapist had not agreed to a long-term treatment, nor did Joe appear to need it to maintain his level of functioning, the therapist determined that sticking to the initial contract outweighed the potential benefits of continuing therapy. Moreover, the therapist also recognized that continuing therapy would involve a departure from IPT to a more psychodynamic transference-based therapy.

The therapist responded to Joe's personal inquiries with pleasant self-disclosure, indicating that he did indeed enjoy fishing and camping. This comment was immediately followed by a statement from the therapist that such activities were clearly important to Joe, and that it would be of benefit to think about other friends with whom Joe could share these, particularly as they would be a great way to continue to build meaningful interpersonal relationships. Thus, the therapist quickly shifted a potential transference encounter to a focus on continuing to develop interpersonal connections outside of therapy. The therapist also reiterated the need to adhere to the therapeutic contract, emphasizing that Joe had both done well in therapy and clearly had the ability to connect well with people.

At session 12, Joe indicated that he felt ready to end treatment. The therapist responded by reiterating that Joe could return for acute treatment in the future if needed – they had already discussed the fact that the death of Joe's mother, among other events, might be a point at which he should return should his symptoms return.

Case example: Penelope

Penelope was a 27-year-old woman who entered IPT for the treatment of an acute and severe episode of postpartum depression. Because she was breastfeeding, she declined her physician's recommendation to use antidepressant medication in addition to starting IPT.

During the course of therapy it became apparent that Penelope had a tendency to be somewhat passive in asking others for help. She tended to expect others to anticipate her needs, and when they did not, she tended to withdraw and isolate herself further. This was evident in her relationship with her husband: she described several instances in which she wanted him to help with household tasks and childcare but had not specifically asked him to do so. When he had not 'read her mind' and done these, she withdrew and described feeling more depressed. In addition, this style was manifest in therapy – early in treatment, she had been quite passive and somewhat difficult to engage as an active participant in solving her problems, often looking to the therapist to 'tell her what to do.'

Despite these tendencies, Penelope had done well in treatment. She had recognized that her communications with her husband were not effectively getting her needs met, and with encouragement, had begun to address her need for help with him directly. He had responded quite positively to her requests, and as she became more direct in her communication, she began to feel more supported and less depressed. With this success, she also changed her in-session behavior, and became more of an active participant in developing new ways to communicate more effectively. She also became involved in a postpartum support group which she found to be of great help.

At the conclusion of sixteen sessions of IPT, she indicated that she was doing well and was somewhat indifferent to continuing in treatment. Despite the transference implications of this statement, the therapist pointed out to her that her depression had been severe, and that both the research on postpartum depression and the therapist's own clinical experience suggested that relapse was a distinct possibility. This was a particular concern given that she was not taking antidepressant medication. The therapist took the initiative to contract for monthly maintenance sessions over the next year, with the understanding that should the depression recur, acute treatment would be re-instituted. Additional discussion focused on the possibility of returning to treatment even after the maintenance treatment was concluded, as Penelope was at risk for depression during subsequent postpartum periods, and she was planning on having more children.

Case example: Jane

Jane was a 35-year-old woman with what appeared to be a relatively straightforward episode of depression resulting from her divorce. She had been married for 5 years, and reported that she had felt that she had been cast adrift when her husband unexpectedly left. She had depended on him as 'her best friend' and had cut off several important relationships with female friends in order to be with him. She initially reported confusion about why he had left, and wanted to understand what had happened. A contract for twelve sessions of IPT was established at the end of the second assessment session.

At session 3, Jane revealed that her ex-husband had been a heavy drinker; session 5 brought the revelation that he had been physically abusive to her. He had also been very adamant that she limit her contacts outside of the marriage, which had resulted in a constriction of her social network. In addition to exploring her ambivalent feelings about her ex-husband, therapy focused on re-establishing her social support network. She contacted several of her female friends and began socializing with them, including one woman who had also recently been through a difficult divorce. As her interpersonal support improved, her symptoms did as well, and she reported at session 10 that she felt she was functioning well and was no longer depressed.

During treatment, Jane's fear that others would not meet her needs was manifest in therapy by a reluctance to disclose personal feelings to her therapist. This was evident in the delayed disclosure of the abusive relationship with her ex-husband, and in her concern that 'therapy might not be of help to someone like me,' a statement she made early in treatment. At that time, the therapist chose to respond to her comment with reassurance that therapy was indeed quite likely to be of help, and that the therapist had previously had great success with other patients with problems similar to Jane's.

Near the end of session 11, when the conclusion of acute treatment was being discussed, Jane revealed to her therapist that she had been a victim of sexual abuse during her childhood. While the therapist appreciated that sticking to the original therapeutic contract was important, she felt that it was far outweighed by the importance of this disclosure, and by the distress that Jane was experiencing in discussing it. Further, given Jane's difficulty in disclosing personal issues and the time invested in building a therapeutic alliance with her, the therapist judged it was best if she worked with Jane on the abuse issues rather than referring her to someone else. The therapist initiated a discussion with Jane about this, and they agreed to end IPT and move to open-ended work on understanding the impact of her abuse experience.

To summarize, it is generally most beneficial to conclude acute treatment as agreed upon by the therapist and patient at the beginning of therapy. The vast majority of well-selected patients will respond within this time frame and will be able to conclude acute treatment without difficulty. There are both theoretical and practical reasons for ending acute treatment as agreed; however, there are circumstances in which patients will clearly benefit from additional treatment, and in which such treatment is indicated. There will also be cases in which the patient has fully engaged in treatment with IPT, has not responded, and continues to need additional treatment, either from the therapist who provided IPT or from another clinician. In such cases, clinical judgment should be used to determine the best course of action.

How to conclude acute treatment

In addition to determining whether to conclude acute treatment, the therapist must also use clinical judgment to decide how to schedule sessions near the end of the acute phase. The clinician should be guided in this matter, as in others, by both clinical experience and empirical data. Unfortunately, there are at present little empirical data to guide this decision, so that there should be more reliance on clinical judgment.

The empirical efficacy studies of acute treatment with IPT have all relied upon protocols which strictly dictate the use of weekly sessions of IPT, followed by an abrupt termination at the conclusion of therapy. In these studies, there is neither latitude for therapists to schedule sessions other than weekly, nor is there latitude regarding termination – no treatment may be offered to patients at the end of the specified number of sessions, even if they remain symptomatic. These protocols have been used solely to maximize the internal validity of the research (i.e., its replicability) rather than because they reflect best clinical practice.

In contrast, clinical experience with IPT, and with other therapies as well, strongly suggests that the best clinical practice is to extend the interval between sessions once the patient is in the recovery stage of acute treatment. Rather than continuing to meet weekly for the duration of treatment, the patient and therapist may choose to meet bi-weekly or even monthly towards the end of treatment if the patient is sufficiently recovered. For more high functioning patients, 6–8-weekly sessions may be sufficient to resolve their acute problems, but they often derive additional benefit from extending session intervals to bi-weekly or monthly once their functioning has improved. This gives them the opportunity to further practice communication skills, reinforce the changes that they have made, and develop more self-confidence while remaining in a supportive relationship – all of which facilitate better and more stable functioning.

It is also helpful to negotiate the number of sessions of therapy, rather than a specified number of weeks of therapy, with a patient during the initial phase of treatment. Meeting weekly until the patient begins to improve, later sessions are scheduled further apart after discussing the change with the patient. Most patients, if doing well, are quite happy to meet less frequently, and often initiate the discussion about doing so when they are feeling better.

In addition to providing more longitudinal care than acute weekly sessions can offer, coming to a gradual conclusion in acute therapy rather than an abrupt termination has a number of other advantages. First, there is less need to focus on the sense of loss that the patient may experience at the conclusion of treatment, as the process is gradual rather than abrupt. Consequently, there is also less concern that problematic transferential issues related to termination will need to be discussed. Second, the graded conclusion more firmly fixes the therapist as a stable attachment figure while encouraging the patient to function independently – the therapist is available, but not necessary, for the patient.

Finally, a graded termination is more consistent with a reasonable rationale for treatment, which fosters the patient's hope for recovery and faith in the treatment. Psychotherapy is the only form of treatment offered by healthcare providers which utilizes an iatrogenically created abrupt end to treatment. Patients expect that they will be provided with help as long as they are suffering – they do not expect that the dictates of a protocol will take precedence over their personal and individual needs. While an abrupt termination can be theoretically justified as a means to increase the intensity of the transference reaction in long-term psychodynamic psychotherapy, there is no theoretical justification for artificially imposing an abrupt and potentially counter-therapeutic termination in time-limited non-transferential treatments such as IPT. The clinician should use his or her clinical judgment to determine if and when to schedule sessions at greater intervals as the patient recovers.

Goals for the conclusion of acute treatment

The ending of the intense therapy relationship which develops in IPT is of utmost importance, particularly as the focus of treatment is the patient's relationships and communication with primary attachment figures. As a result of their attachment styles, many patients will be sensitive to the ending of the therapeutic relationship, and will experience feelings of loss or possibly even rejection. Thus handling the conclusion of therapy well is an essential task for the IPT therapist.

The primary goal of IPT is symptom relief and improvement in interpersonal functioning. A corollary of this is that the specific goals at the time of treatment conclusion are to foster the patient's independent functioning and to enhance his or her sense of competence.

Table 20.1 *Conclusion of Acute Treatment: the Goals*

- Facilitate the patient's independent functioning.
- Enhance the patient's sense of competence.
- Reinforce new communication behavior.
- Reinforce the use of social supports.
- Contract for the provision of continuing maintenance treatment if needed.

The idea is to help the patient appreciate that he or she has resources and skills to manage problems, and to squarely attribute therapeutic gain to the patient. As acute treatment ends, the therapist should make clear that the patient has improved, has made changes, and has the capability to function independently – the therapist is still available in the background should a future emergency arise, but the expectation is that the patient will not only function independently but do so quite capably.

Metaphorically, IPT follows the old adage 'give a man a fish and he will eat for a day, teach a man to fish and he will eat for a lifetime.' Ideally, in IPT patients learn new communication skills, develop insight into how they communicate their needs, and establish more functional social support networks, all in the service of improving interpersonal functioning. These are all new or improved 'fishing skills.'

The metaphor can, however, be extended further in a way consistent with IPT. As with a fishing mentor or teacher, new situations may arise in which the student or patient may again desire some expert help. When a patient is fishing for bass, a shark might appear on the line – if so, asking for additional advice is not only helpful but also a darn good idea. When appropriate, patients should be encouraged to ask for additional therapy, as recognizing when help is needed and asking for it in an appropriate and effective manner is intrinsic to the IPT approach to treatment.

At the conclusion of acute treatment, the therapist should take the stance that he or she is a resource available to the patient should difficulties arise in the future. It is essential for the therapist to be seen by the patient as a stable attachment figure even after acute treatment concludes – an attachment figure that should be called upon for help only when circumstances are dire, but one which is available nonetheless. It should be kept in mind that the therapist is, temporarily at least, an important and appropriate part of the patient's social support network. If future crises arise, the ability to effectively call upon extended social support, including the therapist, should be reinforced.

CONCLUSION OF ACUTE TREATMENT: KEY ISSUES

It is incumbent upon the therapist to discuss specifically a number of issues with the patient prior to concluding acute treatment. These are:

- A maintenance contract.
- The provision of medication.
- The discussion of potential future problems.

The most important among these is a discussion about *future treatment*. There are several alternatives for this, and a *specific contract* should be established with the patient for whichever option is chosen. Options include: specifically scheduling maintenance sessions at monthly or greater intervals; concluding acute treatment with the understanding that the patient will contact the therapist should problems recur; or planning to have the patient contact another provider in the future if needed if the therapist is not available.

Decisions about how to structure future treatment must rely upon clinical judgment. Often, they are guided by logistical and other considerations. For instance, some patients will be receiving medication from a healthcare provider other than the therapist – in this case, there may be less concern about scheduling maintenance sessions as the physician can observe the patient for signs of relapse. Distance is another concern, as is cost – while the benefits of acute treatment may make the investment of time required to travel to appointments and the cost of acute treatment a wonderful investment for the patient, the cost–benefit equation may not support continued maintenance treatment at long distance or great financial cost.

Continued use of medication should also be discussed with the patient. Physicians conducting IPT can do this in the context of the therapy itself. Other mental healthcare providers should emphasize the need to continue medication even after the conclusion of IPT – patients should be firmly directed to continue medication until they have discussed stopping it with their physician.

The last item which should be discussed with the patient is the *recognition of early symptoms of recurrence* which may signal another episode of illness, or which signal a return of interpersonal problems. Along with this, therapists should explicitly discuss future events which may be associated with relapse or recurrence.

Many of these circumstances will be obvious: a woman who experienced postpartum depression who plans to have additional children should be counseled about the possibility of a recurrence; a patient who had difficulty with the death of an elderly parent should discuss the possibility that he or she will meet with difficulty at the death of the surviving parent. Symptoms may also be obvious: a review of the onset of depression may reveal that sleep problems appeared before the full-blown episode occurred – patients should be counseled to watch for such signs and to seek help should they return.

CONCLUSION OF TREATMENT: SPECIFIC TASKS

Table 20.2 *Therapeutic Techniques for Concluding Acute IPT*

- Positive reinforcement of the patient's gains.
- Acknowledgment of the patient's sense of loss/grief/transition.
- Normalization of feelings about conclusion of therapy.
- Therapist self-disclosure of feelings about conclusion.
- Solicitation of feedback from the patient.
- Management of post-therapy contacts.

Several specific techniques can be utilized to great effect during the conclusion of treatment. Primary among these is giving *direct feedback* to patients. In IPT, the therapist should review the progress made in therapy, giving as much positive feedback to patients as is genuinely possible. A review of the problems identified in the Interpersonal Inventory and progress in dealing with these, as well as a review of the associated symptomatic improvement, should be conducted. A specific summary of the positive changes that the patient has made in improving his or her communication and in developing a social support network should also be undertaken. Credit for change should be given primarily to the patient – though the therapist has served as a 'coach,' the patient has done the difficult work and has implemented the changes discussed.

It is also important to *acknowledge the sense of loss* that the patient may be experiencing at the conclusion of treatment. This can be mitigated to a great degree if the conclusion is gradual, as described above, and if the therapist makes clear that the patient can return in the future should the need arise. An iatrogenically created abrupt termination, on the other hand, will lead to a more difficulties at the end of therapy.

Even in cases in which conclusion is handled well, however, the patient may have a significant sense of loss which should be directly discussed. The therapist may be one of the first people who has taken an active interest in the patient, or may be one of the few people who has treated the patient with unconditional positive regard. It is often the case that therapists underestimate the impact of concluding therapy: therapists have many patients, while patients have only one therapist.

The *normalization of the patient's loss experience* is a key technique when concluding IPT. The therapist should reassure the patient that it is normal to feel a sense of loss, and that it signifies both the effort that the patient has put into the work and the relationship that he or she has built with the therapist. The therapist should try to link these feelings with the normal sense of concern that many patients experience as they fear that they will not be able to maintain their gains without the therapist's support.

The therapist should also feel free to use *judicious self-disclosure* when discussing the end of therapy, and can relate his or her personal feelings about ending treatment (assuming that they are positive). This serves three purposes:

1   It further 'normalizes' the patient's experience of loss.
2   It models the direct communication of feelings.
3   It reinforces the patient's ability to connect in a meaningful way with others.

For example, a therapist might state to his or her patient:

> 'I have really enjoyed working with you, and will miss the interaction. I often find it difficult to conclude treatment with the people with whom I work, as I find myself feeling close to them and very invested in their success.'

As IPT does not typically focus directly on the patient–therapist relationship, the discussions about concluding treatment should not include questions to the patient about his or her feelings about the therapist on a transference level, nor should they include questions which invite any speculation by the patient about the therapist. Patients may ask personal questions of the therapist as the conclusion draws near – the therapist should respond openly and honestly with judicious self-disclosure, and may then redirect the patient to relationships outside of the treatment instead of querying the patient about their motives for asking, or interpreting any transference reactions.

For instance, in response to a postpartum patient's question about whether or not the therapist has children, the therapist might say:

> 'Yes I do have children, aged 12, 9, 6, and 3. I found myself identifying with many of the problems you described with newborns, and some of our discussions reminded me of some of my experiences with my own children. I have found that talking with others about experiences like that is a great way to develop deeper relationships – just as you have done with some of your friends while we have been working together.'

Another helpful intervention when concluding therapy is to *ask for feedback from the patient* regarding his or her experiences in therapy. One of the obvious benefits of this is that the therapist obtains important information about what did and did not work well in the treatment – invaluable information for a true scientist-practitioner, and wonderful information to add to one's store of clinical experience. Asking for feedback is also a great way of modeling the behavior, further encouraging the patient to do the same. It also emphasizes the collaborative nature of the therapeutic relationship, and reinforces the value of the patient's input to others.

The last intervention which is of benefit in IPT is a careful *management of post-therapy contacts*. In traditional psychodynamic psychotherapy, such contacts are strictly prohibited. Research protocols also prohibit post-therapy contact of any kind. As the goals at the conclusion of treatment with IPT are to facilitate independent functioning and reinforce the gains made by the patient, being receptive to the patient's request for post-therapy contact, or, in some cases, initiating a discussion about post-therapy contact, may be very helpful.

For example, the therapist may determine that it would be helpful to have the patient call or write the therapist a month or two after the conclusion of treatment to 'check-in' with the therapist. If there is concern about relapse with a patient who is unable to attend maintenance therapy, the therapist may even choose to call the patient a month or two after treatment is concluded. Requests by the patient to call or write (or even e-mail) the therapist can generally be met positively as well. There are no data which support the use of an abrupt termination, and clinical experience clearly indicates that, for many patients, this kind of contact is very helpful.

Several principles must be borne in mind, however. First, post-therapy contact of this kind should be mutually agreed upon, and literally 'contracted' with the patient. The therapist must keep up his or her end of the bargain – if agreeing to call the patient after a month, the therapist must follow through. Second, this type of post-therapy contact should be conceptualized by the therapist as a literal maintenance treatment, meaning that all of the therapeutic boundaries must be maintained as when face-to-face sessions were taking place. The same kind of therapeutic goals and techniques should also be in force. Therapists choosing to utilize this technique will also find that it generally diminishes the intensity of the conclusion, which is consistent with the non-transferential and supportive nature of IPT.

MAINTENANCE TREATMENT

How does maintenance treatment differ from acute treatment?

There are two primary differences between acute and maintenance IPT. The first is simply a quantitative matter – maintenance IPT is less frequent and less intense. In some cases, the therapist may even choose to have maintenance sessions of shorter length – 20- or 30-minute appointments may be sufficient for some patients who are doing well. The other difference is qualitative, as the goals of acute treatment are to resolve an interpersonal crisis, while maintenance treatment is designed to maintain functioning and prevent a return of symptoms.

Goals of maintenance treatment

The specific goals of maintenance treatment are:

1 To review the state of the original presenting problem and the progress the patient continues to make.
2 To consider new problems which do not require acute intervention.
3 To continue to maximize the patient's interpersonal functioning over time.
4 To provide a continuing relationship for the resumption of acute treatment if needed.

The first goal of maintenance IPT is to review the patient's presenting problem and the progress that is being made in that particular area. The therapist can make formal reference to the Interpersonal Inventory, or can simply update the status of the interpersonal problems with which the patient was struggling prior to acute intervention. The purpose of this is both to imply to the patient that he or she should continue working on interpersonal communication, and to ensure that the problem has not resurfaced.

New problems which do not require acute intervention may also arise. The most common (and gratifying) way in which this occurs is when patients bring new interpersonal problems to maintenance sessions after they have already started to resolve them. For instance, a patient who originally presented with a marital conflict may bring a conflict with an employer to a maintenance session. With luck, the patient will have already started to apply some of the IPT problem-solving techniques to the problem, and will simply be informing the therapist about that work or asking for specific advice, as opposed to needing a burst of acute treatment.

In other situations, the therapist may need to reinforce the patient's ability to cope with the new problem without needing to return to an acute treatment mode. More dependent patients, or those with anxious ambivalent attachments, may feel less competent to deal with new problems, and their natural tendency is to flee back to treatment. The therapist should use his or her judgment to determine whether a resumption of acute treatment is needed.

The contract for maintenance treatment should be flexible, but all changes should be specifically discussed with the patient. For instance, a patient may come to a bimonthly maintenance session with a conflict in a new relationship. The therapist and patient may agree that since the patient is already familiar with IPT and has already put into practice some problem-solving skills, three weekly sessions might be helpful. This is in contrast to a resumption of a 'full' course of twelve to twenty sessions of IPT, and also stands in contrast to the bimonthly sessions which had been established in the original maintenance contract.

The primary consideration in such cases is that changes in the contract be specifically discussed and mutually agreed upon. Such changes should always be made if they are in the patient's best interest – it is the patient's needs rather than the dictates of the contract that are paramount. Clinical judgment should be used in making such decisions.

In situations in which the patient continues to function well, the therapist can help the patient to maintain this level of functioning with maintenance sessions. The therapist should be strongly encouraging and positively reinforcing, and should encourage the patient to be as independent as possible. This independence is important not only in the patient's social setting, but should be encouraged in session as well. For instance, rather than taking a more active stance while problem solving, the therapist should guide the patient to apply what has been learned in the acute treatment phase, and to generate his or her own solutions to new problems.

Finally, the provision of maintenance sessions gives the patient and therapist a platform from which they can resume acute treatment if needed. Continued contact, or the possibility of resuming contact if needed, gives the patient a real attachment figure to whom he or she can return during a crisis. Continued contact also allows the therapist to help the patient monitor his or her functioning, and for the therapist to suggest a return to more acute treatment if the patient appears headed for a recurrence of symptoms.

Maintenance treatment: strategies and techniques

The basic techniques used in maintenance IPT are no different from those used in acute treatment. The therapist's stance should be slightly less active, however, as the goal is to maximize the patient's independent functioning. Less activity in problem solving is generally helpful, and encouragement that the patient 'knows how to solve the problem' is usually therapeutic as well.

Case example: Mary

Mary was a 27-year-old woman who presented for treatment following the death of her mother in an automobile accident. Her mother, who had been in good health, had been killed by a drunk driver about 3 months earlier. Mary described increasing problems with low mood, crying spells, feelings of guilt, and poor sleep. Though she continued to function at work, she felt that the quality of her work had deteriorated. The incident that compelled her to seek treatment was her anxiety about facing the driver of the other car for the first time at the upcoming trial.

Mary had no psychiatric history, and described an unremarkable childhood. She had been close to her mother, and had last seen her two days prior to the accident. She was able to relate a number of stories about her mother in great detail, and seemed to have a very balanced picture of her mother as a 'whole' person.

Mary's father had been devastated by the death, and Mary described having for the first time to 'care for' her father. She described him as somewhat distant but strong – he was always there when others needed help. She had never seen him cry before her mother's funeral, and since then he had been unable to go back to work. He appeared to be severely depressed, and Mary felt that she had taken on the role of caring for her father. She noted in the initial session that she felt that her concern for her father had kept her from grieving completely.

Mary had one brother who lived some distance away, and though they were not close, she felt they had connected when he had returned for the funeral. He had, however, returned home, leaving her to care for her father. Mary had been married for about 4 years, and described her husband as very supportive. Her husband attended an early session, and left the same impression with the therapist. Her social support was good – she was very involved in her church and had numerous friends at work and in her neighborhood.

As the Interpersonal Inventory took shape, the therapist began to conceptualize the case as one in which a high functioning, relatively securely attached individual was faced with an overwhelming interpersonal crisis. Mary's interpersonal relationships were good, her insight was quite good, and she seemed securely attached in her relationships.

Mary and the therapist agreed to meet for twelve sessions of IPT, with the goal of helping her to deal with her grief and her anxiety about the upcoming trial. Mary was able to make great progress – she was very in touch with her emotions and could describe them in detail when recounting her experiences with the news of her mother's death and her funeral. With the therapist's encouragement, she talked in more detail about her feelings with her husband, then with several other close friends who were very supportive.

Mary also arranged for psychiatric treatment for her father after having used role playing in the session to work out more fully how she wanted to approach her father. He was willing to go to treatment, and appeared to be responding to antidepressant medication. She felt that she could be less physically involved in his care, and they began to talk about their experiences with her mother's death as well.

The most difficult situation was dealing with the driver who had killed her mother. After much discussion with the therapist and with others, Mary elected not to have any communication with him. She did attend the court proceedings (along with several friends she had asked to attend for support), but did not feel that it would accomplish anything to have further contact after he was sentenced. She spoke with her pastor about the anger she felt about the event, and her anger at God for allowing the accident to happen. Though she did not feel that she had 'resolved' the spiritual question, she seemed to be comfortable with the ambiguity the situation had caused, and continued with her religious activities.

Therapy was conducted once weekly until after the court hearing, and thereafter Mary requested that the therapy be switched to once every 2 weeks. Since she was doing well and seemed to have very supportive relationships, the therapist agreed, and a new contract was established to meet bi-weekly for the remaining five sessions. Towards the end of treatment, maintenance treatment was discussed in detail,

The contract that was mutually established at the end of acute treatment was that Mary would return once monthly for 2 months, and then would return in the future if she felt that she needed to do so. Based on her solid attachments, social support, and lack of previous problems, the therapist was quite comfortable with this plan.

The maintenance sessions were quite unremarkable, with the therapist simply reviewing Mary's general functioning, which continued to be quite good. At the end of the second maintenance session, both agreed that there was no need to schedule further meetings. However, Mary did ask for the therapist's e-mail address, stating that she frequently corresponded with people via e-mail and could envision that e-mail would be a nice way to stay in touch.

The therapist had two reactions to this request. The first was a bit of anxiety and irritation at the fact that she had asked this at the end of the session. There were obvious transferential implications to her request which could not be addressed in therapy at this point. The irritation was also in part due to the fact that the therapist had extensive psychodynamic training, and was literally itching to ask more about Mary's request. The anxiety was largely because of the need for a rapid response.

Holding his psychodynamic tendencies in check, the therapist based his response upon his second reaction. This was that there was likely to be some therapeutic benefit in giving Mary a 'transitional object' – the e-mail address – which she could keep as a concrete way of continuing to feel attached to the therapist. The risks involved seemed to be minimal, and the benefits great. First, the entire therapy had been conducted without directly addressing the therapeutic relationship – now did not seem to be a good time to start. Second, entertaining her request in light of the fact that there were no future contacts planned would increase the likelihood that Mary would contact the therapist if she needed help. Finally, denying her request would run the risk of being perceived as rejecting right at the end of therapy, and would be completely inconsistent with the supportive therapeutic stance that the therapist had maintained throughout treatment.

The therapist did not hear from Mary until about a year later, when he received a short e-mail with the news that she was doing well and that she and her husband were expecting their first child in several months. The therapist replied with a brief personal note that he was glad to have heard from her, congratulated her, and wished her well during the remainder of the pregnancy. A fleeting wish to ask Mary to write back after the delivery to update him about the birth and her new child was quashed on the grounds that an old supervisor wouldn't have approved, but the therapist did recognize that this would also have been consistent with maintenance treatment in IPT.

About 5 months later, Mary called the therapist to set up an appointment. She had delivered a healthy baby boy, but had experienced a profound sense of sadness several weeks after the delivery. Though she did not appear to be depressed, she described that the birth had reactivated her feelings of loss regarding her mother. She stated that she had not expected the reaction, but after the birth had really wanted her mother both to be there to see the baby as well as to provide physical help to her. A good friend of hers had recently also had a child, and Mary felt somewhat envious about the fact that this woman's mother had been there to help for about 2 weeks after the birth.

Mary and the therapist agreed to meet for 4-weekly sessions, during which they discussed Mary's reactions to the new circumstances. Once again, she was very articulate and was able to describe her emotional reactions, and shared these with other friends in detail. On a practical level, she invited her mother-in-law to stay for a week as she was making the transition back to work, which she felt was quite helpful even considering the fact that it was her mother-in-law.

With the acute phase concluded and Mary recovered, Mary and the therapist agreed to continue contact as before.

CONCLUSION

Though there are many similarities, acute treatment and maintenance treatment are best conceptualized in IPT as two distinct phases of therapy. The goals and intensity of each differ significantly: the goal of acute treatment is to resolve a current interpersonal crisis, while the goal of maintenance treatment is to prevent recurrence of problems. While the techniques used in both are the same, maintenance therapy generally allows the therapist to be less active and to encourage the patient to apply the problem-solving skills that he or she has learned. While discussion of maintenance treatment is literally mandatory for all patients, clinical judgment should guide the decisions that need to be made about the frequency and type of contact which will occur following acute treatment.

REFERENCE

1. Frank, E., Kupfer, D.J., Perel, J.M., *et al*. 1990. Three-year outcomes for maintenance therapies in recurrent depression. *Archives of General Psychiatry* **47**, 1093–9.

Section 6

Additional Aspects of IPT

21

Psychodynamic Processes

'As I was going up the stair
I met a man who wasn't there
He wasn't there again today
I wish that man would go away'
Anonymous

INTRODUCTION

All human interactions have psychodynamic determinants. Whether it is a conversation with the milkman or an intensive psychotherapeutic exchange, unconscious processes influence all interpersonal interactions. The interactions which occur in IPT are no exception to this rule, and in many ways the successful delivery of IPT hinges on the ability of the therapist to understand and manage these psychodynamic processes. This demands a great deal of skill as the time limit used in IPT requires that these processes be recognized and dealt with quickly, and the avoidance of discussion about the therapeutic relationship in IPT requires that they be anticipated and managed well.

Psychoanalysis and other psychodynamic approaches to psychotherapy rest on two fundamental principles: psychic determinism; and the proposition that unconscious mental processes are a primary influence on an individual's conscious thoughts and behaviors. In other words, according to psychoanalytic theory, people are largely unaware of the processes that drive their behavior, and it is these unconscious factors that lead to neurosis and psychopathology.[1] Freud emphasized the special therapeutic significance of these elements by stating that the term 'psychoanalysis' could be applied to every type of psychotherapy which recognizes the problems of transference and resistance, the basic importance of the unconscious, and the importance of early developmental history.[2] While recognized as important factors, in IPT these core principles are conceptualized somewhat differently, and are addressed in fundamentally different ways.

TRANSFERENCE

Transference in its most general sense refers to the repetition of early patterns of interpersonal relatedness with current partners.[3] The phenomenon is universal, and takes place in all relationships. Transference in its special application to the therapeutic process involves the patient transferring onto the therapist, as a specific interpersonal partner, his or her early experiences in interpersonal relationships. In either case, transference is assumed to be an unconscious process – it is outside of the awareness of the patient.

The significance of transference in psychodynamic psychotherapy is that the transference of early life relationships onto the therapist can be examined 'as if under a magnifying glass.'[3] The therapeutic task in psychodynamic psychotherapy is to create conditions in which the transference will be enhanced, so that it is more easily recognizable as such to the therapist. A detailed examination of the therapeutic experience of the patient and his or her relationship with the therapist, particularly the transferential experience of the patient, is an essential element of psychodynamic psychotherapy. The therapist, as a neutral observer of the patient's reactions, is able to interpret, or give feedback, to the patient about his or her transferential reactions to the therapist, so that the patient can come to recognize the unconscious determinants of his distorted reactions to others.

A cardinal element of all psychotherapies (including IPT) is that the therapist should develop an understanding of the way in which he or she is perceived by the patient. A major task of the psychodynamic therapist is to help a patient discover how and why he or she experiences the therapist in a particular way.[4] In psychoanalytic therapy, this is the key to unlocking early experiences which have distorted the patient's subsequent relationships.

Further, all of the patient's responses to the therapist are colored by the transference and will therefore affect the outcome of treatment. If the patient's transference to the therapist is positive, the patient will experience the therapist as helpful and well-intended, and is likely to 'comply' with treatment interventions. On the other hand, if the patient's transference is negative or suspicious, all of the therapist's statements and interventions will be perceived in that light, and the patient will not trust the therapist.

David Malan[5] has referred to a 'triangle of insight' in which the past and present experience of relationships are linked through the experience of transference within psychotherapy. In other words, as the patient comes to an understanding of the way in which he or she reacts transferentially to the therapist, this understanding is generalized to other relationships in both the past and the present. It is the therapist's task to bring into the patient's conscious awareness these transferential patterns of behavior.

The concept of transference is quite similar to Sullivan's concept of parataxic distortion.[6] Sullivan also believed that individuals form and maintain relationships with distortions or inaccuracies about the real qualities of the relationships, and that these distortions were the product of relationships that the individual had experienced previously. Like Freud, Sullivan also believed that these distortions were largely unconscious.

Sullivan extended the concept of transference, however, by recognizing and emphasizing that transference, or parataxic distortion, does not occur in a vacuum – it is heavily influenced by the other individual in the relationship. In other words, the transference or distortion is affected by the 'real' qualities of the other individual. Further, Sullivan also recognized that both individuals in a relationship have parataxic distortions (including therapists) and that these reciprocal distortions also influence one another.

Bowlby's model of attachment takes this concept one step further. Bowlby, in framing attachment behavior as a fundamental neurologically and physiologically based drive, largely dismissed the importance of the unconscious in relationships. Bowlby argued that rather than being held in the unconscious, the working model of interpersonal relationships that an individual develops is based on his or her real experiences, and reflect an accurate appraisal – accessible to the patient – of his or her prior relationships.

The implications of Bowlby's model were profound from a theoretical standpoint, but did not lead to a dramatic shift in therapeutic technique. Using Bowlby's approach, the therapist still focuses on the therapeutic relationship as a means of understanding the patient's interpersonal distortions and characteristic pattern of engaging in relationships. This is because the patient's working model of relationships – his or her typical style of relating to others – is imposed upon the therapist, just like it is imposed on all other relationships. In contrast to psychoanalysis, however, the therapist helps the patient appreciate this pattern directly rather than interpreting the underlying unconscious elements of it for the patient.

IPT is based largely upon Bowlby's theories of attachment. While recognizing that there are unconscious elements which influence an individual's interpersonal behavior, IPT focuses on those elements which are accessible to the patient. While a patient may initially have limited insight and not be aware of the patterns of behavior in which he or she engages, these interpersonal patterns are not presumed to be driven primarily by unconscious factors. Thus, the therapist can help the patient to appreciate, and subsequently change, his or her behavior by examining patterns in the patient's relationships without the need to 'interpret' the unconscious motives which lie behind the patient's behavior.

IPT also differs from psychodynamic approaches because it does not utilize the therapeutic relationship as the primary means of examining and understanding the transference, parataxic distortions, or maladaptive working models that the patient imposes upon relationships. Instead, IPT is concerned with the way in which the patient manifests these elements in his or her current interpersonal relationships. This is possible because all of the same factors (i.e., transference, parataxic distortions, and maladaptive working models) are operative in the patient's relationships outside of therapy. Focusing on the patient's current interpersonal relationships is desirable in IPT because it allows the patient and therapist to work on the most immediate problems the patient is experiencing, and allows the therapy to focus primarily on rapid symptom resolution rather than intrapsychic change.

Though IPT focuses on the patient's current social relationships, and though the treatment relationship is not a point of intervention in IPT, it cannot be emphasized enough that the therapeutic relationship is a veritable 'goldmine' of information for the therapist. The therapist's experience of the patient provides information about the patient's attachment and communication style, informs the therapist about potential problems in therapy, about the patient's prognosis in treatment, and about specific problems that the patient is likely to be having with others outside of therapy. Though not directly addressed in therapy, it is crucial in IPT to have an appreciation of these factors.

This can best be understood in IPT as being 'psychodynamically informed' as opposed to being 'psychodynamically focused.' Being psychodynamically informed is to acknowledge and consider psychodynamic processes such as transference without discussing them explicitly with the patient or considering them to be a focus of intervention. Being psychodynamically focused is not only to acknowledge the presence of transference and other unconscious factors within the therapeutic relationship, but also to discuss them explicitly as the primary mode of intervention within the treatment.

The difference between being psychodynamically informed and being psychodynamically focused in treatment can be illustrated metaphorically (Figure 21.1). In this analogy, the sharks represent problematic psychodynamic processes as they relate to the conduct of IPT or any other therapy. The psychodynamically informed swimmer on the surface of the water is aware of the sharks, and if they approach too closely will swim away or take appropriate measures to evade them. The goal of the therapist is to cross to the other side of the harbor while avoiding the sharks if at all possible.

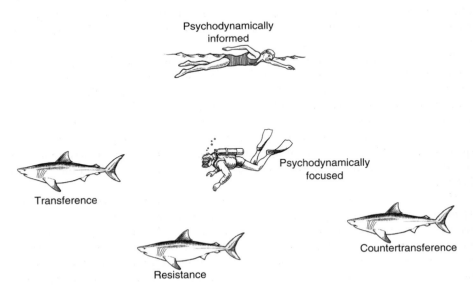

Figure 21.1 *Psychodynamics and IPT.* *Swimming in shark-infested waters is a useful metaphor for conceptualizing the difference between being psychodynamically informed and being psychodynamically focused. To be psychodynamically informed is to swim above the sharks and to be aware of their presence, taking evasive action when necessary. To be psychodynamically focused is to swim with the sharks and to be properly prepared to deal with sharks that attempt to bite!*

The scuba diver, on the other hand, is psychodynamically focused, and is not only prepared to swim with the sharks, but has the goal of seeking them out. To swim with sharks without being consumed takes many years of psychodynamic training and a working knowledge of the proper techniques to deal with them – sharks are notoriously very primitive and instinctual creatures with a nasty aggressive streak. Therapists dealing with Id-driven sharks are well advised to wear a strong protective coat of chain mail!

Metaphorically, the goal of treatment is to cross a harbor full of sharks without becoming a meal. The goal in IPT is to get across the harbor by avoiding the sharks; the goal of psychoanalytic therapy is to root out and destroy the sharks. IPT is well-suited to waters which have a few small sharks; a psychoanalytic approach is necessary in shark-infested waters as there is simply no way to avoid them all.

COUNTERTRANSFERENCE

In his writings about countertransference, Freud [7] conceptualized it as an unconscious interference with the therapist's ability to objectively understand his or her patients. Countertransference is the literal counterpart to transference – it involves the transferring of the therapist's experiences in early childhood relationships onto the therapist's relationship with the patient.[8] As with transference, the process is unconscious. As such, Freud regarded countertransference as at best a nuisance, and at times a barrier to the appropriate conduct of psychotherapy, as it prevented the therapist from objectively understanding the patient.[8] Countertransference, if active, could lead the therapist to make inaccurate interpretations to the patient. The means to eliminate or minimize these countertransferential reactions was for the therapist to undergo analysis him or herself so that these processes could be brought into conscious awareness.

This conceptualization has been broadened by some authors so that it includes all of the reactions of the therapist to the patient, rather than just those that are unconscious and are derived from the therapist's early experiences.[9] Many authors have also recognized that countertransference is as much a factor in therapy as transference, and that the broader countertransferential reactions of therapists must be examined by therapists as part of the therapeutic process.[9,10]

Authors such as Ogden[11] conceptualize countertransference as a psychodynamic phenomenon in which the patient, through the process of projective identification, makes the therapist 'feel' his or her own intrapsychic experience. This process is the basis of some of the interventions used in object relations therapy. Similarly, self-psychology acknowledges countertransference as a pathway to empathy, a concept which is fundamental to some psychotherapies.[12] It is this process of empathic resonance, which is the product of the patient's projection of his or her experience onto the therapist, which forms the basis for the therapeutic relationship and subsequent change. In this model, the process is largely unconscious – the patient's projections upon the therapist are outside of the patient's awareness, and the therapist's task is to bring them into the patient's consciousness.

While recognizing the value of this broader conceptualization of countertransference, in IPT is it most useful to use a more narrow concept. This is important so that a distinction can be made between those reactions which are 'native' to the therapist and those which are elicited by the patient. Those reactions to others which are intrinsic to the therapist or are 'classically' countertransferential do in fact interfere with the therapy, because they cause a distortion of the therapist's perception of the patient and his or her experience.

To put it in an attachment framework, the therapist's working model of relationships – just like the patient's – is influenced by his or her cumulative experience in relationships. If this working model is not an accurate representation of the patient, it will color or distort the relationship between therapist and patient every bit as much as the relationship model imposed by the patient. If a therapist tends to have difficulty trusting others, tends to be self-reliant, or has a need to care for others, these tendencies or models will be played out in the therapy unless the therapist is aware of them and takes steps to counteract them.

The obvious corollary to this is that IPT therapists need to have insight into their own attachment behavior and communication so that they can minimize the distortions in their interpersonal models and more accurately understand the experience of their patients. This also clearly implies that personal psychotherapy should be encouraged for all therapists who wish to deliver IPT.

As a complement to the more narrow view of countertransference, IPT also recognizes and strongly relies on the concept that the patient literally *elicits* reactions in the therapist during the course of therapy. This phenomenon is described in communication theory: the patient's direct and metacommunications in therapy pull for or elicit complementary responses from the therapist. For example, a patient who is hostile will likely elicit a hostile response from the therapist; a patient who is passive will tend to elicit a more dominant response from the therapist (at least initially); a patient who is dismissive will elicit a similar dismissive reaction from the therapist. These reactions are not considered to be countertransferential in IPT; they are natural responses that the patient elicits in the therapist. By extension, the patient is almost certain to be eliciting similar responses in others with whom they interact.

The key distinction in IPT is therefore to distinguish between those reactions that are generated because of the therapist's experiences independent of the patient, and those that are being elicited by the patient directly. The former reactions, native to the therapist, are 'countertransferential' in IPT; the latter are responses elicited by the patient. The former are a barrier to a more accurate understanding of the patient and to developing a therapeutic relationship with the patient; the latter are an extremely important way to more fully understand the patient's attachment and communication style, and to begin to draw hypotheses about the interpersonal problems that the patient is having outside of therapy. Countertransference as it is narrowly conceptualized in IPT actually inhibits the development of empathy because it interferes with understanding, while appreciating the responses the patient is eliciting in the therapist (and by extension the responses they almost certainly elicit in others) forms one of the bases for developing a formulation of the patient's communication problems and for subsequent intervention.

This distinction between 'countertransference' and 'elicited response' is of course somewhat arbitrary and artificial, for the therapist always comes to therapy with parataxic distortions and relationship models which are influenced by his or her previous relationships. These interact with the patient's models and communications, which in turn influence the perception that both individuals have of each other. One can almost envision a spiraling maelstrom of elicited parataxically distorted relationship models whirling around the therapist's office with no possibility of determining whose distortion is whose. Rather than engaging in such therapeutic nihilism, however, it is best in IPT to simplify things to a fundamental principle: individuals (including therapists) can never fully understand one another; but as real people (and therapists) we do the best we can.

As a corollary to these concepts of countertransference and elicited responses, structured, focal, and time-limited treatments such as IPT may offer an intervention that minimizes the impact of the negative responses that patients precipitate in the therapists with whom they work. Patients who are difficult to relate to or work with may benefit from a time-limited intervention in part because the time limit does not allow them to tax the therapist to the point where he or she gets 'burned out' by the patient. An angry borderline patient is much easier to tolerate for fifteen sessions as opposed to four years. Of course, these more difficult patients may ultimately require long-term treatment with heroic therapists. However, the structured nature of IPT often allows the therapist to offer a 'difficult' or 'unlikable' patient the opportunity for a collaborative interaction and perhaps his or her first experience of success in a relationship.

RESISTANCE

In 1892, Freud's case of 'Elizabeth von R' introduced the concept of resistance to psychotherapists.[7] As a construct in psychotherapy, resistance is perhaps best considered as the patient's attempts to maintain his or her intrapsychic status quo. As applied to the therapeutic situation, resistance can be broadly construed as any action or attitude of the patient that impedes the course of the therapy.[13] From a psychoanalytic standpoint, resistance is pervasive in all therapies as all patients always have an unconscious desire to avoid change and to avoid the recognition of painful, shameful, or embarrassing affect, memories, or fantasies.

Fromm-Reichmann[3] defines resistance as 'the reactivation, outside of the patient's awareness, of the motivating powers which were responsible for the patient's original pathogenic dissociative and repressive processes.' In other words, it is an unconscious process which protects individuals from overwhelming or unacceptable anxiety, and is a mechanism of literal 'self-preservation.' Psychological defenses outside of the patient's awareness are responsible for the resistance. In therapy, resistance is manifest in many ways, but all are characterized by avoidance in one form or another of issues which cause the patient to feel anxious.

A primary goal of psychoanalytically oriented psychotherapy is to uncover the genesis of a patient's anxiety – i.e., the unacceptable underlying impulses which the patient is unable to successfully defend against – and it is focused on revealing and understanding the nature of the patient's resistances. In contrast to other therapies that evade or ignore resistance, psychoanalytically oriented therapies seek to uncover the 'cause, purpose, mode, and history' of resistances.[10] Freud stated that the working through of resistances 'is a part of the work which effects the greatest changes in a patient and which distinguishes analytic treatment from any other kind of treatment.'[4]

Though unconscious processes of resistance are acknowledged in IPT, it is the conscious elements of resistance that are therapeutically important. In simple terms, resistance in IPT can be divided into that which is conscious and intentional on the part of the patient, and that which represents a patient's natural inclination to avoid change.

The former has been described as 'intentional blocking'[3] and constitutes active attempts on the part of the patient to undermine or resist therapy.

This type of resistance is most apparent in situations in which treatment is compulsory – patients who are legally required to be in treatment but who do not want to be may intentionally withhold information, refuse to answer questions, or be generally uncooperative with treatment with the fully conscious motive of undermining the treatment. Other examples might include a patient involved in marital therapy who intentionally withholds information about a current affair, an adolescent patient who refuses to speak in a family therapy session, or a patient who intentionally misses an appointment because he or she is angry at the therapist.

The latter type of resistance can be understood as a natural reaction to change that is common to all individuals. This is particularly true of psychotherapy patients, as the fear of the unknown, and the need to take a risk to change, is largely what drives patients to seek treatment. This difficulty in changing behavior is conceptualized in IPT as something that the patient is aware of and has come by honestly – in other words, the patient's real life experiences have led to an understandable fear of particular kinds of change. This is influenced in large part by the patient's attachment experiences and his or her attachment style.

For instance, if the patient has had real experiences of rejection by others, it is completely understandable that he or she would have difficulty in forming new relationships, and would feel that doing so would be very threatening. A patient who has had experiences with others in which they have been abused would have a natural and understandable fear of being in a position in which he or she has to trust others. As with Bowlby's concept of attachment behavior, this kind of resistance is based upon real life experiences, and does not require unconscious processes.

In IPT, the therapeutic response which this conscious fear of change calls forth is very different from that which is indicated in psychodynamic psychotherapy. Rather than intervening by interpreting the patient's unconscious resistance, the IPT therapist can respond to the patient's resistance with empathy. Given the patient's experiences, it is little wonder that he or she finds a particular kind of change difficult. The IPT therapist's job is to understand the difficulty, to empathize with the patient, and to help problem solve and provide positive reinforcement for attempts at change. As a stable attachment figure who provides the patient with unconditional positive regard, the therapist can empathically facilitate change on a conscious level.

In summary, people change for one of two reasons. Either their suffering has become intolerable, or they are able to recognize that they will benefit from the change. The latter requires a fair amount of insight and a high capacity for delayed gratification – changes such as subjecting oneself to graduate school to facilitate a long-term goal would fall into this category. Nearly all psychotherapy patients, however, change because they are in intolerable circumstances – they come to treatment because they are suffering, not because they are seeking greater insight or self-actualization and are willing to undergo a lengthy and expensive process for their greater good. Even in Iowa, the complaint that, 'I'm suffering because I'm having an awful dispute with my spouse' is heard far more frequently in the therapist's office than the statement, 'I'm here for therapy because I have recognized that changing myself proactively will be to my great benefit!'

In medicine, decisions are made with reference to a 'risk–benefit' assessment. In this process, a predetermined clinical outcome, e.g., abolition of a bacterial infection with antibiotics, is pursued using a treatment at a predetermined dose or level, beyond which would be deleterious to the patient. As some patients may be sensitive to usual doses of antibiotics, some patients may also be sensitive to therapeutic interventions which are designed to foster interpersonal change. As the doses of antibiotics may need to be decreased for some patients, so the pacing of therapy may need to be modified for patients for whom change is difficult. This type of 'resistance' or sensitivity to change calls not for interpretation but for empathy, and for positive reinforcement of the change that the patient is able to attempt.

Resistance is an intrinsic part of all therapies, including IPT. Resistance broadly construed should only become a focus of clinical attention if it grossly interferes with therapy. Patients who are interfering with the therapeutic process with intent are generally not good candidates for IPT or any other type of intervention.

CONCLUSION

IPT is subject to the same psychodynamic processes that affect all psychotherapies and all clinical interactions. In IPT these are generally not specifically addressed as part of the treatment unless they appear to threaten the patient's potential benefit from treatment. All of the processes, however, are important as sources of information for the therapist, and understanding them is integral to IPT.

REFERENCES

1. Brenner, C. 1973. *An Elementary Textbook of Psychoanalysis*. New York: Anchor Press.
2. Freud, S. 1938. The history of the psychoanalytic movement. In: Freud, S. (ed.), *The Basic Writings of Sigmund Freud*. New York: Random House.
3. Fromm-Reichmann, F. 1960. *Principles of Intensive Psychotherapy*. Chicago: University of Chicago Press.
4. Freud, S. 1962. Remembering, repeating, and working through. In: Strachey, J. (ed.), *Standard Edition of the Complete Psychological Works of Sigmund Freud*. London: Hogarth Press.
5. Malan, D.H. 1975. *A Study of Brief Psychotherapy*. New York: Plenum.
6. Sullivan, H.S. 1953. *The Interpersonal Theory of Psychiatry*. New York: Norton.
7. Freud, S. 1946. *The Complete Psychological Works*. London: Hogarth Press.
8. Freud, S. 1962. The future prospects of psycho-analytic therapy. In: Strachey, J. (ed.), *Standard Edition of the Complete Psychological Works of Sigmund Freud*. London: Hogarth Press.
9. Abend, S. 1989. Countertransference and psychoanalytic technique. *Psychoanalytic Quarterly* **58**, 374–95.
10. Greenson, R. 1967. *The Technique and Practice of Psychoanalysis*. New York: International Universities Press.
11. Ogden, T.H. 1983. The concept of internal object relations. *International Journal of Psychoanalysis* **64**, 227–35.
12. Kohut, H. 1971. *The Analysis of the Self*. New York: International Universities Press.
13. Strean, H.S. 1994. *Essentials of Psychoanalysis*. New York: Brunner Mazel.

22

Research in IPT

INTRODUCTION

Rather than provide an exhaustive description of the completed and ongoing research studies involving IPT, this chapter focuses on several of the most important, both from a historical perspective and from a clinical practice standpoint. Those studies that have strongly influenced clinical guidelines are described in detail; a list of studies with references is provided at the end of the chapter for readers who wish further information.

The description of the current research in IPT in this chapter also focuses on what is *not known* about the treatment at present. Among other aspects of the treatment, there are many conventions in IPT which have yet to be empirically demonstrated. The use of weekly sessions, for instance, follows clinical tradition rather being based upon empirical data – there are simply no data available which support the use of weekly treatment over bi-weekly, monthly, or even twice-weekly treatment. The use of hour-long sessions, as opposed to half-hour, 15-minute, or 2-hour sessions, is also not an empirically derived practice – there are no data available at present regarding the optimal duration of sessions. A more controversial topic which has also received little study is the training of therapists: while it is assumed that therapists from various professional backgrounds and a variety of levels of training can effectively deliver IPT, this has not been empirically studied. While it is likely that therapists with a wide variety of training experiences can deliver IPT effectively with well-selected patients, more difficult patients probably have better outcomes when they work with therapists who have more experience and more advanced training. This too remains to be empirically tested.

Thus, while there are data available supporting the use of IPT in controlled efficacy studies, many components of IPT simply have not been empirically studied. Many of the conventions followed in IPT (and other psychotherapies for that matter) are based primarily, if not exclusively, on clinical experience and historical precedence.

This makes clear that the clinical practice of IPT must be based on empirical evidence, clinical experience, and clinical judgment. To suggest that empirical data alone should dictate treatment is both naive and unrealistic – there are simply too many aspects of IPT that have not been empirically studied. Further, to insist that the practice of IPT be based solely on empirical data ignores the vast wealth of information that has accumulated from clinical experience with IPT. While the empirical literature support-ing the efficacy of IPT should strongly influence treatment, clinical experience with the treatment and clinical judgment are equally important factors in determining how IPT is delivered.

EARLY STUDIES OF IPT

The first studies regarding IPT were published in the 1970s by Klerman, Weissman, and others.[1,2] In these initial studies, IPT was found to be superior to non-scheduled treat-ment for patients diagnosed with major depression, and was also found to be equivalent to treatment with amitriptyline.[2] A comparison of treatment with IPT or amitriptyline and treatment in which patients received both IPT and amitriptyline demonstrated that the combination of psychotherapy and medication was superior to either alone.[3] Patients in this study reported that the combination treatment was more acceptable and better tolerated.

Though many studies have since confirmed the efficacy of IPT for depression, several of the findings from these studies have not been replicated to date. The finding that combination treatment is superior to treatment with either IPT or medication, for instance, has not been widely tested nor consistently confirmed. In the treatment trials in which IPT was used in combination with imipramine to prevent relapse of recurrent depression, for instance, combined treatment was found to be equivalent to treatment with medication alone.[4] There is simply a paucity of research on the effects of combined treatment with medication and psychotherapy. At present, despite the intuitive appeal of combined treatment and its frequent use for depression and other disorders, there are few data which support the use of combined treatment over treatment with either medication or psychotherapy alone.

Nonetheless, typical clinical practice continues to be the combined use of psychotherapy and medication for depression, despite the lack (at present) of empirical evidence supporting increased efficacy with combined treatment. Clinical experience, however, does support the combined use of medication and IPT in many circumstances. IPT is completely compatible with this practice, and clinical judgment should be used to determine which patients should be treated with both IPT and medication.

Another finding reported in the early studies which has not been replicated is that of differential treatment effects.[5] The notion that treatment with medication would lead to more improvement in the vegetative symptoms of depressive such as insomnia, poor appetite, and energy level, while psychotherapy would lead to greater changes in self-esteem, suicidality, and feelings of guilt has great intuitive appeal. However, there have been no other studies which suggest that there are differential treatment effects from psychotherapy as compared to medication in the treatment of depression. In fact, the NIMH Treatment of Depression Collaborative Research Program (NIMH-TDCRP), which was specifically designed to detect differential treatment effects when comparing imipramine, CBT, and IPT, found none.[6,7]

This discrepancy in results is likely due to two phenomena. First, although there are multiple pathways to recovery from depression, there appears to be a common endpoint. In other words, though the various modalities may initially operate using different mechanisms, the end effect of all treatments appears to be improvement in both the 'psychological' and 'biological' symptoms of depression. The data suggest that this artificial distinction should be re-examined. The second factor which may explain the similarity in outcome when medications and psychotherapy are compared is that the criteria for recovery require that most symptoms be alleviated. Thus, comparing the differential effects of treatment in patients who have recovered is not likely to reflect significant differences, simply because by definition all patients will have relatively few symptoms of any type. Future studies comparing differential treatment effects should focus on those patients who are partial responders, with whom differences may be more evident.

NIMH TREATMENT OF DEPRESSION COLLABORATIVE RESEARCH PROGRAM

Largely because of the success of these early studies, IPT, along with CBT,[8] was chosen as a comparative psychotherapeutic treatment in the National Institute of Mental Health Treatment of Depression Collaborative Research Program[6] (NIMH-TDCRP). The NIMH-TDCRP has been a catalyst for continued research with IPT, as the tremendous publicity given to the study and the weight given the findings in subsequent treatment guidelines and clinical recommendations for treatment helped to make IPT more widely known among clinicians.

The NIMH-TDCRP still stands as the 'gold standard' for psychotherapy efficacy studies, as the research design emphasized clearly specified treatments (including the placebo intervention) and also included extensive training and pilot work which ensured that the therapists delivered the treatments both competently and with a high degree of adherence. Moreover, patients were extensively evaluated prior to inclusion, and both self-report and independent measures of symptoms and change were carefully chosen as outcome measures.

In the TDCRP, a total of 256 subjects was randomized to receive either imipramine, IPT, CBT, or placebo. There was no combined treatment cell. All subjects met DSM-III criteria for major depression, with complex comorbid problems leading to exclusion from the study. All patients were evaluated with a variety of instruments, with the primary outcome measures being the Beck Depression Inventory (BDI)[9] and the Hamilton Rating Scale for Depression (HRSD).[10]

Both psychotherapies were compared to treatment with imipramine and with placebo over sixteen weeks. IPT was found to be superior to treatment with placebo, and was equal to imipramine and CBT for mild to moderate depression.[6] There was some evidence that IPT was more effective than CBT for severe depression (as defined as a

HRSD score >20), but neither psychosocial treatment was shown to be as effective as imipramine for severe depression. The consensus from the NIMH-TDCRP study was that IPT and CBT were effective for mild to moderate depression, but that antidepressant medication should remain the first-line treatment for patients with severe depression.

In the NIMH-TDCRP study, 43 per cent of patients who began treatment with IPT achieved remission of depression, and 55 per cent of patients who completed a full course of IPT achieved remission. Some 23 per cent of patients terminated prematurely, and early terminators were, on average, more severely depressed at intake. In addition, 33 per cent of the patients who remitted when treated with IPT relapsed within eighteen months after treatment was concluded.[11] Both this relapse rate, and the general response rate to acute treatment, were equivalent to that of patients who were treated with CBT or imipramine.

The TDCRP has not been without controversy, however, with advocates of each of the treatments seeming to bring strong biases to the interpretation of the data.[12,13] The debate rages to this day, with advocates of the respective psychotherapeutic and psychopharmacologic schools arguing either that a specific treatment was not provided in a satisfactory fashion, or that the data were not analyzed correctly, each offering a slightly different spin on the results 'proving' the superiority of their treatment.

With respect to IPT in particular, the study design of the NIMH-TDCRP has profoundly influenced the development of the treatment. IPT was chosen for the trial in part because it was distinct from CBT.[14] The study was designed so that each of the treatments would be as different as possible, in particular the psychotherapies, so that the purported mechanisms of action could be explored further.[14] In order to maximize the distinctions, differences in approach and technique were emphasized. For instance, the focus on internal cognitions in CBT was contrasted with the focus on external relationships in IPT. The establishment of a specific agenda for each psychotherapy session, which was required to occur in the beginning of each session of CBT, was contrasted with the manualized dictate in IPT that the opening of each session was to be relatively non-directive. Since the 1984 IPT manual[15] was written largely for this project, these distinctions became codified in the original IPT manual at least in part because they made IPT more distinct from CBT, as opposed to being based solely on clinical experience with the treatment or because these approaches and techniques were theory-driven.

An additional way in which the TDCRP has had an impact on both IPT and CBT is that the manuals for each reflect the methodology used for medication trials for depression that largely drove the development of the TDCRP. Both therapies were chosen because they were time-limited – a consideration which was necessary because of the desire to compare the therapies to medication. At the time, data supported the hypothesis that 16 weeks was an adequate trial of medication – if a patient had not responded to an adequate dose in 16 weeks, it was unlikely that he or she would respond at all to that medication. On the other hand, there were no data available supporting the hypothesis that 16 weeks was the optimum length of treatment for either CBT or IPT. Rather, a 16-week trial was chosen because it was desirable to have equal durations of treatment to compare with the medication trial. It is quite conceivable that providing therapy beyond the 16-week point would lead to continuing improvement, and that some patients who had not responded by that time would have responded at 20 or 24 weeks. There still are no data available regarding the optimum length of treatment for either CBT or IPT, yet nearly all of the acute treatment trials have continued to utilize a sixteen-week course of treatment – despite a lack of empirical evidence supporting that duration.

The most profound effect of the constraints of the medication treatment trial paradigm was that IPT was explicitly based on the 'medical model.' This was a reflection of the prevailing psychiatric milieu at the time, with its emphasis on medical disorders and the 'medicalization of psychiatry,'[16] as well as the desire to make IPT amenable to comparison with antidepressant medication. This narrow model, codified largely for this reason, has persisted to some degree despite the fact that most mental health professionals acknowledge a more complex biopsychosocial model of mental health.[17] Given that IPT is directed specifically at interpersonal factors and social support, the biopsychosocial model certainly describes more accurately the theoretical basis of IPT and the practical approach taken by IPT therapists.

Another major influence on the development of IPT as a result of its inclusion in the TDCRP and the medication trials of Klerman *et al.* was that the major outcome measures of IPT were symptomatic. Because medications for depression are targeted specifically at DSM symptoms, the efficacy of IPT as a comparison treatment was measured by the reduction it brought about in these same depressive symptoms. The implication is that the 'value' of IPT is restricted to the narrow focus of relieving a predefined cluster of symptoms, which is based on a simplistic analogy to medication and the use of the 'drug metaphor.'[18]

While there is no doubt that symptom relief is a highly desirable goal, and little doubt from efficacy studies that IPT does lead to a reduction in symptoms, this narrow focus has displaced attention from the other possible benefits of IPT. These include changes in insight, satisfaction with social relationships, general life satisfaction and well-being, or an 'acceptance' of life circumstances which is more congruent with the patient's current condition. Though these concepts are very difficult to quantify and to measure, neglecting them as possible changes in IPT, and focusing narrowly on symptomatic outcome alone, runs the risk of missing some of the most powerful and beneficial aspects of the therapy – changes which would be unique to psychotherapy as opposed to the use of medication.

The lasting effect of the NIMH-TDCRP on IPT is that IPT was designed, and frequently continues to be used, in a fashion that is dictated by adherence to the medical model. IPT continues to be primarily focused narrowly on symptomatic relief. Most research in IPT continues to examine it as it is narrowly applied to well-circumscribed DSM psychiatric disorders, rather than examining its impact on interpersonal problems in general. As a consequence of this disorder-based approach, a literal 'alphabet soup' of IPT manuals has been developed, each modified slightly for a particular DSM diagnosis. Rather than recognizing that there are general principles of IPT that can be learned and applied to patients with a variety of diagnoses, the impractical implication is that therapists must learn a completely different form of IPT for each diagnosis. In addition, rather than recognizing that comorbidity is the rule rather than the exception in clinical practice, these specific manuals have focused on single discreet disorders.

The upshot is that the clinical dissemination of IPT has been greatly limited by these factors. As only empirical efficacy data are accepted as justification for use of a treatment in some circles, *there often continues to be an insistence that IPT be delivered exactly as it was in the NIMH-TDCRP in order to carry the imprimatur of a validated treatment.* Finding this rigid application of IPT both impractical and non-applicable to their clinical work, many non-research therapists have eschewed the treatment. New techniques based on clinical experience are dismissed, eliminating potentially effective innovative interventions.

The NIMH-TDCRP is an excellent example of the way in which empirical studies have affected psychotherapy development. It is also an excellent example of the reasons empirical research can inform, but should not dictate, clinical practice. The TDCRP was a superbly designed study, and its limitations have been readily acknowledged by its authors. The data should heavily influence the way in which therapies for depression are chosen and applied. It is also clear however, that because of the limitations of the study, clinical experience and clinical judgment should continue to play a major role in the application of IPT in a clinical setting.

MAINTENANCE TREATMENT OF RECURRENT DEPRESSION

Kupfer, Frank, Reynolds, and colleagues at the University of Pittsburgh have conducted several elegant studies using IPT as a maintenance treatment for patients with recurrent major depression. In one of the primary studies of IPT as maintenance treatment, acutely depressed patients who had suffered at least three prior episodes of depression were treated during an index episode with a combination of imipramine and IPT over sixteen weeks. Those patients who recovered following this acute treatment were then assigned to one of five maintenance treatment cells: (i) imipramine alone; (ii) imipramine plus monthly IPT; (iii) monthly IPT alone; (iv) monthly IPT plus placebo; or (v) placebo alone. The patients were then followed to determine the length of time until they experience a relapse of their depression.

The mean depression-free survival time was significantly longer for those patients who received imipramine alone or imipramine plus IPT as compared to IPT alone or placebo.[4] Over a 3-year period, the mean survival time before relapse of depression was about 120–130 weeks for patients who received imipramine with or without IPT as an adjunct treatment. The patients who received IPT alone or IPT plus placebo had a mean survival time of about 75–80 weeks. Though significantly longer than the mean depression-free interval experienced by patients who received only placebo (roughly 40 weeks), treatment with IPT without medication clearly was not as beneficial as treatment with maintenance antidepressant medication. It is from this study that the current consensus that recurrent depression should be treated with maintenance antidepressant medication derives.[19, 20] Maintenance IPT is considered a viable alternative for patients who do not want to take medication, or who cannot tolerate it.

The Pittsburgh study, like the TDCRP, is also subject to some limitations. First, the study was a straightforward efficacy study, with well-selected patients with little co-morbidity, utilizing highly trained therapists who were required to adhere stringently to a treatment manual. While these efficacy data should strongly influence clinical practice, there are at present no data available about the effectiveness of either IPT or imipramine in general clinical settings. While there is little doubt that the findings likely hold true for most patients, clinical experience and clinical judgment should continue to inform treatment decisions with the unique individuals that are encountered in therapy.

Another critique of the Pittsburgh study has been that the 'dosing' of IPT and medication were not equal. In other words, the once-monthly use of IPT was not comparable in strength to the dose of imipramine, which was continued at the same dose required to resolve the acute episode of depression. In contrast, the dose of IPT was one-fourth that provided to bring about remission of depression.

Leaving aside concerns about the validity of the 'dosing' paradigm – which derives directly from the medical model and antidepressant treatment trials – it is important to recognize that little is known about the clinical application of IPT as a maintenance treatment. For instance, it is not known whether non-research patients who seek treatment for acute episodes of depression want to continue with maintenance treatment once the problem is resolved. Therapists are all too familiar with patients who decline further treatment once their immediate concerns are resolved, despite the fact that the therapist strongly recommends continuing treatment. In addition, nothing is known about the feasibility of monthly sessions – in clinical practice, what is typical is that the patient and therapist work together to determine when maintenance or follow-up sessions will occur. This common clinical practice of having individual patients and therapists develop their own unique treatment contracts rather than having treatment dictated to them by a study protocol has yet to be examined empirically. It is, however, nearly always the way in which the treatment is provided, and is supported by a great deal of clinical experience.

Sequential treatment with medication and IPT

Frank and colleagues compared two groups of women with recurrent unipolar depression.[21] In the first group, a combination of IPT and pharmacotherapy was initiated at the outset of treatment. In the second group, IPT alone was provided first; those women who did not remit with IPT alone were then offered the combination treatment. In the group in which the combination was initiated at the outset of treatment, the remission rate was 66 per cent, comparable to the remission rate observed in most outpatient treatment studies of major depression. In contrast, the remission rate was 79 per cent in the group of women treated sequentially, which was significantly greater than that observed in the group that received combination treatment from the outset. Time to recovery was longer in the sequentially treated group however, as combined treatment was not initiated until a full course of IPT had failed. Results suggest that the strategy of offering IPT to women with recurrent depression followed by antidepressant medication can be a highly effective treatment. It is also one that may be particularly attractive to women during childbearing years. The efficacy of this strategy remains to be examined in patients with single episodes of depression, as does the effectiveness of the treatment.

PHYSIOLOGICAL STUDIES OF IPT

Thase and colleagues[22] examined the relationship between EEG sleep profiles and response to IPT in 91 outpatients with recurrent depression. Patients with abnormal sleep profiles had significantly poorer clinical outcomes, and rates of remission from depression were significantly lower than for those patients with more normal sleep profiles. Overall, 48 per cent of patients achieved remission with 16 weeks of IPT alone, but remission rates were 58 per cent in the group of patients with normal sleep profiles as compared to 37 per cent in the group with abnormal sleep profiles.

A second group of studies utilized newer neuroimaging technologies to study physiologic changes associated with treatment with IPT. Martin and coworkers[23] studied twenty-eight patients with major depression who were randomly assigned to treatment with either IPT alone or with 37.5 mg, twice-daily doses of venlafaxine. Single photon emission computed tomography (SPECT) imaging was conducted prior to treatment and after 6 weeks of treatment. Right posterior cingulate blood flow was increased after 6 weeks in the IPT group, while both treatment groups had increased right basal ganglia blood flow. Overall, patients had significant improvements on the HRSD score and the BDI. There was a consistent trend, however, toward a better outcome for the venlafaxine group.

Brody and coworkers[24] obtained positron emission tomography (PET) scans in twenty-four subjects with major depression before and after treatment with paroxetine or IPT alone, and also obtained PET scans of sixteen control subjects. Depressed patients were assigned to treatment on the basis of their personal preference. Patients with depression had regional brain metabolic abnormalities at baseline that appeared to change in the direction of normalization with treatment. Relative prefrontal cortex and left anterior cingulate gyrus metabolism decreased and relative left temporal lobe metabolism increased in both treated groups. Only the paroxetine-treated group, however, had a significant decrease in right ventrolateral prefrontal cortex metabolism. Although both groups improved over the 12 weeks of treatment, those subjects treated with paroxetine showed a greater improvement in HRSD score than did subjects treated with IPT.

FUTURE RESEARCH

IPT has been demonstrated to be efficacious with a number of psychiatric disorders in both open and controlled treatment trials. There are as yet no studies examining the use of IPT in general clinical settings – in other words, all of the data supporting IPT are based on efficacy studies rather than on effectiveness studies. References for these studies are noted below.

There is much that remains unknown about the use of IPT. Fundamental questions such as what the optimum duration of IPT should be, what the optimum length of sessions should be, and the effect of setting (i.e., research versus clinical practice) remain to be studied. There are, however, four basic questions which are absolutely crucial to the use of IPT which remain to be addressed, as follows.

Which patients are best suited for IPT as opposed to other treatments?

This is a fundamental question about when IPT should be applied, and for whom. The research to date provides very little information regarding treatment selection for specific patient's, leaving clinicians to use their intuition and clinical judgment.

One intriguing idea which has yet to be tested is that the way in which patients conceptualize their problems may predict differential outcomes across treatments. For example, if a patient, in his or her presenting complaint, largely conceptualizes his or her problem in interpersonal terms such as conflicts in relationships or role transitions, he or she may benefit more from IPT. Conversely, a patient who presents his or her problems in more cognitive terms, such as having thoughts of failure or unrealistic expectations for performance, might benefit more from treatment with CBT.

Is strict adherence to the IPT manual better than allowing clinicians to use their clinical judgment with individual cases?

Clinical experience strongly suggests that allowing clinicians to use their clinical judgment leads to better outcome. This is, however, ultimately an empirical question. Several critics of psychotherapy efficacy studies in general have supported this assertion, arguing that one of the most effective aspects of therapy is that it is self-correcting, and that therapist judgment allows the therapist to adapt the treatment so that it is more effective for a given individual.[25] To use a medication comparison, a pharmacologist does not continue to adhere to a strict medication protocol when the patient develops side effects or the medication is causing worsening of symptoms – the physician shifts to another medication or method of treatment. Yet strict adherence to a psychotherapy manual in a clinical setting requires therapists not to deviate, even when it is clear that the therapy is not working.

In more subtle ways, the requirement that therapists strictly adhere to a manual also prevents therapists from exercising therapeutic creativity. For instance, a therapist may believe that adding a cognitive therapy technique, such as activity scheduling, to a course of IPT will help a particular patient. However, only a therapist who is 'allowed' to do so rather than 'required' to follow a rigid protocol will be able to use this kind of technique. There is little doubt based on clinical experience that patients do in fact benefit from a variety of techniques, and that a 'mix and match' approach is often taken in therapy. While intuitively appealing and widespread in private practice, this idea has not been tested empirically.

An interesting set of studies is currently underway at the University of Iowa. In these studies, the traditional efficacy design, based on the NIMH-TDCRP, has been modified to include some aspects of clinical judgment. In one study, a course of 'standard' IPT, in which therapy is delivered to depressed patients in twelve weekly sessions over 12 weeks, is being compared to treatment with IPT in which the patient and therapist are able to determine when and how frequently to meet. This test of therapist judgment is a small but important step in moving towards more effectiveness testing – i.e., measuring the effects of IPT as it is used in a clinical setting.

What are the necessary elements of IPT?

Most empirical studies of IPT continue to be based on the original manual developed by Klerman *et al.*[15] While efficacy is documented for the entire 'treatment package' of IPT as described in the manual, there are still no data regarding which parts of the package are essential to the conduct of the therapy. For instance, is the medical model necessary as the basis for the treatment, or can other models be used more effectively? Is a specification of the problem areas necessary in order for the treatment to work well? Should interpersonal sensitivity be considered a problem area, or is it best conceptualized as a personality or attachment variant? For that matter, are the problem areas fully inclusive, or are there additional areas that should be added?

The latter point is particularly important, as it has spawned a plethora of subtypes of IPT treatments for which additional problem areas have been added. IPT for adolescents,[26] for instance, has added the problem area of 'single-parent families' to the original problem areas; IPT for depressed pregnant women[27] has added the problem area of complicated pregnancy to the mix. In contrast, IPT could be conceptualized as a more universally applicable treatment rather than having multiple IPT variants, and could be more broadly understood as interpersonally focused, with the problem areas framed as general principles instead of necessary specifics of the treatment. This is, ultimately, a question that can be addressed empirically, although at present no empirical evidence exists to support either position. However, clinical experience suggests that IPT can easily be used as a more broadly based treatment, and that dissemination of IPT may be hindered by an insistence that each of the subtypes is a distinct entity.

There has also been little research conducted on what might be added to IPT to make it more effective. Would adding relaxation techniques make IPT more effective in some circumstances? What about regular assignment of homework, or using the 'empty chair' technique to practice new communication skills? In essence, a strict adherence to an empirical model may do great harm because it strongly discourages creativity[28] and may hinder more effective techniques from being incorporated into the IPT model.

What level of training is required to effectively deliver IPT?

IPT has been largely confined to research settings in the United States, though its dissemination as a clinical intervention has been more widespread in Europe and Australasia. As a consequence, most IPT in the US is delivered by highly trained Ph.D. or M.D. level therapists, while elsewhere it is delivered by therapists with similar levels of training as well as by therapists with less extensive training. In neither instance has there been much research regarding the level of training required to deliver the treatment proficiently. While it is generally accepted that 'well-trained' therapists with psychodynamic experience can deliver IPT, no data currently exist to support the proposition that this kind of training is necessary. Moreover, the current recommendations for research level training (i.e., 40 hours of didactic training and two supervised cases) have not been tested as to their effects on therapist proficiency and outcome in clinical settings.

An important corollary to this question involves its relationship with the use of therapist judgment. Specifically, is IPT best delivered 'by the book,' or is it – in the hands of a competent and experienced therapist – better utilized as a framework for treatment with the expectation that the therapist can improve outcomes by using his or her therapeutic judgement? Conversely, for therapists with little experience, perhaps it is best to have more strict adherence to a manual, as their lack of experience limits the effectiveness of their clinical judgment.

CONCLUSION

There is no doubt that IPT is one of the most thoroughly studied psychotherapies. There are a number of very high-quality efficacy studies which clearly demonstrate the benefit of IPT when used in controlled settings. These data should heavily influence the practice of IPT in non-research settings. Although there is a lack of empirical data at present regarding the clinical use of IPT, clinical experience clearly indicates that it is also effective in this setting.

REFERENCES

1. Klerman, G.L., DiMascio, A., Weissman, M.M., Prusoff, B.A., Paykel, E.S. 1974. Treatment of depression by drugs and psychotherapy. *American Journal of Psychiatry* **131**, 186–91.
2. Weissman, M.M., Prusoff, B.A., DiMascio, A. 1979. The efficacy of drugs and psychotherapy in the treatment of acute depressive episodes. *American Journal of Psychiatry* **136**, 555–8.
3. Weissman, M.M., Klerman, G.L., Prusoff, B.A., Sholomskas, D., Padian, N. 1981. Depressed outpatients: results after one year of treatment with drugs and/or interpersonal psychotherapy. *Archives of General Psychiatry* **38**, 51–5.
4. Frank, E., Kupfer, D.J., Perel, J.M., *et al*. 1990. Three-year outcomes for maintenance therapies in recurrent depression. *Archives of General Psychiatry* **47**, 1093–9.
5. DiMascio, A., Weissman, M.M., Prusoff, B.A. 1979. Differential symptom reduction by drugs and psychotherapy in acute depression. *Archives of General Psychiatry* **36**, 1450–6.
6. Elkin, I., Shea, M.T., Watkins, J.T., *et al*. 1989. National Institute of Mental Health Treatment of Depression Collaborative Research Program: general effectiveness of treatments. *Archives of General Psychiatry* **46**, 971–82.
7. Imber, S.D., Pilkonis, P.A., Sotsky, S.M., *et al*. 1990. Mode-specific effects among three treatments for depression. *Journal of Consulting and Clinical Psychology* **58**, 352–9.
8. Beck, A.T., Rush, A.J., Shaw, B.F., Emery, G. 1979. *Cognitive Therapy of Depression*. New York: Guilford Press.
9. Beck, A.T., Ward, C.H., Mendelson, M., Mock, J., Erbaugh, J. 1961. An inventory for measuring depression. *Archives of General Psychiatry* **4**, 561–71.
10. Hamilton, M.A. 1967. Development of a rating scale for primary depressive illness. *British Journal of Social and Clinical Psychology* **6**, 278–96.
11. Shea, M.T., Elkin, I., Imber, S.D., *et al*. 1992. Course of depressive symptoms over follow-up. Findings from the National Institute of Mental Health Treatment of Depression Collaborative Research Program. *Archives of General Psychiatry* **49**, 782–7.
12. Klein, D.F., Ross, D.C. 1993. Reanalysis of the National Institute of Mental Health treatment of depression collaborative research program general effectiveness report. *Neuropsychopharmacology* **8**, 241–51.
13. Jacobson, N.S., Hollon, S.D. 1996. Cognitive-behavior therapy versus pharmacotherapy: Now that the jury's returned its verdict, its time to present the rest of the evidence. *Journal of Consulting and Clinical Psychology* **64**, 74–80.
14. Elkin, I., Parloff, M.B., Hadley, S.W., Autry, J.H. 1985. NIMH Treatment of Depression Collaborative Treatment Program: background and research plan. *Archives of General Psychiatry* **42**, 305–16.
15. Klerman, G.L., Weissman, M.M., Rounsaville, B.J., Chevron, E.S. 1984. *Interpersonal Psychotherapy of Depression*. New York: Basic Books.
16. Detre, T. 1987. The future of psychiatry. *American Journal of Psychiatry* **144**, 621–5.
17. Engel, G.L. 1980. The clinical application of biopsychosocial models. *American Journal of Psychiatry* **137**, 535–44.

18. Stiles, W.B., Shapiro, D.A. 1989. Abuse of the drug metaphor in psychotherapy process-outcome research. *Clinical Psychology Review* **9**, 521–44.

19. Kupfer, D.J., Frank, E., Perel, J.M. 1992. Five year outcomes for maintenance therapies in recurrent depression. *Archives of General Psychiatry* **49**, 769–73.

20. Frank, E., Spanier, C. 1995. Interpersonal psychotherapy for depression: overview, clinical efficacy, and future directions. *Clinical Psychology: Science and Practice* **2**, 349–69.

21. Frank, E., Grochocinski, V.J., Spanier, C.A., *et al.* 2000. Interpersonal psychotherapy and antidepressant medication: evaluation of a sequential treatment strategy in women with recurrent major depression. *Journal of Clinical Psychiatry* **61**, 51–7.

22. Thase, M.E., Buysse, D.J., Frank, E., Cherry, C.R. 1997. Which depressed patients will respond to interpersonal psychotherapy? The role of abnormal EEG sleep profiles. *American Journal of Psychiatry* **154**, 502–9.

23. Martin, S.D., Martin, E., Rai, S.S., Richardson, M.A., Royall, R. 2001. Brain blood flow changes in depressed patients treated with Interpersonal Psychotherapy or venlafaxine hydrochloride: preliminary findings. *Archives of General Psychiatry* **58**, 641–8.

24. Brody, A.L., Saxena, S., Stoessel, P., *et al.* 2001. Regional brain metabolic changes in patients with major depression treated with either paroxetine or interpersonal therapy: preliminary findings. *Archives of General Psychiatry* **58**, 631–40.

25. Edelson, M. 1994. Can psychotherapy research answer this psychotherapist's questions? In: Talley, P.F., Strupp, H.H., Butler, S.F. (eds), *Psychotherapy Research and Practice: Bridging the Gap*. New York: Basic Books.

26. Mufson, L., Moreau, D., Weissman, M.M., Klerman, G.L. 1993. *Interpersonal Psychotherapy for Depressed Adolescents*. New York: Guilford Press.

27. Spinelli, M.A. 2001. Interpersonal psychotherapy for antepartum depressed women. In: Yonkers, K., Little, B. (eds), *Management of Psychiatric Disorders in Pregnancy*. New York: Oxford University Press, 105–21.

28. Henry, W.P. 1998. Science, politics, and the politics of science: the use and misuse of empirically validated treatment research. *Psychotherapy Research* **8**, 126–40.

FURTHER READING

NIMH-TDCRP

Ablon, J.S., Jones, E.E. 1999. Psychotherapy process in the National Institute of Mental Health Treatment of Depression Collaborative Research Program. *Journal of Consulting and Clinical Psychology* **67**, 64–75.

Agosti, V. 1999. Predictors of persistent social impairment among recovered depressed outpatients. *Journal of Affective Disorders* **55**, 215–19.

Agosti, V., Stewart, J.W. 1998. Social functioning and residual symptomatology among outpatients who responded to treatment and recovered from major depression. *Journal of Affective Disorders* **47**, 207–10.

Agosti, V., Ocepek-Welikson, K. 1997. The efficacy of imipramine and psychotherapy in early-onset chronic depression: a reanalysis of the National Institute of Mental health Treatment of Depression Collaborative Research Program. *Journal of Affective Disorders* **43**, 181–6.

Barber, J.P., Muenz, L.R. 1996. The role of avoidance and obsessiveness in matching patients to cognitive and interpersonal psychotherapy: empirical findings from the Treatment for Depression Collaborative Research Program. *Journal of Consulting and Clinical Psychology* **64**, 951–8.

Blatt, S.J., Quinlan, P.A., Pilkonis, P.A., Shea, M.T. 1995. Impact of perfectionism and need for approval on the brief treatment of depression: the National Institute of Mental Health Treatment of Depression Collaborative Treatment Program revisited. *Journal of Consulting and Clinical Psychology* **63**, 125–32.

Blatt, S.J., Quinlan, D.M., Zuroff, D.C., Pilkonis, P.A. 1996. Interpersonal factors in brief treatment of depression: further analyses of the National Institute of Mental Health Treatment of Depression Collaborative Research Program. *Journal of Consulting and Clinical Psychology* **64**, 162–71.

Blatt, S.J., Sanislow, C.A., Zuroff, D.C., Pilkonis, P.A. 1996. Characteristics of effective therapists: further analyses of data from the National Institute of Mental Health Treatment of Depression Collaborative Research Program. *Journal of Consulting and Clinical Psychology* **64**, 1276–84.

Blatt, S.J., Zuroff, D.C., Bondi, C.M., Sanislow, C.A., Pilkonis, P.A. 1998. When and how perfectionism impedes the brief treatment of depression: further analyses of the National Institute of Mental Health Treatment of Depression Collaborative Research Program. *Journal of Consulting and Clinical Psychology* **66**, 423–8.

Blatt, S.J., Zuroff, D.C., Bondi, C.M., Sanislow, C.A. 2000. Short- and long-term effects of medication and psychotherapy in the brief treatment of depression: further analyses of data from the NIMH TDCRP. *Psychotherapy Research* **10**, 215–34.

Crits-Christoph, P., Connolly, M.B., Shappell, S., Elkin, I., Krupnick, J. 1999. Interpersonal narratives in cognitive and interpersonal psychotherapies. *Psychotherapy Research* **9**, 22–35.

Elkin, I., Pilkonis, P.A., Docherty, J.P., Sotsky, S.M. 1988. Conceptual and methodological issues in comparative studies of psychotherapy and pharmacotherapy, I: Active ingredients and mechanisms of change. *American Journal of Psychiatry* **145**, 909–17.

Elkin, I., Pilkonis, P.A., Docherty, J.P., Sotsky, S.M. 1988. Conceptual and methodological issues in the comparative studies of psychotherapy and pharmacotherapy, II: nature and timing of treatment effects. *American Journal of Psychiatry* **145**, 1070–6.

Elkin, I., Gibbons, R.D., Shea, M.T., *et al.* 1995. Initial severity and differential treatment outcome in the National Institute of Mental Health Treatment of Depression Collaborative Research Program. *Journal of Consulting and Clinical Psychology* **63**, 841–7.

Gibbons, R.D., Hedeker, D., Elkin, I., *et al.* 1993. Some conceptual and statistical issues in analysis of longitudinal psychiatric data. Application to the NIMH Treatment of Depression Collaborative Research Program. *Archives of General Psychiatry* **50**, 739–50.

Hill, C.E., O'Grady, K.E., Elkin, I. 1992. Applying the Collaborative Study Psychotherapy Rating Scale to rate therapist adherence in cognitive-behavior therapy, interpersonal therapy, and clinical management. *Journal of Consulting and Clinical Psychology* **60**, 73–9.

Krupnick, J.L., Sotsky, S.M., Simmens, S., *et al.* 1996. The role of the therapeutic alliance in psychotherapy and pharmacotherapy outcome: findings in the National Institute of Mental Health Treatment of Depression. *Journal of Consulting and Clinical Psychology* **64**, 532–9.

O'Malley, S.S., Foley, S.H., Rounsaille, B.J., *et al.* 1988. Therapist competence and patient outcome in interpersonal psychotherapy of depression. *Journal of Consulting and Clinical Psychology* **56**, 496–501.

Rounsaville, B.J., Chevron, E.S., Weissman, M.M. 1984. Specification of techniques in interpersonal psychotherapy. In: Williams, J.B., Spitzer, R.L. (eds), *Psychotherapy Research: Where are We and Where Should We Go?* New York: Guilford Press.

Rounsaville, B.J., Chevron, E.S., Prusoff, B.A., *et al*. 1987. The relation between specific and general dimensions of the psychotherapy process in interpersonal psychotherapy of depression. *Journal of Consulting and Clinical Psychology* **55**, 379–84.

Shea, M.T., Pilkonis, P.A., Beckham, E., *et al*. 1990. Personality disorders and treatment outcome in the NIMH Treatment of Depression Collaborative Treatment Program. *American Journal of Psychiatry* **147**, 711–18.

Sotsky, S.M., Simmens, S.J. 1999. Pharmacotherapy response and diagnostic validity in atypical depression. *Journal of Affective Disorders* **54**, 237–47.

Sotsky, S.M., Glass, D.R., Shea, M.T., *et al*. 1991. Patient predictors of response to psychotherapy and pharmacotherapy: findings in the NIMH Treatment of Depression Collaborative Research Program. *American Journal of Psychiatry* **148**, 997–1008.

Stewart, J.W., Garfinkel, R., Nunes, E.V., Donovan, S., Klein, D.F. 1998. Atypical features and treatment response in the National Institute of Mental Health Treatment of Depression Collaborative Research Program. *Journal of Clinical Psychopharmacology* **18**, 429–34.

Sullivan, P.F., Joyce, P.R. 1994. Effects of exclusion criteria in depression treatment studies. *Journal of Affective Disorders* **32**, 21–6.

Watkins, J.T., Leber, W.R., Imber, S.D., *et al*. 1993. Temporal course of change of depression. *Journal of Consulting and Clinical Psychology* **61**, 858–64.

Whisman, M.A. 2001. Marital adjustment and outcome following treatments for depression. *Journal of Consulting and Clinical Psychology* **69**, 125–9.

Zlotnick, C., Shea, M.T., Pilkonis, P.A., Elkin, I., Ryan, C. 1996. Gender, type of treatment, dysfunctional attitudes, social support, life events, and depressive symptoms over naturalistic follow-up. *American Journal of Psychiatry* **153**, 1021–7.

Zlotnick, C., Elkin, I., Shea, M.T. 1998. Does the gender of a patient or the gender of a therapist affect the treatment of patients with major depression? *Journal of Consulting and Clinical Psychology* **66**, 655–9.

Zuroff, D.C., Blatt, S.J., Sanislow, C.A., Bondi, C.M., Pilkonis, P.A. 1999. Vulnerability to depression: reexamining state dependence and relative stability. *Journal of Abnormal Psychology* **108**, 76–89.

Zuroff, D.C., Blatt, S.J., Sotsky, S.M., *et al*. 2000. Relation of therapeutic alliance and perfectionism to outcome in brief outpatient treatment of depression. *Journal of Consulting and Clinical Psychology* **68**, 114–24.

Neurophysiological studies

Brody, A.L., Saxena, S., Stoessel, P., *et al*. 2001. Regional brain metabolic changes in patients with major depression treated with either paroxetine or interpersonal therapy: preliminary findings. *Archives of General Psychiatry* **58**, 631–40.

Brody, A.L., Saxena, S., Mandelkern, M.A., Fairbanks, L.A., Ho, M.L., Baxter, L.R. 2001. Brain metabolic changes associated with symptom factor improvement in major depressive disorder. *Biological Psychiatry* **50**, 171–8.

Buysse, D.J., Tu, X.M., Cherry, C.R., *et al*. 1999. Pretreatment REM sleep and subjective sleep quality distinguish depressed psychotherapy remitters and nonremitters. *Biological Psychiatry* **45**, 205–13.

Martin, S.D., Martin, E., Rai, S.S., Richardson, M.A., Royall, R. 2001. Brain blood flow changes in depressed patients treated with Interpersonal Psychotherapy or venlafaxine hydrochloride: preliminary findings. *Archives of General Psychiatry* **58**, 641–8.

Thase, M.E., Buysse, D.J., Frank, E., Cherry, C.R. 1997. Which depressed patients will respond to interpersonal psychotherapy? The role of abnormal EEG sleep profiles. *American Journal of Psychiatry* **154**, 502–9.

Geriatric depression

Buysse, D.J., Reynolds, C.F., Houck, P.R., *et al*. 1997. Does lorazepam impair the antidepressant response to nortriptyline and psychotherapy? *Journal of Clinical Psychiatry* **48**, 426–32.

Dew, M.A., Reynolds, C.F., Houck, P.R., *et al*. 1997. Temporal profiles of the course of depression during treatment. Predictors of pathways toward recovery in the elderly. *Archives of General Psychiatry* **54**, 1016–24.

Dew, M.A., Reynolds, C.F., Mulsant, B., *et al*. 2001. Initial recovery patterns may predict which maintenance therapies for depression will keep older adults well. *Journal of Affective Disorders* **65**, 155–66.

Frank, E., Prigerson, H.G., Shear, M.K., Reynolds, C. 1997. Phenomenology and treatment of bereavement-related distress in the elderly. *International Clinical Psychopharmacology* **2** (suppl. 7), S25–9.

Hinrichsen, G.A. 1997. Interpersonal psychotherapy for depressed older adults. *Journal of Geriatric Psychiatry* **30**, 239–57.

Hinrichsen, G.A. 1999. Treating older adults with interpersonal psychotherapy for depression. *Journal of Clinical Psychology* **55**, 949–60.

Miller, M.D., Wolfson, L., Frank, E., *et al*. 1997. Using interpersonal psychotherapy (IPT) in a combined psychotherapy/medication research protocol with depressed elders. A descriptive report with case vignettes. *Journal of Psychotherapy Practice and Research* **7**, 47–55.

Miller, M.D., Cornes, C., Frank, E., Ehrenpreis, L., Silberman, R., Schlernitzauer, M.A., Tracey, B., Richards, V., Wolfson, L., Zaltman, J., Bensasi, S., Reynolds, CF, III. 2001. Interpersonal psychotherapy for late-life depression: past, present, and future. *Journal of Psychotherapy Practice and Research* **10**, 231–8.

Mossey, J.M., Knott, K.A., Higgins, M., Talerico, K. 1996. Effectiveness of a psychosocial intervention, interpersonal counseling for subdysthymic depression in medically ill elderly. *Journal of Gerontology* **51A**, 172–8.

Opdyke, K.S., Reynolds, C.F., Frank, E., *et al*. 1996. Effect of continuation treatment on residual symptoms in late-life depression: how well is 'well'? *Depression and Anxiety* **4**, 312–19.

Reynolds, C.F., Frank, E., Perel, J.M., *et al*. 1994. Treatment of consecutive episodes of major depression in the elderly. *American Journal of Psychiatry* **151**, 1740–3.

Reynolds, C.F., Frank, E., Perel, J.M., Mazumdar, S., Kupfer, D.J. 1995. Maintenance therapies for late-life recurrent major depression: research and review circa 1995. *International Psychogeriatrics* **7** (suppl.), 27–39.

Reynolds, C.F., Frank, E., Houck, P.R., *et al*. 1997. Which elderly patients with remitted depression remain well with continued interpersonal psychotherapy after discontinuation of antidepressant medication? *American Journal of Psychiatry* **154**, 958–62.

Reynolds, C.F., Dew, M.A., Frank, E., *et al*. 1998. Effects of age at onset of first lifetime episode of recurrent major depression on treatment response and illness course in elderly patients. *American Journal of Psychiatry* **155**, 795–9.

Reynolds, C.F., Frank, E., Dew, M.A., *et al*. 1999. Treatment of 70(+)-year-olds with recurrent major depression. Excellent short-term but brittle long-term response. *American Journal of Geriatric Psychiatry* **7**, 64–9.

Reynolds, C.F., Frank, E., Perel, J.M., *et al*. 1999. Nortriptyline and interpersonal psychotherapy as maintenance therapies for recurrent major depression: a randomized controlled trial in patients older than fifty-nine years. *Journal of the American Medical Association* **281**, 39–45.

Reynolds, C.F., Miller, M.D., Pasternak, R.E., *et al*. 1999. Treatment of bereavement-related major depressive episodes in later life: a controlled study of acute and continuation treatment with nortriptyline and interpersonal psychotherapy. *American Journal of Psychiatry* **156**, 202–8.

Taylor, M.P., Reynolds, C.F., Frank, E., *et al*. 1999. Which elderly depressed patients remain well on maintenance interpersonal psychotherapy alone?: report from the Pittsburgh study of maintenance therapies in late-life depression. *Depression and Anxiety* **10**, 55–60.

Wolfson, L., Miller, M., Houck, P., *et al*. 1997. Foci of interpersonal psychotherapy (IPT) in depressed elders: clinical and outcome correlates in a combined IPT/nortriptyline protocol. *Psychotherapy Research* **7**, 45–56.

Maintenance treatment of depression

Feske, U., Frank, E., Kupfer, D.J., Shear, M.K., Weaver, E. 1998. Anxiety as a predictor of response to interpersonal psychotherapy for recurrent major depression: an exploratory investigation. *Depression and Anxiety* **8**, 135–41.

Frank, E. 1991. Interpersonal psychotherapy as a maintenance treatment for patients with recurrent depression. *Psychotherapy* **28**, 259–66.

Frank, E., Kupfer, D.J. 1987. Efficacy of combined imipramine and interpersonal psychotherapy. *Psychopharmacology Bulletin* **23**, 4–7.

Frank, E., Jarrett, D.B., Kupfer, D., Grochocinski, V. 1984. Biological and clinical predictors of response in recurrent depression: a preliminary report. *Psychiatry Research* **13**, 315–24.

Frank, E., Kupfer, D.J., Perel, J.M., *et al*. 1990. Three-year outcomes for maintenance therapies in recurrent depression. *Archives of General Psychiatry* **47**, 1093–9.

Frank, E., Kupfer, D.J., Wagner, E.F., McEachran, A.B., Cornes, C. 1991. Efficacy of interpersonal psychotherapy as a maintenance treatment of recurrent depression. Contributing factors. *Archives of General Psychiatry* **48**, 1053–9.

Frank, E., Grochocinski, V.J., Spanier, C.A., *et al*. 2000. Interpersonal psychotherapy and antidepressant medication: evaluation of a sequential treatment strategy in women with recurrent major depression. *Journal of Clinical Psychiatry* **61**, 51–7.

Kamlet, M.S., Paul, N., Greenhouse, J., Kupfer, D., Frank, E., Wade, M. 1995. Cost utility analysis of maintenance treatment for recurrent depression. *Controlled Clinical Trials* **16**, 17–40.

Kupfer, D.J., Frank, E. 2001. The interaction of drug- and psychotherapy in the long-term treatment of depression. *Journal of Affective Disorders* **62**, 131–7.

Kupfer, D.J., Frank, E., Perel, J.M. 1989. The advantage of early treatment intervention in recurrent depression. *Archives of General Psychiatry* **46**, 771–5.

Kupfer, D.J., Frank, E., Perel, J.M. 1992. Five year outcomes for maintenance therapies in recurrent depression. *Archives of General Psychiatry* **49**, 769–73.

Pilkonis, P.A., Frank, E. 1988. Personality pathology in recurrent depression: nature, prevalence, and relationship to treatment response. *American Journal of Psychiatry* **145**, 435–41.

Spanier, C., Frank, E., McEachran, A.B., Grochocinski, V.J., Kupfer, D.J. 1996. The prophylaxis of depressive episodes in recurrent depression following discontinuation of drug therapy: integrating psychological and biological factors. *Psychological Medicine* **26**, 461–75.

Perinatal depression

Depression and HIV

Markowitz, J.C., Spielman, L.A., Scarvalone, P.A., Perry, S.W. 2000. Psychotherapy adherence of therapists treating HIV-positive patients with depressive symptoms. *Journal of Psychotherapy Practice and Research* **9**, 75–80.

Swartz, H.A., Markowitz, J.C., Spinelli, M.G. 1997. Interpersonal psychotherapy of a depressed, pregnant, HIV-positive woman. *Journal of Psychotherapy Practice and Research* **6**, 165–78.

Swartz, H.A., Markowitz, J.C. 1998. Interpersonal psychotherapy for the treatment of depression in HIV-positive men and women. In: Markowitz, J.C. (ed.), *Interpersonal Psychotherapy. Review of Psychiatry Series*. Washington, DC: American Psychiatric Press, 129–55.

Dysthymia

Markowitz, J.C. 1993. Psychotherapy of the post-dysthymic patient. *Journal of Psychotherapy Practice and Research* **2**, 157–63.

Markowitz, J.C. 1994. Psychotherapy of dysthymia. *American Journal of Psychiatry* **151**, 1114–21.

Markowitz, J. 1998: *Interpersonal Psychotherapy for Dysthymic Disorder*. Washington, DC: American Psychiatric Press.

Mason, B.J., Markowitz, J.C., Klerman, G.L. 1993. Interpersonal psychotherapy for dysthymic disorders. In: Klerman, G.L., Weissman, M.M. (eds), *New Applications of Interpersonal Psychotherapy*. Washington, DC: American Psychiatric Press, 225–64.

Group treatment of depression

Levkowitz, Y., Shahar, G., Native, G., *et al.* 2000. Group interpersonal psychotherapy for patients with major depressive disorder – pilot study. *Journal of Affective Disorders* **60**, 191–5.

MacKenzie, K.R., Grabovac, A.D. 2001. Interpersonal psychotherapy group (IPT-G) for depression. *Journal of Psychotherapy Practice and Research* **10**, 46–51.

Wilfley, D.E., MacKenzie, K.R., Welch, R.R., Ayres, V.E., Weissman, M.M. 2000. *Interpersonal Psychotherapy for Group*. New York: Basic Books.

Depression: general

Blanco, C., Lipsitz, J., Caligor, E. 2001. Treatment of chronic depression with a 12-week program of interpersonal psychotherapy. *American Journal of Psychiatry* **158**, 371–5.

Blom, M.B., Hoencamp, E., Zwaan, T. 1996. Interpersoonlijke Psychotherapie voor depressie: een pilot-onderzoek. *Tijdschrift voor Psychiatrie* **38**, 398–402.

Browne, G., Steiner, M., Roberts, J., *et al.* Sertraline and interpersonal psychotherapy, alone and combined, in the treatment of patients with dysthymic disorder in primary care: a 2 year comparison of effectiveness and cost. *Journal of Affective Disorders* (in press).

Cornes, C.L. 1993. Interpersonal psychotherapy of depression (IPT): a case study. In: Wells, R., Gianetti, V. (eds), *Casebook of the Brief Psychotherapies*. New York: Plenum Press, 53–64.

Deykin, E., Weissman, M., Tanner, J., Prusoff, B. 1975. Participation in therapy. A study of attendance patterns in depressed outpatients. *Journal of Nervous and Mental Disease* **160**, 42–8.

DiMascio, A., Weissman, M.M., Prusoff, B.A. 1979. Differential symptom reduction by drugs and psychotherapy in acute depression. *Archives of General Psychiatry* **36**, 1450–6.

Dorrepaal, E., van Nieuwenhuizen, C., Schene, A., de Haan, R. 1998. The effectiveness of cognitive and interpersonal psychotherapy in the treatment of depression: a meta-analysis. [in Dutch]. *Tijdschrift voor Psychiatrie* **40**, 27–39.

Foley, S.H., Rounsaville, B.J., Weissman, M.M. 1989. Individual versus conjoint interpersonal psychotherapy for depressed patients with marital disputes. *International Journal of Family Psychiatry* **10**, 29–42.

Frank, E., Spanier, C. 1995. Interpersonal psychotherapy for depression: overview, clinical efficacy, and future directions. *Clinical Psychology: Science and Practice* **2**, 349–69.

Frank, E., Grochocinski, V.J., Spanier, C.A., *et al.* 2000. Interpersonal psychotherapy and antidepressant medication: evaluation of a sequential treatment strategy in women with recurrent major depression. *Journal of Clinical Psychiatry* **61**, 51–7.

Gillies, L.A. 2001. Interpersonal psychotherapy for depression and other disorders. In: Barlow, D.H. (ed.), *Clinical Handbook of Psychological Disorders: A Step-by-Step Treatment Manual.* 3rd edition. New York: Guilford Press.

Herceg-Baron, R.L., Prusoff, B.A., Weissman, M.M., DiMascio, A., Neu, C., Klerman, G.L. 1979. Pharmacotherapy and psychotherapy in acutely depressed patients: a study of attrition patterns in a clinical trial. *Comprehensive Psychiatry* **20**, 315–25.

Klerman, G.L. 1989. Evaluating the efficacy of psychotherapy for depression: the USA experience. *European Archives of Psychiatry and Neurological Sciences* **238**, 240–6.

Klerman, G.L., Weissman, M.M. 1993. *New Applications of Interpersonal Psychotherapy.* Washington, DC: American Psychiatric Press.

Klerman, G.L., DiMascio, A., Weissman, M.M., Prusoff, B.A., Paykel, E.S. 1974. Treatment of depression by drugs and psychotherapy. *American Journal of Psychiatry* **131**, 186–91.

Markowitz, J.C. 1998. *Interpersonal Psychotherapy.* Washington, DC: American Psychiatric Press.

Markowitz, J.C. 1999. Developments in interpersonal psychotherapy. *Canadian Journal of Psychiatry* **44**, 556–61.

Markowitz, J.C., Schwartz, H.A. 1997. Case formulation in interpersonal psychotherapy of depression. In: Eels, T.D. (ed.), *Handbook of Psychotherapy Case Formulation.* New York: Guilford, 192–222.

Paykel, E.S., DiMascio, A., Klerman, G.L., Prusoff, B.A., Weissman, M.M. 1976. Maintenance therapy of depression. *Pharmakopsychiatrie Neuropsychopharmakologie* **9**, 127–36.

Perez, J.E. 1999. Integration of cognitive-behavioral and interpersonal therapies for Latinos: an argument for technical eclecticism. *Journal of Contemporary Psychotherapy* **29**, 169–83.

Rounsaville, B.J., Weissman, M.M., Prusoff, B.A., Herceg-Baron, R. 1979. Process of psychotherapy among depressed women with marital disputes. *American Journal of Orthopsychiatry* **49**, 505–10.

Stuart, S. 1997. Use of interpersonal psychotherapy for depression. In: *Directions in Psychiatry.* Volume 17. New York: Hatherleigh Company, 263–74.

Thase, M.E., Greenhouse, J.B., Frank, E., *et al.* 1997. Treatment of major depression with psychotherapy or psychotherapy-psychopharmacology combinations. *Archives of General Psychiatry* **54**, 109–15.

Weissman, M.M., Klerman, G.L. 1973. Psychotherapy with depressed women: an empirical study of content themes and reflection. *British Journal of Psychiatry* **123**, 55–61.

Weissman, M.M., Klerman, G.L., Paykel, E.S. 1974. Treatment effects on the social adjustment of depressed patients. *Archives of General Psychiatry* **30**, 771–8.

Weissman, M.M., Prusoff, B.A., Klerman, G.L. 1978. Personality and the prediction of long-term outcome of depression. *American Journal of Psychiatry* **135**, 797–800.

Weissman, M.M., Klerman, G.L., Prusoff, B.A., Sholomskas, D., Padian, N. 1981. Depressed outpatients: results after one year of treatment with drugs and/or interpersonal psychotherapy. *Archives of General Psychiatry* **38**, 51–5.

Weissman, M.M., Markowitz, J.W., Klerman, G.L. 2000. *Comprehensive Guide to Interpersonal Psychotherapy*. New York: Basic Books.

Zuckerman, D.M., Prusoff, B.A., Weissman, M.M., Padian, N.S. 1980. Personality as a predictor of psychotherapy and pharmacotherapy outcome for depressed outpatients. *Journal of Consulting and Clinical Psychology* **48**, 730–5.

Bipolar disorder

Frank, E., Kupfer, D.J., Ehlers, C.L., *et al*. 1994. Interpersonal and social rhythm therapy for bipolar disorder: integrating interpersonal and behavioural approaches. *Behavioural Therapist* **17**, 143–6.

Frank, E., Hlastala, S., Ritenour, A., *et al*. 1997. Inducing lifestyle regularity in recovering bipolar disorder patients: results from the maintenance therapies in bipolar disorder protocol. *Biological Psychiatry* **41**, 1165–73.

Frank, E., Swartz, H.A., Mallinger, A.G., Thase, M.E., Weaver, E.V., Kupfer, D.J.1999. Adjunctive psychotherapy for bipolar disorder: effects of changing treatment modality. *Journal of Abnormal Psychology* **108**, 579–87.

Frank, E., Swartz, H.A., Kupfer, D.J. 2000. Interpersonal and social rhythm therapy: managing the chaos of bipolar disorder. *Biological Psychiatry* **48**, 593–604.

Miklowitz, D.J., Frank, E., George, E.L. 1996. New psychosocial treatments for the outpatient management of bipolar disorder. *Psychopharmacology Bulletin* **32**, 613–21.

Robertson, M. 1999. Interpersonal psychotherapy for patients recovering from bipolar disorder. *Australasian Psychiatry* **7**, 329–31.

Swartz, H.A., Frank, E. 2001. Psychotherapy for bipolar depression: a phase-specific treatment strategy? *Bipolar Disorders* **3**, 11–22.

Eating disorders

Agras, W.S., Walsh, T., Fairburn, C.G., Wilson, G.T., Kraemer, H.C. 2000. A multicenter comparison of cognitive-behavioral therapy and interpersonal psychotherapy for bulimia nervosa. *Archives of General Psychiatry* **57**, 459–66.

Birchall, H. 1999. Interpersonal psychotherapy in the treatment of eating disorders. *European Eating Disorders Review* **7**, 315–20.

Fairburn, C.G., Jones, R., Peveler, R.C. 1991. Three psychological treatments for bulimia nervosa: a comparative trial. *Archives of General Psychiatry* **48**, 463–9.

Fairburn, C.G., Jones, R., Peveler, R.C. 1993. Psychotherapy and bulimia nervosa: the longer-term effects of interpersonal psychotherapy, behavioural psychotherapy, and cognitive behaviour therapy. *Archives of General Psychiatry* **50**, 419–28.

Fairburn, C.G., Norman, P.A., Welch, S.L. 1995. A prospective study of the outcome in bulimia nervosa and the long-term effects of three psychological treatments. *Archives of General Psychiatry* **52**, 304–12.

Fernandez, M.L. 1998. Interpersonal therapy applied to a group of family patients with eating disorders. *Revista de Psiquiatria Infanto-Juvenil* **4**, 238–44.

Jones, R., Peveler, R.C., Hope, R.A., Fairburn, C.G. 1993. Changes during treatment for bulimia nervosa: a comparison of three psychological treatments. *Behaviour Research and Therapy* **31**, 479–85.

McIntosh, V.V., Bulik, C.M., McKenzie, J.M., Luty, S.E., Jordan, J. 2000. Interpersonal psychotherapy for anorexia nervosa. *International Journal of Eating Disorders* **27**, 125–39.

Wilfley, D.E., Agras, W.S., Telch, C.F., *et al*. 1993. Group cognitive-behavioral therapy and group interpersonal psychotherapy for the non-purging bulimic individual: a controlled comparison. *Journal of Consulting and Clinical Psychology* **61**, 296–305.

Wilfley, D.E., Frank, M.A., Welch, R., Spurrell, E.B., Rounsaville, B.J. 1998. Adapting interpersonal psychotherapy to a group format (IPT-G) for binge eating disorder: toward a model for adapting empirically supported treatments. *Psychotherapy Research* **8**, 379–91.

Anxiety disorders

Lipsitz, J.D., Marshall, R.D. 2001. Alternative psychotherapy approaches for social anxiety disorder. *Psychiatric Clinics of North America* **24**, 817–29.

Lipsitz, J.D., Markowitz, J.C., Cherry, S., Fyer, A.J. 1999. Open trial of interpersonal psychotherapy for the treatment of social phobia. *American Journal of Psychiatry* **156**, 1814–16.

Interpersonal counseling

Dieguez, P.M., Rodriguez, V.B., Fernandez, L.A. 2001. Psychotherapy in primary health care: interpersonal counselling for depression. *Medifam-Revista de Medicina Familiar y Comunitaria* **11**, 156–62.

Klerman, G.L., Budman, S., Berwick, D., *et al*. 1987. Efficacy of a brief psychosocial intervention for symptoms of stress and distress among patients in primary care. *Medical Care* **25**, 1078–88.

Lave, J.R., Frank, R.G., Schulberg, H.C., Kamlet, M.S. 1998. Cost-effectiveness of treatments for major depression in primary care. *Archives of General Psychiatry* **55**, 645–51.

Mossey, J.M., Knott, K.A., Higgins, M., Talerico, K. 1996. Effectiveness of a psychosocial intervention, interpersonal counseling for subdysthymic depression in medically ill elderly. *Journal of Gerontology* **51A**, 172–8.

Schulberg, H.C., Scott, C.P., Madonia, M.J., Imber, S.D. 1993. Applications of interpersonal psychotherapy to depression in primary care practice. In: Klerman, G.L., Weissman, M.M. (eds), *New Applications of Interpersonal Psychotherapy*. Washington, DC: American Psychiatric Press.

Schulberg, H.C., Block, M.R., Madonia, M.J. 1996. Treating major depression in primary care practice. *Archives of General Psychiatry* **53**, 913–19.

Physical medicine

Stuart, S., Cole, V. 1996. Treatment of depression following myocardial infarction with interpersonal psychotherapy. *Annals of Clinical Psychiatry* **8**, 203–6.

Stuart, S., Noyes, R. 1999. Attachment and interpersonal communication in somatization disorder. *Psychosomatics* **40**, 34–43.

Substance abuse

Carroll, K.M., Rounsaville, B.J., Gawin, F.H. 1991. A comparative trial of psychotherapies for ambulatory cocaine abusers: relapse prevention and interpersonal psychotherapy. *American Journal of Drug and Alcohol Abuse* **17**, 229–47.

Carroll, K.M., Rounsaville, B.J., Gordon, L.T., *et al*. 1994. Psychotherapy and pharmacotherapy for ambulatory cocaine abusers. *Archives of General Psychiatry* **51**, 177–87.

Rounsaville, B.J., Glazer, W., Wilber, C.H., Weissman, M.M., Kleber, H.D. 1983. Short-term interpersonal psychotherapy in methadone-maintained opiate addicts. *Archives of General Psychiatry* **40**, 629–36.

Adolescents

Moreau, D., Mufson, L., Weissman, M.M., Klerman, G.L. 1991. Interpersonal psychotherapy for adolescent depression: description of modification and preliminary application. *Journal of the American Academy of Child and Adolescent Psychiatry* **30**, 642–51.

Mufson, L., Dorta, K.P. 2000. Interpersonal psychotherapy for depressed adolescents: theory, practice, and research. In: Esman, A.H., Flaherty, L.T. (eds), *Adolescent Psychiatry: Developmental and Clinical Studies. Volume 25. The Annals of the American Society for Adolescent Psychiatry*. Hillsdale, NJ: The Analytic Press.

Mufson, L., Fairbanks, J. 1996. Interpersonal psychotherapy for depressed adolescents: a one-year naturalistic follow-up study. *Journal of the American Academy of Child and Adolescent Psychiatry* **35**, 1145–55.

Mufson, L., Moreau, D., Weissman, M.M., Klerman, G.L. 1993. *Interpersonal Psychotherapy for Depressed Adolescents*. New York: Guilford Press.

Mufson, L., Moreau, D., Weissman, M.M. 1994. The modification of interpersonal psychotherapy with depressed adolescents (IPT-A): phase I and phase II studies. *Journal of the American Academy of Child and Adolescent Psychiatry* **33**, 695–705.

Mufson, L., Weissman, M.M., Moreau, R.G. 1999. Efficacy of interpersonal psychotherapy for depressed adolescents. *Archives of General Psychiatry* **56**, 573–9.

Rosselo, J., Bernal, G. 1999. The efficacy of cognitive-behavioral and interpersonal treatments for depression in Puerto Rican adolescents. *Journal of Consulting and Clinical Psychology* **55**, 379–84.

Santor, D.A., Kusumakar, V. 2001. Open trial of interpersonal psychotherapy in adolescents with moderate to severe major depression: effectiveness of novice IPT therapists. *Journal of the American Academy of Child and Adolescent Psychiatry* **40**, 236–40.

Miscellaneous

Chevron, E.S., Rounsaville, B.J., Rothblum, E.D., Weissman, M.M. 1983. Selecting psychotherapists to participate in psychotherapy outcome studies. Relationship between psychotherapist characteristics and assessment of clinical skills. *Journal of Nervous and Mental Disease* **171**, 348–53.

Donnelly, J.M., Kornblith, A.B., Fleischman, S., *et al*. 2000. A pilot study of interpersonal psychotherapy by telephone with cancer patients and their partners. *Psycho-oncology* **9**, 44–56.

Feske, U., Frank, E., Kupfer, D.J., Shear, M.K., Weaver, E. 1998. Anxiety as a predictor of response to interpersonal psychotherapy for recurrent major depression: an exploratory investigation. *Depression and Anxiety* **8**, 135–41.

Foley, S.H., O'Malley, S., Rounsaville, B., Prusoff, B.A., Weissman, M.M. 1987. The relationship of patient difficulty to therapist performance in interpersonal psychotherapy of depression. *Journal of Affective Disorders* **12**, 207–17.

Luty, S.E., Joyce, P.R., Mulder, R.T., Sullivan, P.F., McKenzie, J.M. 1998. Relationship between interpersonal psychotherapy problem areas with temperament and character: a pilot study. *Depression and Anxiety* **8**, 154–9.

Markowitz, J.C. 1995. Teaching interpersonal psychotherapy to psychiatric residents. *Academic Psychiatry* **19**, 167–73.

Markowitz, J.C. 1997. The future of interpersonal psychotherapy. *Journal of Psychotherapy Practice and Research* **6**, 294–9.

Markowitz, J.C., Svartberg, M., Swartz, H.A. 1998. Is IPT time-limited psychodynamic psychotherapy? *Journal of Psychotherapy Research and Practice* **7**, 185–95.

Markowitz, J.C., Leon, A.C., Miller, N.L., Cherry, S., Clougherty, K.F., Villalobos, L. 2000. Rater agreement on interpersonal psychotherapy problem areas. *Journal of Psychotherapy Practice and Research* **9**, 131–5.

Rounsaville, B.J., Chevron, E.S., Weissman, M.M. 1984. Specification of techniques in interpersonal psychotherapy. In: Williams, J.B., Spitzer, R.L. (eds), *Psychotherapy Research: Where are We and Where Should We Go?* New York: Guilford Press.

Rounsaville, B.J., Chevron, E.S., Weissman, M.M., Prusoff, B.A., Frank, E. 1986. Training therapists to perform interpersonal psychotherapy in clinical trials. *Comprehensive Psychiatry* **27**, 364–71.

Rounsavillle, B.J., O'Malley, S.S., Foley, S., Weissman, M.M. 1988. Role of manual-guided training in the conduct and efficacy of interpersonal psychotherapy for depression. *Journal of Consulting and Clinical Psychology* **56**, 681–8.

Sole'-Puig, J. 1997. The European launch of interpersonal psychotherapy in the Tenth World Congress of Psychiatry. *European Psychiatry* **12**, 46–8.

Stuart, S. 1997. Use of interpersonal psychotherapy for other disorders. In: *Directions in Mental Health Counseling*. New York: Hatherleigh Company, 4–16.

Weissman, M.M. 1997. Interpersonal psychotherapy: current status. *Keio Journal of Medicine* **46**, 105–10.

Weissman, M.M. 1998. The many uses of interpersonal therapy. *Harvard Mental Health Letter* **14**, 4–5.

Weissman, M.M., Markowitz, J.C. 1994. Interpersonal psychotherapy. Current status. *Archives of General Psychiatry* **51**, 599–606.

Weissman, M.M., Rounsaville, B.J., Chevron, E. 1982. Training psychotherapists to participate in psychotherapy outcome studies. *American Journal of Psychiatry* **139**, 1442–6.

Integrated Case Example: Allan

INTRODUCTION

This chapter is a synthesis of all of the components discussed throughout this book. The use of IPT with 'Allan,' a 42-year-old man who presented for treatment of an episode major depression, is described.

PART I: CLINICAL ASSESSMENT

Background

Allan was a 42-year-old married father of two teenage daughters. He worked as a proof reader and had done so for the previous 10 years. He had initially presented to his family physician complaining of insomnia and some abdominal pain. His family physician, after closer assessment, had diagnosed a Major Depressive Disorder and had instituted treatment with an antidepressant medication. After 3 weeks, Allan had failed to derive any substantial benefit from this medication, and a referral was made to a psychiatrist.

Initial interview with the psychiatrist

Allan arrived half an hour early for his appointment, whereupon he was informed by the psychiatrist's secretary that the psychiatrist was running approximately 5–10 minutes behind schedule. This appeared to irritate Allan, though he did not directly communicate his annoyance.

Allan described having difficulty sleeping over the previous 3–6 months. He reported feeling irritable and frustrated, and also had complaints of non-specific abdominal pain and headaches. In her referral letter, Allan's family physician had reported that he had been experiencing depressed mood for most of the day with a tendency for his mood to lift through the afternoon. She had noted both initial and terminal insomnia characterized by daily early morning wakening at approximately 4:00 a.m. Allan had further described having a reduction in the level of interest in his usual activities, and a reduced capacity for enjoyment. Allan also reported that he had been experiencing difficulty with concentration which had impaired his ability to perform his job. Allan had divulged to his family physician that he had intermittent suicidal thoughts, and had contemplated overdosing on his medication and alcohol.

The psychiatrist inquired specifically about psychotic symptoms, which did not appear to be present, and then further clarified Allan's suicidal ideation. Though Allan reported that he had at times had thoughts that he might be better off dead, he had no specific thoughts of suicide nor any intent. Further, he noted that he would never attempt such an action as it would be devastating for his family.

As the interview progressed, the psychiatrist asked about Allan's social situation. Allan remarked that he had been increasingly unhappy in his marriage, and that he had conflicts with both of his teenage daughters, Eliza, aged 17, and Anna, aged 14. As the psychiatrist asked more about the problems with his wife, Allan replied:

'Pam doesn't have much time for me any more. She seems to have fallen out of love and I don't think she wants to be with me any more. I don't think I am a particularly nice person to be with at the moment. I see things falling apart.'

On further inquiry, it became apparent that Allan and Pam had been arguing excessively, and that their relationship had become 'cold and stale' in Allan's words. When the psychiatrist inquired further about Allan's relationship with his daughters, Allan reported that he had some form of a 'falling out' with his older daughter Eliza, and that Anna had become increasingly difficult in her behavior at home, annoying both Allan and his wife.

When asking about Allan's interests and activities outside of the workplace, the psychiatrist found that there was very little evidence of a social support network. Indeed, Allan had little or no contact with anybody outside of his immediate family, and he seemed quite socially isolated and unsupported.

Allan had been prescribed antidepressant medication at a modest dose, but had not obtained any real symptomatic benefit. Allan's family doctor had also prescribed a benzodiazepine as a night-time sedative, and Allan had become increasingly dependent upon this medication and had trebled the dose of these tablets on his own. Allan denied that he consumed alcohol or other illicit substances, and denied that he had been obtaining prescriptions for sedatives elsewhere apart from his family physician.

Past psychiatric history

Allan denied previous consultation with any healthcare professional regarding his mental health. On closer inquiry, it appeared that Allan had suffered prolonged periods of dysphoria, and it was likely that there had been one or two occasions throughout his early adolescence and young adulthood where he had periods of significant depression that lasted for months. He had, however, never sought any form of psychiatric treatment or counseling.

Past medical history

Allan reported being in good health, with no known physical problems. His only medications included the antidepressant and the benzodiazepine prescribed by his family doctor.

Family psychiatric history

Allan was the only child of his parents' marriage. His mother had been hospitalized recurrently throughout his childhood with episodes of severe, possibly psychotic, depression. It was likely that the first onset of her depression was after Allan's birth. He told the psychiatrist that he had been raised by a variety of caregivers throughout his childhood, and that his father became detached from him and his mother. Allan did not recall feeling particularly affectionate or close to any of his caregivers, nor was he able to recall fondly any relationships with school teachers or peers. Allan reported that his mother had recently suffered another episode of severe depression and had been hospitalized again:

> 'She tends to spend a long time in the hospital. I am not sure she ever really gets better. I have never known her to be "normal."'

Allan was unaware of any other family members who had experienced psychological problems.

Social and developmental history

Allan was carried to term in an uncomplicated pregnancy and delivery. There was no evidence that his mother had been depressed antenatally. He was not aware of any delay in reaching his developmental milestones. Allan described few meaningful attachments as a child, and recalled that he was generally anxious and avoidant in his behavior. He reported that he was isolated at school with few if any friends, and was described by his teachers as a 'shy but pleasant child.' There was no evidence of separation anxiety or somatizing symptoms as a child. Allan completed 5 years of secondary education before leaving to join the Civil Service where he worked in a low-level administrative capacity for the next 10 years. Throughout his employment in the Civil Service he had few if any social contacts, but did involve himself in solitary physical activities such as attending a gymnasium and joining running clubs.

Allan and Pam had met at a church function during his early 20s. Pam had been on a holiday from abroad, and after meeting Allan they formed a relationship which he described as 'initially close, more of a friendship than lovers.' Pam migrated to live with Allan and they were married after a 2-year courtship. Eliza was born after they had been married for 12 months, and Anna 3 years later. Allan described being happy in his role of father, particularly with Eliza, with whom he felt very close. He recalled spending a lot of time with Eliza when she was younger, and he particularly enjoyed going on long runs with her. He had been less close to Anna, but still felt that their relationship was good. Allan described that as his relationship with Pam had deteriorated over the years he had grown closer to Eliza.

Eliza had begun to spend increasing amounts of time away from the family home, and had seemed to Allan to have been avoiding contact with him – particularly over the previous 6 months. Allan stated that approximately 9 months ago he became aware of a relationship that Eliza was developing with an older woman, which he believed was sexual. Allan felt that her sexual choices were a manner of 'punishing' him.

Allan summed up his social relationships by stating,

'I now feel completely alone – there is nobody for me.'

Premorbid personality

Allan described a longstanding difficulty with intimate relationships. He reported that he found strong emotional states such as anger and sadness intolerable. He described a pattern of exploding in torrents of rage, only to become deeply ashamed at losing control. This difficult cycle of rage and shame was greatly distressing to him. The therapist noted, however, that when explored in detail, this 'rage' was quite limited. In fact, the therapist observed that what Allan labeled "rage" would have been labeled as simple anger by most people. It appeared that Allan was most concerned about losing control of his emotions, and felt that any display of anger was a 'rage.'

The psychiatrist came to the view that Allan had a tendency to rely on obsessional and perfectionistic coping strategies, such as working longer hours, trying to atone for his perceived failings by repetitively attending to tasks, and by over-emphasizing order and goal achievement. There seemed to be a tendency for him to view the world in an 'all or nothing' way, focusing primarily upon the negative aspects of life. The psychiatrist felt there was clear evidence that this was a stable pattern of personality functioning that had likely been present since childhood.

Mental state examination

Allan presented as a fit-looking, middle-aged man who was casually attired in jeans and a collared shirt. He wore a neatly trimmed beard with glasses, and had short, cropped hair. The psychiatrist had great difficulty establishing rapport with Allan, and found him to have little or no warmth. Very little eye contact was evident. Allan's affect was flat and he described his mood as 'quite depressed.' While there was no disorder of thought, there appeared to be significant self-reproach and hopelessness in his thought content, which did not appear to be delusional in intensity. There were no perceptual disturbances evident. Allan had only limited insight into the severity of his problems – he acknowledged that some of his vegetative symptoms were excessive and might be indicative of an illness, but he was unable to recognize his problems as a 'depression.'

Diagnostic formulation

The psychiatrist made the following DSM-IV multi-axial diagnoses:

- *Axis I*   Major depressive disorder
                     Dysthymic disorder (rule out)
- *Axis II*   Obsessive-compulsive personality traits
- *Axis III*   None
- *Axis IV*   Family and marital disputes
                     Illness of mother
                     Social isolation
- *Axis V*   GAF = 55

Initial management

The psychiatrist first clarified that Allan was not acutely suicidal and in need of inpatient care. Because of the failure to achieve symptom relief, the psychiatrist increased the dose of the antidepressant medication. A non-addictive sedative medication was prescribed, and Allan was provided with a schedule to safely taper the benzodiazepine he was taking. The psychiatrist sought the results of the laboratory investigations ordered by Allan's family physician, all of which were normal. The psychiatrist was also informed that Allan's physical examination was unremarkable.

The psychiatrist considered a number of potential psychotherapeutic treatment approaches to Allan's problems. The psychiatrist was mindful of the likely presence of an avoidant style of attachment as evidenced by the account of Allan's early environment, his current interpersonal functioning, and his interaction with the psychiatrist in the first interview. Another consideration was the likely presence of significant personality traits, as evidenced by Allan's description of his long-term pattern of social relationships.

The psychiatrist considered the following possible therapeutic interventions:

1 *Cognitive behavior therapy* (CBT): this psychotherapeutic approach had merit for a number of reasons. The first was its focal and structured nature. While not engaging problematic aspects of attachment and psychodynamics, CBT would still be likely to help Allan address the dysfunctional nature of his cognitive schema, particularly the obsessional aspects of his thoughts and behavior.
2 *Self-psychology*: it was clear to the psychiatrist that Allan had what could be considered as a life-long history of 'empathic failures' by caregivers. Allan's account of his childhood, particularly his relationship with his chronically ill mother and distant father, his history of multiple caregivers, and his description of few if any nurturing relationships as a child, suggested to the psychiatrist that a therapeutic relationship which was validating and provided him with some experience of empathic understanding would be beneficial.
3 *Family therapy*: Allan's account of his family functioning highlighted significant problems in the realm of his relationships with his wife and daughters. There was certainly evidence that the family system was not effectively adapting to Allan's illness, and there were clear implications for the family's long-term functioning and its effect upon Allan's depressive illness and vice-versa.
4 *Interpersonal psychotherapy*: while there were clear biological and psychological reasons for Allan to have developed depression at this point in his life, perhaps the most compelling aspect of his presentation was the relationship difficulties he was

experiencing in his marriage and with his daughters, as well as his significant social isolation. This suggested that a treatment which was interpersonally focused would offer Allan the best chance of achieving symptom relief, in combination with medication.

In addition, the therapist was also guided to a degree by the extant empirical literature. First, efficacy studies suggested that IPT would be a suitable treatment for the depression Allan was experiencing. IPT would also be a suitable and empirically validated treatment for dysthymia. Second, there was evidence from the NIMH-TDCRP that IPT might be better suited to patients with more obsessive traits, as opposed to treatment with CBT. Though there was little empirical evidence that combined treatment with both medication and therapy would be of additional benefit to Allan, the psychiatrist nonetheless elected to continue with both the antidepressant and with therapy on the basis of his clinical experience, which suggested that the combined treatment was likely to be very helpful in this case.

The potential for a problematic therapeutic relationship, given Allan's history of relationship failures, suggested to the psychiatrist that his approach with IPT would need to be modified given Allan's avoidant attachment style. First, the therapist recognized that he needed to spend more time to carefully develop a therapeutic alliance with Allan, and would need to take special care to listen reflectively and to communicate empathy to Allan. Second, the pacing of the therapy would need to be modified, as Allan would likely need more time to develop a sense of trust in the therapist and to be able to disclose information more freely. Finally, the therapist recognized that he would need to work very carefully to convey to Allan that he was interested in truly understanding him, and that he needed to be flexible in the therapeutic agenda so that Allan did not perceive that the therapist was imposing an agenda upon him.

Interpersonal formulation

The interpersonal formulation for Allan is shown in Figure 23.1.

The therapist provided the following feedback to Allan in both a verbal and written form:

'Allan, it appears you have developed an episode of major depression. The clinical features that you describe, as well as the severity of your symptoms, convince me that this is more than just sadness. It is clear that there are a number of factors that have interacted to produce this episode at this point in your life. Severe depression is due in part to genetic factors, and the history of your mother's severe depression suggests to me that you have almost certainly inherited a vulnerability to this illness. Fortunately, there do not appear to be other physical factors that have contributed at this point, as you appear to have been quite well physically over the years.'

'I also think that there are a number of psychological vulnerabilities that have led you to become depressed. While you are clearly a hard-working and detail-oriented man – indeed this has helped you achieve much in your work – I suspect that these traits have also been an "Achilles heel" for you in dealing with other aspects of your life. While it has worked well for you in the past to deal with problems by working harder, things recently have come to a point at which this strategy doesn't seem to be working any longer.'

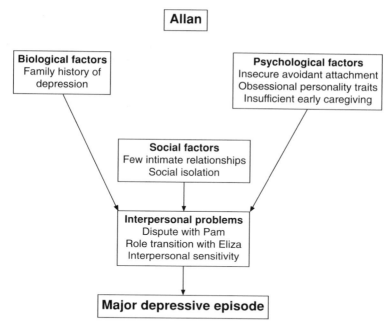

Figure 23.1 *Interpersonal Formulation.*

'Most compelling for me, however, is the context in which you have become depressed. You have described to me how your marriage with Pam has deteriorated to the point where you feel it is failing. You have also told me that your "special" relationship with Eliza has also changed, and this seems to have been a great loss for you as well.'

'While I feel that medication has an important place in your treatment, I believe that we need to address many of these issues using psychotherapy. Psychotherapy, like medication, has many varieties. For example, some treatments might examine your thinking patterns, or perhaps the way in which your family is interacting. I feel, however, that because of the interpersonal context of your depression, that Interpersonal Psychotherapy, or IPT, will be the most helpful for you.'

'IPT is a focal treatment that looks primarily at your current relationships. It has been shown in numerous scientific studies to be beneficial in the acute treatment of depression, and this seems to be because it helps individuals deal with their unique interpersonal problems. I believe that we can make the best use of the psychotherapy by focusing on your interpersonal relationships and helping you to make changes in them. What are your thoughts about this?'

Allan responded to the psychiatrist that he thought that the formulation was 'fairly accurate,' and that perhaps there was some hope in working with his relationships. While he was a bit skeptical about the value of talking with someone about his problems, he agreed to start IPT.

The therapist was careful to frame the formulation in a way that was likely to be acceptable to Allan. First, it was framed in Allan's language – the therapist consistently talked about his thoughts rather than his feelings, and asked Allan to respond in the same way by asking about his thoughts about the summary as opposed to asking about his feelings about it. Second, the therapist also highlighted Allan's strengths rather than framing the formulation as a summary of his weaknesses, which Allan would likely take as criticism. Finally, the therapist also framed the formulation as a hypothesis rather than as a definitive interpretation, and carefully invited Allan's feedback about it.

The therapeutic contract

Allan and the psychiatrist agreed to meet for twelve 50-minute sessions of IPT over the next several months. They initially agreed to begin by meeting weekly, with an explicit discussion of the possibility of meeting less frequently as Allan improved. Allan agreed to be prompt in attendance and to give at least 24 hours notice should he wish to change appointments. Allan agreed that the focus of treatment would be on interpersonal issues, and that after he and the therapist had compiled the Interpersonal Inventory a specific interpersonal focus would be developed. The therapist provided Allan with an information sheet regarding IPT (see Appendix A). In addition to a written version of the interpersonal formulation, the psychiatrist also provided Allan with a copy of the interpersonal formulation diagram for him to consider. The psychiatrist also agreed that any medication management issues could be briefly discussed at the beginning or end of each session, but that the bulk of the time should be dedicated to interpersonal issues. Mindful of Allan's expectations of treatment, the therapist felt that a formal written contract was worthwhile, and he provided this to Allan at the next session.

PART II: THE COURSE OF TREATMENT WITH IPT

Interpersonal Inventory

During sessions 1 and 2, Allan and the therapist compiled the Interpersonal Inventory (see Appendix B). The Interpersonal Inventory is displayed in Figure 23.2.

While compiling the Interpersonal Inventory, the following three areas were discussed in greater depth.

1. ALLAN'S RELATIONSHIP WITH PAM

Pam and Allan had met while she was visiting on a working holiday. Allan had said that he had enjoyed spending time with Pam, particularly given that 'she was better at social contact.' Allan described that Pam had been solely responsible for organizing the couple's social life, and that he would 'go along for the ride' so long as Pam 'was prepared to break the ice.' While Allan did not feel he was excessively socially anxious, he felt more comfortable in this passive role.

Allan reported that recently Pam had become increasingly 'fed up with my behavior.' He reported that Pam consistently 'would not do what I requested, particularly around the house, and I would often argue with her about this.' Allan reported that their conversations frequently became arguments, and that things were now at the point where nothing could really be discussed.

Interpersonal Inventory

Patient Name: Allan
Date of Birth: × × × × × ×
Other Clinicians: × × × × × ×
Insurance Details: × × × × × ×
Date of First Consultation: × × × × × ×
Contracted Number of Sessions: 12

Name of Other: Pam
Relationship: Wife
Patient's Account of Problem: Says 'she hates me' – reports that they were always
'friends' Tends to communicate in a demanding and
angry way – she then responds by doing the opposite,
eg not take out the trash He goes to work at 4pm she
arrives home at 5pm – she is in bedwhen he gets home
In role play: unable to really alter tone Seems to get
into a cycle of anger and more obsessionality

Areas Requiring Further Clarification: Previous attempts to solve problems
with Pam and how he communicated

Agreed Problem Area: Disputes   Role   Grief and   Interpersonal
                                   Transition   Loss   Sensitivity
                      Impasse

Special Issues:

Figure 23.2 Interpersonal Inventory.

Allan told the therapist that Pam was now spending more time with her own friends and was increasing the number of hours she was at work. Over the past several years, Allan had been working afternoon shifts and Pam working during the day. The only contact they now had was for a few moments in the evening, after Allan had arrived home from work, at which time he would usually find Pam already asleep. On weekends, Pam continued to make arrangements 'with the girls,' from which Allan was obviously excluded. Allan reported that their sexual relationship had all but ceased, and that there was now little affection between the couple.

The therapist asked for some specific Interpersonal Incidents in which the couple came into conflict. Allan reported the following interaction:

Therapist: Can you tell me about the last time you and Pam argued?
Allan: Yes, just the other night we had a fight.
Therapist: Tell me more about what was happening at the time.
Allan: I had arrived home, the trash had not been put out, and there were dirty dishes in the sink.
Therapist: What happened then that led to the conflict?
Allan: I reminded her that I had specifically told her to take out the trash and clean up the dishes.
Therapist: Can you tell me how you asked her to do that?
Allan: What words exactly?
Therapist: Yes – I'd really like to understand better how you communicate with her.
Allan: I said, 'Pam, I have asked you before to put the garbage out. The house is

becoming a mess. You know that just drives me crazy.'
Therapist: And how did Pam respond?
Allan: She didn't say anything.
Therapist: What was the emotional message you conveyed? Were you upset, angry, neutral?
Allan: Well, mostly I was angry. I even let my voice get pretty loud, and then I felt guilty afterwards because I lost my temper. I need to do a better job of controlling my emotions.

From this and several other Interpersonal Incidents the therapist inferred that there was very poor communication at present between Allan and Pam, and that there was a need to specifically focus upon this within the treatment. Having reviewed the various problem areas, Allan felt that his problems with Pam were best characterized as an interpersonal dispute, which he described as at the impasse phase.

2. ALLAN'S RELATIONSHIP WITH ELIZA

Allan and Eliza had enjoyed a close relationship until approximately nine months before, when she decided to leave school in the 5th year of High School in order to join the workforce. This had disappointed Allan, as he had wanted Eliza to complete her final exam at school and join a profession. Allan reported that his relationship with Eliza was, in many ways, closer than that with Pam. He fondly recalled jogging and swimming with Eliza, and having a friendly competition to 'improve our personal bests.'

The therapist noted that as Allan was discussing the loss of his relationship with Eliza, his affect became more bland and restricted, despite the clearly significant loss he was describing. When the therapist asked about Allan's views of Eliza's relationship with an older woman, he responded:

'I can't understand why she's doing this to me. Where did I go wrong with this?'

At this point, the therapist felt a great temptation to explore the cognitive processes underlying Allan's belief that Eliza's apparent sexual choices were a way of 'punishing' him. Despite the significance of this, the therapist reminded himself that the focus of IPT in this particular problem area was to examine the interpersonal implications of the changes in Allan's relationship with Eliza. The therapist stated to Allan:

Therapist: Allan, I can see that you have a number of significant conflicts about some of Eliza's choices, and you clearly feel that these are in some way a punishment. What I'd like to focus on is more clearly understanding what is happening to your relationship with Eliza, and how it affects you and the depression from which you are suffering. We need to consider whether you view this as a dispute in the same way that you categorize the problem area with Pam, or whether it is more accurate to think of it within another area such as grief, where there is a loss to be mourned. I can also imagine that thinking of it as a role transition would acknowledge not only the loss of the old relationship with Eliza, but also the challenges of developing a new relationship with her.
Allan: I certainly feel a loss, so I guess grief fits. Can you tell me more about role transitions again?
Therapist: Well, role transition looks at changes in relationships and how they affect each person differently. Many people who have developed psychological symptoms

in the context of a role transition have had a loss experience, and they often feel great sadness or anxiety about it. There is also usually a need to adapt to a new role which they may feel ill equipped to deal with. While I can see that grief certainly reflects how you are feeling at the moment, role transition may also fit well. I think that either grief or role transition would work, but I also think that it needs to be your decision.
Allan: Well, I guess that I have to still be her dad, so perhaps looking at this as a role transition would probably work best.
Therapist: In that case we need to talk about the old role or the old relationship as something you have lost, and also the new role as something you have gained.
Allan: That would help make things simpler for me, yes.

Following this, the therapist and Allan set about discussing the old role and new role in both positive and negative lights.

3. THE ISSUE OF INTERPERSONAL SENSITIVITY

The therapist was concerned that Allan's social isolation and inability to utilize any social support network were significant factors in the genesis of his mood symptoms, and were likely to represent ongoing vulnerabilities. The therapist felt that this area was a significant problem, and therefore initiated the following interaction:

Therapist: Allan, in addition to the family conflicts we've discussed, I wanted to talk more about the general sense of isolation you are feeling.
Allan: Yes – it is a problem.
Therapist: You told me earlier that you tended to rely on Pam to 'break the ice with people.'
Allan: That's right.
Therapist: In what way do you find it difficult to do this yourself?
Allan: Well, I've never really tried, I guess.
Therapist: Why do you think that is?
Allan: I've never had much luck in relationships. Not since I was a kid, and certainly not as an adult.
Therapist: Do you think that there is a particular problem that comes up time and time again?
Allan: I haven't really thought about it in that way.
Therapist: Perhaps we could look at a few examples of relationships in which you felt this has been a problem, and see if there is a pattern.
Allan: You mean like dragging over old ground?
Therapist: Well, even though we are working on your current relationships, I think we can learn about your current problems by paying some attention to what has happened in the more recent past.

Following this exchange, Allan and the therapist discussed a few examples of instances in which Allan had tried and failed to initiate interpersonal contact. It appeared that the common theme throughout all of these relationship failures had been Allan's tendency to place high expectations upon those around him, only to find that they did not follow up with further contact. Allan described that if a particular social contact had not followed through with a request or not met an expectation, then Allan would express disapproval. Typically, Allan would not initiate further contact and ultimately the relationship would dissolve. The therapist provided the following feedback to Allan:

> **Therapist:** The problems you are describing are fairly common among people who suffer from depression and anxiety. In IPT, we talk about this kind of interpersonal sensitivity as a problem area in its own right. Interpersonal sensitivity refers to the particular vulnerability that individuals have in initiating and maintaining social support. There is a lot of evidence to support the idea that people who are vulnerable to psychological distress have difficulties initiating and maintaining social support. When using interpersonal sensitivity as a problem area, the idea is to try to help people clarify exactly what their difficulties are in this regard, and help them to learn new ways of overcoming their difficulties in relationships. While it isn't expected that people will change who they are, it is often very helpful to identify one or two vulnerabilities and to work on improving or consolidating social skills.

Allan and the therapist agreed that within the Interpersonal Inventory there were three problem areas that Allan felt needed the most attention:

- An *interpersonal dispute* in the impasse phase with Pam.
- A *role transition* with Eliza.
- *Interpersonal sensitivity.*

Session 3

Session 3 began with Allan arriving 15 minutes before the start of the appointment. The therapist invited Allan to take a seat and stated:

> **Therapist:** Allan, we are now going to change pace, and for the next seven or eight sessions you will be largely directing where we take the discussion. As you recall we discussed three specific problem areas from the Interpersonal Inventory. Which one of those would you like to start discussing today?

Following this invitation, Allan elected to talk about his interpersonal dispute with Pam. The therapist then made use of the technique of Interpersonal Incidents to further elaborate other examples of disagreements between Allan and Pam. The therapist was able to highlight two factors which were related to the dispute. The first was that the way in which Allan was communicating his needs to Pam may not have been conveying his message adequately. Second, the therapist felt that Allan's expectations of Pam were not realistic.

Allan made the general statement that 'Pam never listens to me' and described feeling angry, disappointed, and frustrated. The therapist was able to introduce the possibility that Pam may have also felt angry and frustrated by Allan's requests, possibly because of the way in which the two of them were communicating. Allan acknowledged the possibility that this might be the case, but was still of the view that his expectations of Pam were not unreasonable, although he admitted that he might need to look at alternative ways of discussing them with her.

At the end of the session, Allan still felt that the relationship dispute was at an impasse, but was less convinced that it was insoluble.

Session 4

The session began with the therapist focusing the discussion on the interpersonal issues discussed the week previously:

> **Therapist:** Allan, last week we discussed your dispute with Pam in some detail. Can you tell me what has happened with that relationship during the week?

Allan responded that there had been two or three further arguments along similar lines to those already reported. The therapist asked Allan to provide more examples of some specific communications. Allan gave numerous verbatim examples of his statements such as '*you never do what I ask, you don't show me any respect*' and '*Pam, I've told you a thousand times to take the trash out on Monday nights.*' Several specific incidents were discussed, each of which was in essence a repetition of the initial incident that Allan reported.

The therapist suggested to Allan that there might be some alternative ways of approaching the subject with Pam, and that by utilizing a role play, there might be some opportunities to work on modifying the problematic communication. The rest of the session was spent with the therapist and Allan role playing an instance in which he was unhappy with some aspects of Pam's home care. The therapist and Allan initially conducted the role play with Allan playing himself. However, Allan consistently communicated in an accusatory and rather irritable way. Rather than directly giving feedback to Allan about this communication style, the therapist suggested that they try an alternative approach in which the therapist played Allan and Allan played Pam. The therapist was particularly concerned about being perceived by Allan as too critical, given Allan's rather avoidant style and the early stage in therapy.

In this reverse role play, the therapist attempted to model non-confrontative ways of communicating with Pam, including statements such as '*Pam, how about we talk over a cup of coffee about getting on top of this housework*' or '*Pam, what ways do you see that we can make this house run more smoothly.*' Allan saw potential merit in this approach, but continued to externalize the problem, though he did acknowledge that his communication style could be improved.

Session 5

Session 5 began late, as the therapist ran over time with a previous patient and needed to take an urgent phone call. When Allan entered the room he sat down and appeared quite angry. He then stated:

> 'I can't believe you are this disorganized! You finished four minutes early at the end of the last session and today you are running fifteen minutes late. I bet you still charge me the same fee!'

The therapist was quite taken aback by this exchange and was initially at a loss as to how to respond. The therapist finally stated:

> 'Allan, I am sorry that you feel that I don't value your time. I do my best to stick to my schedule, but sometimes my day gets out of control with phone calls and other people running over time. Despite that, I can certainly understand why you are angry with me, and appreciate the fact that you let me know how you feel.'

As the therapist was responding, Allan began to cry. This was startling for the therapist, as this was the first time Allan had shown any real affect. After Allan had regained his composure, the therapist attempted to link this affect with what Allan was thinking at the time by examining his process affect. Allan responded:

'I can't believe that just happened. Everybody I ever deal with lets me down, and the relationship goes nowhere. You are the only person who has been able to make any sense to me and now this is going to go bad as well.'

The therapist tried to validate Allan's concerns by checking his understanding of what Allan had said, and then responded:

'Allan, I hear your concerns and your frustration. I wonder if what has just happened here tells us in some way about what is happening in your other relationships, particularly with your dispute with Pam. I have not been aware of your concerns about time pressure, although I know you have expectations about this. I am wondering if the same pattern that leads to problems with Pam is evolving here. If we can trace how this emerged with Pam, I think we can better understand your conflict with her.'

The therapist considered a number of options in using the therapeutic relationship. One possibility would have been to examine the ways in which Allan had communicated his expectations to the therapist. Although he was mindful of how distressed Allan had become, the therapist felt that this was better not dealt with directly, particularly given Allan's insecure attachment style. The therapist therefore moved to an exploration of the similarities in Allan's relationship with Pam. Allan, presumably motivated by his new affective experience, was able to finally link his expectations with the consistent dispute with Pam.

The session ended on time with the therapist stating:

'Allan, I think this has been one of the most productive sessions we have had thus far. I appreciate how difficult it was for you to give me feedback about being late, but I think that taking that risk really helped me to understand you much better. I also appreciate the reminder to keep my schedule in order.'

Sessions 6 and 7
Session 6 began on time with Allan apologizing again for his previous behavior. The therapist acknowledged the apology, and again reinforced the fact that Allan's comments had been helpful in understanding him better. For Allan, the experience of addressing his frustration and resolving it with the therapist seemed to have reassured him that it was possible with Pam. He reported to the therapist that he had discussed his expectations with Pam, following his role-playing rehearsal in session 4. Allan stated that he felt that the problem had improved, and that he would like to concentrate on the problems with Eliza.

The therapist referred to the Interpersonal Inventory and reacquainted Allan with his statements about the 'positive' and 'negative' aspects of both the old role and the new role. The therapist asked questions about Allan's happier memories of Eliza's childhood which seemed to lead to a discernible shift in Allan's affect.

Session 7 began where session 6 had finished. The therapist picked up the thread of the discussion in session 6 and moved the focus of discussion on to an exploration of the new role:

Therapist: It is very clear to me that you feel that you have lost something significant with Eliza's growing up.

Allan: It's hard to describe really. She continues to change, and I guess I do as well, but we just aren't close like we used to be.

Therapist: Change leaves a lot of us vulnerable at times.

The therapist and Allan then discussed the particular difficulties he faced in dealing with Eliza's relationship with the 'older woman.' Rather than being concerned about her sexuality, Allan was concerned that Eliza was going to be exploited by this older woman and 'get hurt.' The therapist stated that he had talked with many patients about the difficulty parents have dealing with the changes that occur as their children become adults, and that this was a frequent source of distress. The therapist felt that his relationship with Allan had progressed to a point where he could also disclose some of his own life experiences.

Therapist: I think I can understand your difficulty. I can remember when my kids were growing up, it was always hard to strike a balance between giving them their freedom, their own choices and knowing when to come in to bail them out. You never stop worrying though, do you?

Allan: You've got that right. I seem to be constantly worried about Eliza, though I can't seem to bring myself to tell her why I am concerned.

The psychiatrist then suggested a homework task for Allan: he could have a conversation with Eliza about her relationship, but rather than focus on his concerns, he could ask her how her relationship with the older woman had evolved, and where she saw things going, in a friendly and interested way rather than as a concerned parent.

Sessions 8 and 9

Session 8 began with Allan reporting that the homework assignment, which he completed the evening following the previous session, was very successful. He had finally talked with Eliza about her relationship, and had also invited her partner over to visit as well. He stated:

> 'I guess my relationship is going to be this way. I still miss my little girl but she isn't a little girl anymore. I guess I am going to have to deal with her as a young woman.'

The therapist asked Allan how this impacted his relationship with Emma, his younger daughter, to which Allan replied:

> 'It seems that she has been responding to a lot of what is going on around her. I think that as things have settled down with Pam and Eliza and myself that she has felt more calm and things have sorted themselves out.'

The discussion then moved to the issue of interpersonal sensitivity. During the Interpersonal Inventory, the therapist had noted a consistent pattern in which Allan's expectations of others were often unrealistic and poorly communicated, leading to failures in his social relationships. Allan appeared to developing some understanding of this problem, however, the therapist was concerned that introducing this concept might undermine Allan's improving self esteem. Rather than giving direct feedback to Allan about his social skills, the therapist chose to focus on Allan's general social support.

> Therapist: As we discussed some time earlier, people who don't have good social supports are often vulnerable to develop psychological distress. What are some ways you could get some additional support outside of your family?

The therapist used the technique of problem solving to help Allan generate potential ways to increase his social support. Allan listed three possibilities:

- Approaching a colleague for a drink after work.
- Joining a hiking club.
- Attending a church function.

Allan agreed to a homework assignment to consider which option looked best for him and to make some preliminary inquiries.

In session 9, Allan told the therapist that he had made some inquiries about hiking clubs and had some contact details. He said that he had chosen to approach a colleague at work with whom he felt some connection. The rest of the session was devoted to Allan rehearsing potential communication strategies through role playing. A homework task was set for Allan to approach the colleague and invite him out for a beer after work.

Session 10

Session 10 began with Allan reporting that he had invited a colleague out, and had an enjoyable drink after work. He said that this colleague had then invited Allan and Pam to his place for a barbecue the following weekend. The therapist noted a considerable improvement in Allan's mood, although Allan reported some ongoing difficulties with his sleep. Allan agreed that he was improving, noting that he felt less stressed about his relationships and that his marriage was improving.

The therapist then returned to the previous discussion and asked about the possibility of joining a hiking club. The rest of the session was then devoted to Allan practicing his communication meeting the members of the group who had been planning a hike in the bush outside of the city that weekend.

The therapist then reminded Allan that there were two sessions left that would be devoted to ending acute treatment. As Allan was doing well, the therapist asked Allan about his thoughts about meeting bi-weekly or monthly. Allan stated that he was comfortable in spacing out the meetings, as he also felt that he was doing well. He added, however, that he was not prepared to stop therapy at this point, and liked to know that he would still be able to see the therapist even though it would be a while before the next appointment. Allan and the therapist specifically agree to meet on a monthly basis for the last two sessions.

Session 11

A month later, Allan reported that he was continuing to do well. He had continued with social contacts at work, and though they were limited, he felt that they were of benefit. Allan expressed some surprise that he was able to initiate some of these, and felt pleased that he had begun to develop some new confidence in his social skills. His relationship with Pam had also continued to improve, as had his relationship with Eliza. After a review of progress to date, the following dialogue ensued:

> Therapist: Allan this is the first of our last two sessions. Traditionally, this has been called 'termination,' which sounds a little dramatic to me. I prefer to think of these as

sessions devoted to 'tying things together' in order to set the scene for the next phase of treatment. There is a quote from Winston Churchill I always like to use here: "this is not the beginning of the end, this is the end of the beginning. . . ."

Allan: You didn't do the accent that well, but I think I know what you mean.

Therapist: Allan, what are your thoughts about finishing up with therapy soon?

Allan: Oh, I think that I'll do fine – I'm not really concerned.

Therapist: That's good – I think your confidence is warranted. What I am getting at, though, is more about your thoughts about ending our relationship.

Allan: I really hadn't given it much thought. After all, you will still be prescribing my medications, and we had talked about meeting every three months or so to check on that, so it isn't as if I'll never see you again.

Therapist: I'm also glad that we will have the chance to meet periodically too – I like to keep track of the people I've worked with to make sure that they are doing well. I have worked with a lot of patients, though, who still felt that finishing up the 'therapy' part of the treatment, and especially meeting much less frequently, was hard for them.

Allan: I suppose that it will be a bit hard for me – I do enjoy talking to you now – at least after we got over the time when you were late. I probably will miss this – it's been a good way to talk through some problems. And I never really thought that talking about things was all that helpful before.

Therapist: I wanted to let you know that I will also miss meeting with you. I have really enjoyed working with you, and it's been great to see you make so much progress.

At this point, the therapist considered continuing this line of questioning about Allan's reactions to the impending conclusion of treatment. However, based on Allan's responses, the therapist felt that pressing the issue further would not be productive, particularly given Allan's attachment style. Further, to continue to press Allan for more reactions would move the therapy into a discussion of the therapeutic relationship, which would be a move strongly against the precedence set in the treatment thus far. The therapist could see no particular point in doing this, especially since Allan was doing so well. Moreover, the therapist had intentionally structured the therapy so that the conclusion would be less abrupt – both the spacing of the later sessions and the specific contract for provision of medication in the future were designed to lessen the impact of the conclusion.

The therapist therefore decided to return to the original Interpersonal Inventory and highlighted the ways in which the problem areas discussed had been formulated, and the progress that Allan had made in each of them. The therapist reminded Allan that the interpersonal dispute had originally been at an impasse, but had been brought back to the renegotiation phase as he had addressed his communication and also looked critically at his expectations of Pam. Allan reported that he and Pam had enjoyed a significant improvement in their relationship, and that Pam had even asked to accompany Allan on one of his hikes.

The therapist then looked at the role transition affecting Allan's relationship with Eliza and reminded Allan that he had experienced a loss of the relationship with his young daughter, but had also acquired a new relationship with his adult daughter. He praised Allan for his ability to adapt to the circumstances and also his courage in inviting his daughter's partner to the family home for a meal. Allan reported that he felt quite happy with his progress in this area and was more confident that Eliza would be able to come and 'talk to me father to daughter, but as a woman rather than my little girl.'

The therapist also praised Allan for his ability to initiate new social contacts. The therapist noted that Allan's improving ability to communicate had led in part to his recovery.

The therapist gave Allan one final homework task for their final session, which was to develop a list of problems which might arise in the future.

Session 12

The final session occurred 1 month later, and began with Allan admitting he was feeling a little sad about the end of treatment. The therapist replied by stating that while the acute and intense treatment phase would conclude at the end of this session, there would be continuing clinical contact as treatment with psychotropic medication was ongoing, and that depression was a relapsing and remitting condition. Since the clinical contact was continuing, the therapist encouraged Allan to contact him should problems emerge, at which point they would renegotiate a new treatment contract.

Allan then reported a number of potential future problems following the homework task set in session 11. One of those included the recurrence of his problematic communication with Pam. The therapist and Allan then discussed how he might apply his new skills in this regard.

When discussing potential problems with Eliza, Allan felt that there could be further complications in her relationship with her partner, but that continuing to treat her as an adult was the best way to help her to deal with this.

Allan and the therapist then went on to discuss the issue of Allan's general social supports. Allan was aware that his tendency to isolate himself could reemerge, and stated that he would try to pay attention to how he communicated his needs and expectations with his friends and acquaintances.

The therapist then concluded:

'Allan, when we first met I was very concerned about how much distress you were experiencing, and to be perfectly honest I was very worried about you and your safety. I was also concerned that psychological treatment may have been a problem because of your initial reluctance to talk to someone about your problems and your relationships in particular. Despite my concerns, you have done extremely well – I have been impressed not only with the way in which you have dealt with Pam and Eliza, but with the way in which you have been able to discuss things with me. This has been a very rewarding psychotherapeutic experience for me, particularly as you have worked so hard and have made so much progress.'

Characteristically, Allan blushed and smiled. He stood, shook the therapist's hand and left – exactly 50 minutes after he had entered.

Appendices

Appendices

Patient Information for IPT

Your clinician has recommended that you receive treatment with Interpersonal Psychotherapy (IPT). This document is designed to answer the frequently asked questions that patients or clients have about IPT.

WHAT IS IPT?

IPT is a structured form of psychotherapy or counseling that examines the ways in which problems in human relationships contribute to psychological stress, and the ways in which psychological problems affect human relationships. Counseling comes in many forms, each having a particular focus and emphasis. IPT differs from other forms of treatment because it focuses primarily on relationship problems. When a person is able to deal with relationship problems more effectively, his or her psychological symptoms frequently improve. IPT is designed to help people recognize the interpersonal problems they face, and to make changes in their relationships. Many scientific studies have demonstrated the benefit of this approach using IPT.

WHAT IS TALKED ABOUT IN IPT?

Your therapist will likely spend a few sessions talking with you about your current relationships as a way of understanding how they are connected with your symptoms. Your therapist will generally keep the discussion focused upon these kinds of problems. The relationship issues described by most people usually fall into one of the following areas:

- *Interpersonal disputes*: disagreements or arguments with others, and unmet expectations.
- *Role transitions*: circumstances in which your life changes, such as retiring or having a baby.

- *Grief and loss*: an emotional reaction to a major loss, such as when someone close to you has died. Loss of relationships or health status may also fall into this category.
- *Interpersonal sensitivity*: difficulty initiating or maintaining relationships with others.

WHAT ARE THE 'RULES' IN IPT?

Your therapist will discuss a few important matters with you. The first is the number of sessions and their length. This varies somewhat, but there are usually no more than twenty sessions. In IPT, the time limit is important as it helps move the treatment forward more quickly. Your therapist will keep to the number of sessions and the length of sessions you have agreed upon, unless you both explicitly agree to do otherwise. Your therapist will also discuss the arrangements for lateness or missed sessions, and will give you information about what to do in case of emergencies.

WHAT ABOUT MEDICATION?

The practice of combining IPT and medications such as antidepressants is common, and for some people this may have advantages over receiving either treatment alone. If your therapist is a doctor, it is likely he or she will discuss the role of medication with you and spend time during your sessions discussing your medication. If medication is being prescribed for you by a doctor other than your therapist, please be sure to inform your therapist about the medications and any changes to them.

WHAT CAN I EXPECT TO HAPPEN OVER THE COURSE OF TREATMENT?

In the initial sessions of IPT you and your therapist will spend some time surveying the important relationships in your life and identifying those which should be discussed in more detail. Your therapist will work with you to complete an Interpersonal Inventory, which is a register of your key relationships and the problems associated with them. This inventory provides a reference for you and your therapist, and will be a focus of discussion during the course of treatment. While you and your therapist should try to complete the Interpersonal Inventory as thoroughly as possible in the first few sessions of treatment, there will be opportunities to further develop the inventory throughout all of the sessions.

During the middle sessions of treatment, you and your therapist will discuss your specific interpersonal problems and work on generating solutions to them. Some types of activity that may take place include 'brainstorming' solutions to problems, working on improving communication, and discussing your emotional reactions to your relationships problems.

When concluding therapy, you and your therapist will discuss the progress you have made during the treatment. You should also spend some time planning ahead for any other problems you anticipate coming in the future. You and your therapist should also make specific plans for any future treatment you may require.

Interpersonal Inventory Form

Patient name:

Date of birth:

Other clinicians:

Insurance details:

Date of first consultation:

Contracted number of sessions:

Name of other:

Relationship:

Patient's account of problem:

Areas requiring further clarification:

Agreed problem area: Disputes   Role Transition   Grief + Loss   Interpersonal
                                                                    Sensitivity

Special issues:

IPT Formulation Sheet

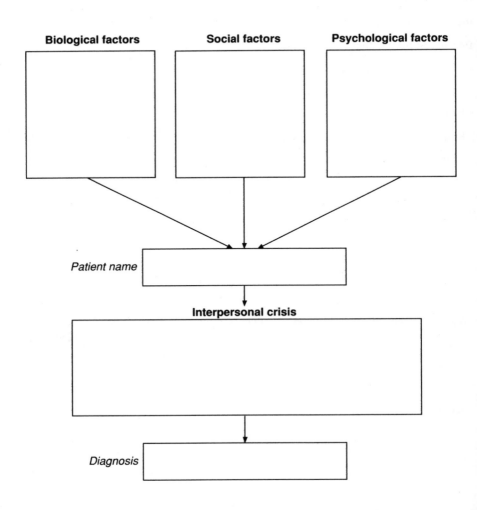

The International Society of Interpersonal Psychotherapists (ISIPT)

In May 2000, clinicians and researchers from around the world resolved to create an international association in order to more effectively disseminate IPT as a clinical and research treatment. The International Society of Interpersonal Psychotherapists (ISIPT) was formed as a not-for-profit organization for that purpose.

The goals of the ISIPT are to:

1 Promote awareness of IPT as an efficacious and effective treatment for psychiatric and psychological problems.
2 Monitor training and accreditation of IPT therapists.
3 Provide a format for regular exchanges of ideas between clinicians and researchers, particularly regarding new research and clinical initiatives using IPT.

At present, the ISIPT has three regional chapters – The Americas, Oceania, and Europe. Each chapter has a Regional Chair and oversees IPT activity in its region. The ISIPT runs and maintains a website which can be found on the world wide web at www.interpersonalpsychotherapy.org. Anyone can visit the public domain of the website, which provides information about IPT and describes current research. Information about how to join the ISIPT can also be found at this site.

Training and Certification in IPT

The authors of the 1984 IPT textbook[1] suggested that prospective IPT therapists should come from a counseling or medical background, attend a specified number of hours of didactic training in the theory and practice of IPT, and be supervised by a recognized expert in at least two IPT cases. These guidelines were essentially the same as those utilized in the NIMH-TDCRP.[2] These guidelines are currently accepted by most experts in the field as the standard for designation as a 'research quality' therapist.

When the International Society for Interpersonal Psychotherapy was established in 2000, the issue of training and accreditation emerged as one of its key concerns. The current view of ISIPT is that clinical training in IPT should consist of at least:

1 General training in mental health, including the fields of medicine, psychology, social work, occupational therapy, or psychiatric nursing.
2 Attendance at a training program approved by ISIPT that includes at least 16–24 hours of didactic instruction. The course should highlight the theoretical and practical aspects of IPT, and should include opportunities for interaction via role plays and discussion of clinical material.
3 Supervision of at least one case with a supervisor recognized by the ISIPT, which includes audio or videotaped treatment sessions.

A consensus regarding clinical accreditation has not been reached at the time of this writing. Clinicians interested in further training in IPT should make contact with ISIPT via its website at: www.interpersonalpsychotherapy.org.

REFERENCES

1. Klerman, G.L., Weissman, M.M., Rounsaville, B.J., Chevron, E.S. 1984. *Interpersonal Psychotherapy of Depression*. New York: Basic Books.
2. Elkin, I., Parloff, M.B., Hadley, S.W., Autry, J.H. 1985. NIMH Treatment of Depression Collaborative Treatment Program: background and research plan. *Archives of General Psychiatry* **42**, 305–16.

Adapting IPT to a Research Setting

Interpersonal Psychotherapy: A Clinician's Guide is designed primarily to serve as a guide to the use of IPT in clinical settings. Throughout the book, we have emphasized the use of clinical judgment, and have also emphasized the flexibility of the treatment, as well as its applicability to a wide variety of psychiatric and psychological problems. Our goal is to disseminate IPT, which we believe to be an efficacious and effective treatment which is of great benefit to many patients.

In addition to facilitating the clinical use of IPT, there continues to be a need for empirical studies investigating both the effectiveness and the efficacy of IPT.[1,2] Effectiveness, which refers to the value of a treatment in uncontrolled clinical settings, is in essence a combination of the 'real-life' utility of the treatment and its feasibility. Efficacy, on the other hand, refers to research in which the replicability of the study is the primary concern, and such studies usually involve random assignment to the various treatments being compared. Both types of studies are needed with IPT and with other psychotherapies.

IPT: A Clinician's Guide can literally be used off the shelf as a guide or manual for effectiveness studies. In such studies, the aim is to examine the benefit of IPT as it is applied in clinical settings, and the role of therapist judgment and the need to be flexible in treatment delivery are important factors to include in such protocols, as they should reflect what happens in clinical practice. A larger range of patient problems can also be examined in this setting, as clinical populations are fraught with comorbidity and complicated social situations.

While *IPT: A Clinician's Guide* can also potentially be used as a manual for efficacy studies, a number of modifications are required in order to do so. First, the patient population to be studied needs to be specifically defined. In contrast to the *Guide*, which emphasizes the use of IPT for a variety of patient problems not limited to diagnosis, most efficacy studies are disorder-based, and require that subjects be well described. Second, specific requirements for therapist training need to be provided and must be met by the therapists who deliver the IPT in efficacy studies. Third, specific outcome measures must be selected and applied to all patients – traditionally, these have been primarily symptom-based, as opposed to the approach advocated for general clinicians, in which social functioning and general well-being are emphasized as treatment goals in addition to symptom relief.

The extent of therapeutic flexibility must also be clearly specified in efficacy studies. In contrast to the flexibility inherent in the clinical use of IPT, the number of allowable sessions must be specified in efficacy studies, as well as the format and scheduling of the sessions. The division between acute and maintenance sessions must also be operationally defined in efficacy studies.

The most import factor in the adaptation of this guide to efficacy studies is that the techniques which are to be used, and those which are to be prohibited, must be specifically defined in efficacy studies. The degree of therapist judgment which is permitted, such as scheduling extra sessions, must be described. The primary concern is to describe the protocol in detail and in operational terms, so that the efficacy study can potentially be reproduced.

In summary, researchers conducting efficacy studies must be detailed in their descriptions of the patients with whom they work, the specifics of the therapy that is being used, and the training which is provided to research therapists. Those conducting effectiveness studies must do the same, though the degree to which factors such as therapist judgment and patient homogeneity are allowed to vary is much greater.

Our primary goal is to facilitate the dissemination and clinical use of IPT. We also hope that *IPT: A Clinician's Guide* will inspire researchers to continue to examine both the efficacy and the effectiveness of IPT in a variety of research and clinical settings.

REFERENCES

1. Barlow, D.H. 1996. Health care policy, psychotherapy research, and the future of psychotherapy. *American Psychologist* **51**, 1050–8.
2. Nathan, P.E., Stuart, S., Dolan, S. 2000. Research on psychotherapy efficacy and effectiveness: between Scylla and Charybdis? *Psychological Bulletin* **126**, 964–81.

Index